THE EPIDEMIOLOGY OF HUMAN MYCOTIC DISEASES

THE EPIDEMIOLOGY OF HUMAN MYCOTIC DISEASES

Edited by

YOUSEF AL-DOORY, Ph.D.

Associate Professor
Epidemiology and Infectious Diseases
Associate Professor of Pathology
(Laboratory Medicine)
George Washington University
School of Medicine
Washington, D. C.

With a Foreword by

Michael L. Furcolow, M.D.

Professor of Community Medicine
and Pediatrics
University of Kentucky Medical School
Lexington, Kentucky

CHARLES C THOMAS • PUBLISHER
Springfield • Illinois • U.S.A.

Published and Distributed Throughout the World by

CHARLES C THOMAS • PUBLISHER
Bannerstone House
301-327 East Lawrence Avenue, Springfield, Illinois, U.S.A.

ISBN 0-398-03380-3

Library of Congress Catalog Card Number 74 30107

With THOMAS BOOKS *careful attention is given to all details of manufacturing and design. It is the Publisher's desire to present books that are satisfactory as to their physical qualities and artistic possibilities and appropriate for their particular use.* THOMAS BOOKS *will be true to those laws of quality that assure a good name and good will.*

Library of Congress Cataloging in Publication Data

Al-Doory, Yousef, 1924-
The epidemiology of human mycotic diseases.
Includes index.
1. Medical mycology. 2. Epidemiology. I. Title.
[DNLM: 1. Mycoses—Occurrence. WC450 D691e]
RC117.A48 614.5'5'9 74-30107
ISBN 0-398-03380-3

Printed in the United States of America

X-11

This book is dedicated to the memory of those who have suffered and died needlessly from mycotic diseases; due mainly to a slow acceptance of the importance and magnitude of these diseases by the health profession, especially of those entrusted with the keeping of the mind of future practitioners.

CONTRIBUTORS

L. AJELLO, Ph.D.
Director
Mycology Division
Bureau of Laboratories
Center for Disease Control
Department of Health, Education and Welfare
Atlanta, Georgia

Y. AL-DOORY, Ph.D.
Associate Professor
Department of Epidemiology and Environmental Health and
Department of Pathology (Laboratory Medicine)
George Washington University School of Medicine
Washington, D C.

R. D. BAKER, M.D.
Armed Forces Institute of Pathology
Washington, D. C.
Professor of Pathology, Emeritus
College of Medicine and Dentistry of New Jersey
Rutgers Medical School
Piscataway, New Jersey

E. W. CHICK, M.D.
Professor
Department of Community Medicine and
Department of Cell Biology
College of Medicine
University of Kentucky and
Research Laboratory in Mycology
Veterans Administration Hospital
Lexington, Kentucky

B. M. CLARK, M.B., B.S., M.R.C., Path. Reader
Professor
Department of Medical Microbiology
University College Hospital
University of Ibadan
Ibadan, Nigeria

M. L. DILLON, JR., M.D.
Professor and Chief
Department of Surgery (Cardiothoracic)
Veterans Administration Hospital and
University of Kentucky Medical Center
Lexington, Kentucky

N. L. GOODMAN, Ph.D.
Associate Professor
Department of Community Medicine
College of Medicine
University of Kentucky
Lexington, Kentucky

M. A. GORDON, Ph.D.
Director, Laboratories for Mycology
Division of Laboratories and Research
New York State Department of Health
Albany, New York

D. L. GREER, Ph.D.
Associate Professor
International Center for Medical Research
University of Valle
Cali, Colombia

H. W. LARSH, Ph.D.
Research Professor and Chairman
Department of Botany and Microbiology
University of Oklahoma
Norman, Oklahoma

R. LOPEZ-MARTINEZ, M.D.
Instituto Mexicano del Seguro Social
Servicio de Dermatologia y Micologia Medica
Medica
Hospital General del Centro Medico Nacional
Mexico

E. MACOTELA-RUIZ, M.D., F.A.C.P.
Professor
Department of Dermatology
University of Mexico School of Medicine and
Head of the Service
Centro Medico Nacional y
Hospital General
Servicio de Dermatologia y Micologia Medica
Mexico

A. RESTREPO, M., Ph.D.
Department of Microbiology and Parasitology
School of Medicine
University of Antioquia
Medellin, Colombia

G. D. ROBERTS, Ph.D.
Section of Clinical Microbiology
Mayo Clinic and Mayo Foundation
Rochester, Minnesota

J. T. SINSKI, Ph.D.
Associate Professor
Department of Microbiology and Medical Technology
University of Arizona
Tucson, Arizona

J. M. SLACK, Ph.D.
Professor
Department of Microbiology
West Virginia University
Morgantown, West Virginia

R. F. SPROUSE, Ph.D.
Associate Professor
Department of Microbiology
School of Medicine and
Department of Veterinary Microbiology
College of Veterinary Medicine
University of Missouri
Columbia, Missouri

F. E. SWATEK, Ph.D.
Professor and Chairman
Department of Microbiology
California State University
Long Beach, California

H. I. WINNER, M.D., F.R.C.P., F.R.C.Path.
Professor
Department of Microbiology
Charing Cross Hospital
Medical School
University of London
London, England

FOREWORD

For a long time there has been a need for a comprehensive summary of the epidemiology of the human mycotic diseases. All the workers in the field have proceeded with individual diseases and sometimes are advanced quite far in unraveling the complex problems of the epidemiology of these most interesting infections; however, no place in the literature has there been a comprehensive attempt to get together the epidemiology of all the various diseases in one place for the use of the medical scientist and student. Dr. Al-Doory's book seems to fill that need. He has collected together a number of world famous experts who have written on each disease and the result is presented herewith. I know that everyone concerned with epidemiology and with the various mycotic diseases will find it a treasure of most interesting data and rewarding information.

Dr. Al-Doory and the authors are to be congratulated on the efforts put forth to bring together in one volume all this information. I am certain that it will prove to be a popular and enlightening book. I am certain that many interesting comparisons will be made of the epidemiology of the various mycotic diseases to discern their similarities and differences. Indeed, it appears now that many of the diseases have quite different epidemiology and means of spreading, and it is hoped that this book will serve as a focus for further knowledge in the planning of new studies.

Michael L. Furcolow

PREFACE

SIXTY YEARS AGO the serious study of Medical Mycology was considered a novel endeavor. Mycotic diseases, when properly diagnosed, were limited to scattered case reports. It was normal procedure for mycoses sufferers to be treated for dermatological or parasitological disorders.

Today, however, case reports involving the mycoses reveal an entirely different epidemiologic pattern. Refined research techniques and diagnostic procedures have enabled medical mycologists to trace mycoses involvements in cases of so-called tuberculosis, carcinoma, heart and liver disease, and many more.

Increased knowledge of the role which fungi play in the health and disease patterns of man has enlarged the scope of Medical Mycology significantly, adding to its stature as a major medical science.

But knowledge of the mycoses gained through epidemiologic surveys and procedures cannot be of benefit to the consumer of medical services, the patient, unless medical students, practitioners, and others in the health field, expose themselves to available information. Likewise, mycologists must become more aware of the importance of epidemiologic studies to the field and schedule research in this area.

Therefore, the purpose of this volume is the publication of available epidemiologic data on mycotic diseases, by authorities in the field, thus highlighting potentialities for future study and/or research. This book will be a first as far as the mycoses are concerned, but it is our aim that it serve as a valuable reference source and a nucleus for future epidemiologic studies.

More importantly, we hope it may serve as a useful guide to medical practitioners and others, on the prevalence of the mycoses, relating this work to the health field in general.

Our sincere thanks and appreciation are due to the contributors to this volume, for the tremendous amount of time and effort involved, and, more importantly, the interest and cooperation required to complete it. We owe a special thanks to: Dr. Michael L. Furcolow for his Foreword; to the Department of Epidemiology and Environmental Health of the George Washington University School of Medicine for the handling of all correspondence; to the George Washington University Committee on Research for a Grant-in-aid for preparation of the book manuscript; to Charles C Thomas for valuable suggestions and publication of the volume; and to my wife for editorial aid and encouragement during those trying times which must draw sympathy from all those who, at one time or another, have undertaken such a project. To this unique group—a special gratitude.

Yousef Al-Doory

CONTENTS

THE EPIDEMIOLOGY OF HUMAN MYCOTIC DISEASES

Chapter 1

INTRODUCTION

YOUSEF AL-DOORY

THE NATURAL HISTORY OF DISEASE, epidemic and endemic infectious and noninfectious, consists of interaction between the agent, the host, and the environment. Furthermore, all three possess characteristics which influence the origin, distribution, and frequency of a particular disabling interaction.

At one time the concept of the term *epidemiology* was "the science of studying epidemics." Literally translated from the Greek, *epidemiology* means "study upon people" (epi=upon, demos=people, logos=study). The modern definition however, is the study of the distribution and dynamics of disease in human populations.

In the context of this definition, the frequency of a disorder based on comparisons of the affected with the unaffected in the population under study must be considered together with any notable geographic boundaries and population characteristics, such as sex, age, race, ethnic group, marital and socioeconomic status, and occupation. It also includes population distributions ranging from families to entire countries, or continents, and temporal relations for diurnal, seasonal, annual, and even centennial epochs.

What is the purpose and value of epidemiologic data? Although the major goal is clarifying etiologic agents which influence health care at many levels, various groups and agencies also benefit from the collection of such data. Health and social program planners need this data for valid estimates of the cost of illness for both the diseased person and the expense of providing care, as well as the influence upon his family and productivity.

Schematics of health care centers are dependent to a large degree upon accurate estimates of the frequency and outcome of diseases. In addition, public health workers need all available epidemiologic data to determine the extent and nature of illness in the community, to outline and establish departures from baseline experience, to put into perspective past experience in relation to future trends, and finally, to devise and carry out any environmental control or genetic counseling measures as needed to attack the problems at hand.

The major source of epidemiologic information on diseases is the physician; he is also the principal user of epidemiologic data. The role of the physician is to determine the effects upon patients of a course of illness, to seek ways to alter the course of the disease within the development of preventive and/or treatment measures, and to define the disease in groups of patients.

SCOPE AND DEFINITION OF EPIDEMIOLOGY

Investigation of disease characteristics in populations to provide new information concerning etiology, and the development and testing of new methods of disease control and prevention are the main roles for epidemiology. Three aspects of epidemiology are commonly identified: descriptive, analytic, and experimental.

The descriptive aspect of epidemiology refers to the identification of persons affected and unaffected in a population, and the circumstances in time and place under which the disease occurs.

An understanding of descriptive epidemiology is essential for conducting analytic epidemiology, where results may generate specific hypotheses for analytic measures. On the other hand, the experimental aspect of epidemiologic studies consists of research under conditions which permit the investigator to control variables involved.

The epidemiologist's role is to seek answers to questions related to cause, cure, and prevention. Information sought is generally not readily available, and its value always must be weighed against time and expense. Because of this, the descriptive phase of epidemiology is certainly influenced by data from sources such as hospital records, physician's offices, clinic centers, morbidity and mortality reports, vital statistics, census records, journal publications, and other sources. In studying such information, the main variables to be considered are time, place, and individual.

The element is an essential ingredient for any epidemiologic investigation. Incubation period depends upon the rate of growth of the infectious agent and the portal of entry. In noninfectious diseases, the incubation period is much longer and usually measured in periods of months or years, instead of days, as in the infectious diseases. The lengthy incubation period of some diseases, such as cancer and radiogenic leukemia, is believed to be contributed to independent and multiple etiologic factors. This has been termed, recently as the *multihit* theory of causation in noninfectious diseases.

In certain instances sudden outbreaks of disease occur by having a number of people exposed to one causative agent, microbiological or chemical. In these kinds of outbreaks, usually the agent is transferred by a common vehicle such as water, food, or air. These point-source outbreaks are generally characterized by short incubation periods.

A change in disease that occurs gradually over a period of years or decades, is called a *secular change*. Observation of death certificate data accumulated for the last half century indicates that mortality from certain diseases has changed. One of the most marked changes has been the decline in mortality of cancer of the stomach in the United States. Prior to 1930, the age-adjusted death rate from stomach cancer was more than twenty-five per 100,000 population, while the corresponding annual mortality rate in 1970 was less than ten per 100,000 population.

As to the mycoses, statistical data are limited in this area, but the general impression is that the frequency of cases with opportunistic fungal infection (mucormycosis, aspergillosis, cryptococcosis and candidosis) has increased dramatically within the United States over the last ten years.

Observations of such changes in disease frequency or mortality from disease over a period of time have initiated interest for many epidemiologic studies seeking reasons or clues for the change. Many investigators believe that these changes in rates reflect basic changes that have occurred in the human environment, or improved methods of diagnosis, or possibly a combination of both. An example, pertinent to the study of fungal disease, is that improvement in medical technology, such as open heart surgery, has created the possibility for an increase in individuals "at risk" for opportunistic fungal diseases.

Seasonal changes have a striking effect on many diseases. For example, diseases contracted through vectors show marked variations corresponding to the period of feeding activities of the vector or of their breeding functions. Human activities, whether recreational or occupational, account for variations in exposure to sources of different infections leading to seasonal fluctuations in frequency of disease. Cutaneous mycoses are examples of diseases that occur more frequently during the summer.

In determining the epidemiologic characteristic of a population, sex, age, race, occupation, education, marital status, parity, and ethnic background compose the main variables to be considered.

Age is an important descriptive variable for the distribution of disease. Disease frequency differs in different age groups, and variations in frequency with age is more than that which occurs with any other descriptive variable. For example, incidence of degenerative diseases increases progressively throughout the life span, due to the body changes which occur with age. In certain instances, the change of disease frequency with age is dependent upon exposure to environmental situations. For example, in infancy there is high protection and minimum exposure but potential exposure increases with age, and is highest in school age groups. In adulthood, occupational and sexual exposure lead to certain diseases. From the mycologic point of view, the incidence of most mycoses is much higher among the middle-aged population, twenty to forty years of age, than among the younger or the older populations.

Another important epidemiologic observation is the variation in disease according to sex. The predominance of diseases in one sex over the other is believed to be due to exogenous factors (environmental), endogenous (constitutional) or the interaction of both. In the United States as an example, more males are born than females, in a ratio of 106 to 100; but death rates of males are higher than those of females for the majority of diseases.

Morbidity rates, on the other hand, are higher in women than in men for most diseases, with the exception of a few predominant diseases of males such as peptic ulcer, accidents, and lung cancer. In chromomycosis, which is a subcutaneous mycotic disease, the ratio as reported, reaches twenty males infected for every one female.

Socioeconomic status, as a parameter by which people can be divided in order to study distribution of disease, is indicated by income, occupation, and education. It is evident from many studies that infant mortality rates, malnutrition, and morbidity rates of infectious diseases are high in low socioeconomic groups.

Risk factors of many diseases have been identified to be due to physical, chemical or mental environmental exposure related to specific occupations. For example, professionals have higher mortality rates from coronary heart disease when compared with those unskilled. Most cases of silicosis occur among those in the mining, brick, and glass industries. Occupational dermatoses are the most important of the occupational diseases in the United States and are responsible for more than one half of all occupational disease compensation cases.

The race factor is another variable which affects the distribution of diseases; white and black populations in the United States are examples. Death rates in certain diseases such as coccidioidomycosis are much higher in nonwhites, occurring more frequently among blacks and, from some reports, even higher among the Philippinoes. Differences in disease frequency according to race may be due to genetic make-up specific for the race.

However, even where a genetic factor is deemed critical to the expression of disease, environmental conditions may have an effect upon the time of onset of the disease, the rapidity of its progression, and perhaps even the development of new mutations.

The manifestation of disease may be determined by the interplay of the complex elements of environment upon the genetic background of the individual. Under natural conditions, it often becomes difficult to distinguish genetic from environmental factors.

DIAGNOSIS OF DISEASE

Many factors may influence the identification of diseases or syndromes basic to the epidemiologic study of an illness. The presence of pathognomonic physical signs or specific laboratory test results, current nomenclature, diagnostic fashions, medical standards, and the frequency of the disease are among such factors. Also the intensity of the disease from the "subclinical" or clinically unapparent to the clinically apparent case, or to the initial recognition of the disease as the cause of death or as an incidental finding at autopsy, are major factors.

In assessing mortality statistics diagnostic criteria are of special importance in the United States, where only a small proportion of those who die are autopsied. Results from attempts at validation of mortality statistics with autopsy material have been discouraging. Where the majority of deaths are not subject to pathologic verification, it is expected that a high rate of error in clinical diagnosis may occur; generally it is the unusual or the uncertain cause of death for which autopsy is performed.

Review of clinical records as verification to validate death data is diagnostic consensus, rather than diagnostic proof. The clinical impression with whatever laboratory support exists, is what is found in these records. But, as a matter of fact, most of the information utilized in population studies rests upon the diagnostic impression of practicing physicians.

EPIDEMIOLOGIC DATA

Any discussion of the frequency of disease is commonly based on the following: case series, relative frequencies, and rates.

A consecutive list of cases observed in a hospital, clinic, physician's practice, or any medical center is known as a *case series*. The absence of bias in such a series is supposedly dependent upon the consecutive basis for selection, but such a listing may not relate the subjects to any clearly defined population; it may serve mainly to identify the presence of the disease. Because of the factors influencing selection from clinic to clinic, or center to center such a series rarely represents an identifiable population.

Autopsy series are compiled from only a fraction of hospital cases with all their potential biases. They are limited to selection among those who die; therefore, they are not representative of all who have been affected with the illness under study.

It is unfortunate, however, that pathologists and clinicians persist in comparing clinical or autopsy series, and speculating upon reasons for observed differences. This often happens without consideration of the fact that the subjects of the cases might have originated from different populations.

Another common misinterpretation in medical analysis is the assumption that the most frequent age group of persons in the series is representative of the age of greatest risk for that disease. It is almost impossible to determine from distribution of cases alone, whether a disease is really common to an age, sex, or group, more than any other. In spite of these shortcomings, however, both the case series and the *relative frequency* study continue to provide bases for hypotheses as to cause or risk factors, leading to intensive, refined, and more definitive population oriented studies.

Relative frequency refers to a comparison of clinical cases, hospital deaths, or autopsies performed in a medical center, to the total number of admitted patients. Relative frequency varies with both the number of diagnosed or verified cases in the numerator, and the number of deaths or autopsies in the denominator. Both of these figures (denominator and numerator) are affected by the type of practice or admission policies of the hospital, the combined influences leading to all causes of death, and the social and medical factors concerning autopsy practices. But the ratio is not necessarily affected in the same way throughout different studies.

Three types of population-based rates can be used in epidemiologic studies: incidence, prevalence and mortality. Each of these has a numerator and a denominator, and each can be expressed in appropriate units; howover, each is subject to a certain amount of error. Formulas are as follow:

$$\text{Incidence rate: } \frac{\text{Cases occurring during a stated interval of time}}{\text{Population at risk}}$$

$$\text{Prevalence rate: } \frac{\text{Cases present on a given date}}{\text{Population at risk}}$$

$$\text{Mortality rate: } \frac{\text{Deaths during a stated interval of time}}{\text{Population at risk}}$$

The number of new cases that develop during a certain interval of time per unit of population, usually expressed as cases per 100,000 population per year, is called *incidence* or *attack risk.* This ratio is concerned mainly with the time of onset of the disease, and is the preferred measure for etiologic studies.

The population at risk (denominator) may be the entire population; or both cases and denominator may refer to a specific segment in a population, i.e. those of certain age, sex, etc. When onset is uncertain in a disease, it is more practical to measure incidence based on the earliest date of diagnosis, which may vary with the individual's readiness to seek medical services, as well as the availability and quality of such services.

Prevalence rate is strictly the ratio of the affected to the population at risk at a given time. Prevalence may be a more useful statistic than incidence for a relatively uncommon disease with an insidious onset and a prolonged course. The prevalence rate of a chronic disease such as coccidioidomycosis, for example, represents the accumulation of cases over several years, which will provide a larger and more stable numerical value for comparisons than does annual incidence. Also, this rate may be expressed as cases per unit of population.

In other words, prevalence reflects the number of living patients residing in the specified geographic area, which includes affected immigrants but not former residents who emigrated before prevalence day. Therefore, with the assumption of no change in annual incidence or survival over time, the interrelation of incidence and prevalence for a chronic disease can be expressed as:

Prevalence rate = average duration (in years) X average annual incidence rate.

The number of persons who die each year from the specified disease per 100,000 population is known as mortality or death rate. For a uniformly fatal disease, especially one of short duration (such as mucormycosis), the death rate is also a reflection of the incidence rate. Here again, sex-, age-, and race-specific rates can be used.

The case-fatality rate is the frequency of death among the afflicted. If, for example, forty of one hundred patients with cryptococcal meningitis die in a year, the case-fatality rate would be 40 percent, whereas if these forty were part of a community of 10,000,000 people, the annual mortality rate for this disease would be 0.4 per 100,000 population.

Morbidity and mortality rates vary with such characteristics as age, and, for some ailments, race or sex. Therefore, the population "at risk" must be taken into account in developing suitable comparisons. This is particularly important if the frequency of a disease in two populations with different age distributions, are compared.

The choice of the rate to be used in a population study is determined by many factors. When a disease has a low incidence, for example, then case finding through individual examinations of the population, as well as prospective studies comparing subsequent hypothetical risk factors, are impractical. Usually, most information on population and relevant composition is derived from the census; while cases in most studies are obtained from either surveys or populations or from records of physicians or other medical resources in the community. Census information is subject to error (enumerations are usually lower) varying as to age, sex, ethnic group, and marital status of the population under study.

Numerator is the element most subject to error in epidemiologic studies; i.e. failure of the physician to record or recall the diagnosis observed, inaccuracies of diagnosis, and variations among physicians in diagnostic criteria or definition of a disease or syndrome. However, published mortality rates are useful if the disease has a high case fatality rate and therefore is likely to be reported as the underlying cause of death. Both incidence and prevalence data are useful, if properly applied, in determining measures of the impact of a disease on a population.

It should be noted, however, that incidence implies recognition of a date of onset, or a date of diagnosis. Prevalence is more useful in comparing the frequency of a slowly progressive disease, whose duration does not vary appreciably in different populations.

Selection of a particular rate, therefore, depends upon not only the clinical characteristics of the disease under study, but also the source of information, the delineation of the population "at risk," and the point the investigator is trying to present or stress.

Seldom do epidemiologic studies attain the status of a carefully controlled experiment; rather, most remain observational. Therefore, when differences in results are statistically significant at a given probability level, often the conclusion is that either a rare event has occurred, or the series are truly different, or there is hidden bias so that the series are not truly comparable.

On the other hand, in a carefully controlled experiment, when results obtained are not significantly different, then we can conclude that any true difference which exists is not sufficiently large to be detected by an experiment of this size. The conclusion in observational studies can be that there is no difference, or that the sample size was too small to detect whatever true difference existed, or that noncomparability of the two series has masked the difference. Readers with further interest in this aspect of epidemiology are referred to standard textbooks of statistics for a description of test procedures.

Chapter 2

THE EPIDEMIOLOGY OF ACTINOMYCOSIS

JOHN M. SLACK

ISRAEL (53) IN 1878 relates a description of a case of actinomycosis observed by von Langenbeck in 1845 which is the earliest recorded case of the disease. He then goes on to give a very complete history of two cases and he is the first to apply the name actinomycosis.

Actinomycosis (13, 16, 18, 38, 109) is a chronic granulomatous disease characterized by suppuration, abscess formation, and draining sinuses. It occurs throughout the world without relation to age, sex, race, seasons or occupation and is not an opportunistic disease. A specific diagnosis is expedited by a high degree of clinical suspicion, nevertheless, there is often delay because of: 1) failure to clinically consider actinomycosis and to alert the Pathology and Microbiology laboratories of this possibility; 2) the collection of inadequate samples or failure to maintain the specimens under anaerobic conditions; and 3) the lack of awareness that the direct fluorescent antibody technique (62, 103, 105) can be used to identify *Actinomyces* in a clinical specimen or from a culture. Clinically, the disease (13) is frequently divided into cervicofacial (60%), thoracic (15%), abdominal (20%) and other types (5%). This terminology of disease types will be followed in the subsequent discussions.

CERVICOFACIAL: This is a subacute or chronic granulomatous disease in which the onset may go unnoticed until a persistent swelling develops (usually in the parotid or mandibular region)

(23, 29, 43, 44, 45, 80). Then one or more draining sinuses develop discharging a yellowish, thick to serous, exudate which if carefully examined usually contains the diagnostic sulfur granules. These granules should be examined microscopically for the presence of gram-positive filaments and hyaline clubs although the latter are not always present (45, 115). The overlying skin often has a reddish-purple cast. There is rarely involvement of the regional lymphatics but the infection may spread by direct continuity or via the blood stream (36, 44). A periostitis may develop but direct invasion of the bone is rare although it has been reported for the maxilla, mandibles, and cranium (35, 80). There is frequently a history of dental decay, tooth extraction, fracture of the jaw, other types of trauma or basically any circumstance which breaks the normal epithelial surface providing devitalized tissue and anaerobic conditions for the growth of the *Actinomyces*. In brief, the clinical characteristics are: 1) pain (some are painless), 2) trismus, 3) firm swelling, 4) fistulas, and 5) yellowish granules.

THORACIC: This form may result from: 1) inhalation or aspiration of the *Actinomyces* present in the oral cavity (in plaque, calculus or tonsillar crypts) via the tracheobronchial tree, 2) organisms being carried into the lung by a foreign body, 3) hematogenous extension, 4) extension of an existing infection such as cervicofacial actinomycosis spreading down tissue planes of the neck to the mediastinum or abdominal actinomycosis perforating the diaphragm (11, 26, 90, 106, 113). The primary lesion, which is seldom seen, may be in the bronchioles, peribronchial tissue or in the lung parenchyma. The infection may spread through the chest wall producing multiple sinuses which tend to heal and then reopen discharging more pus. Sulfur granules may be observed in such exudate as well as in the sputum. The disease is sometimes divided into broncho, pleuro or pneumo-actinomycosis with the common principal symptoms being chest pains, fever, cough with expectoration, and weight loss. Clinically it may resemble tuberculosis, pulmonary abscess or bronchiogenic carcinoma (75, 91). If sulfur granules are not demonstrable a differential diagnosis is often impossible without an exploratory thoractomy. Nevertheless, the *Actinomyces* should be considered as a possible etiological agent in any chronic lung disease (40).

ABDOMINAL: This type of infection usually develops as a result of an acute, perforative gastrointestinal disease or after trauma (surgical or accidental) (1, 85, 92). The gastrointestinal disease could include any one of a variety of ulcerative diseases or appendicitis. One report (92) indicated that 72 percent of 122 cases of abdominal actinomycoses were preceded by an attack of acute appendicitis, usually perforative. Thus, actinomycotic infections develop more frequently in the right lower quadrant of the abdominal wall. Extension from such foci is usually by direct continuity intra-abdominally (could be hematogenous) to involve any tissue or organ including muscle, liver, spleen, kidney, fallopian tubes, ovaries, uterus, testes, bladder or rectum (*J. Urol. 103*:126, 1970; *87*:567, 1962; 119). The patient becomes aware of such a complication usually through the development of an indurated mass (which may stimulate carcinoma) at the site of the operation or in the flank or pelvis which then begins to soften and develop one or more draining sinuses. These sinuses are sometimes the first reported symptom. The systemic symptoms are initially mild with a slow but progressive development of fever, malaise, weakness, and pain.

BONE INVOLVEMENT: Primary bone infection is rare and then is usually an extension from an adjacent soft tissue infection. Periostitis results with a stimulation of new bone formation causing a thickening of the bone which may be the only X-ray finding. If the bone is actively invaded there are usually localized areas of bone destruction surrounded by increased bone densities. The foci may be interconnected by sinus tracts. The actual mechanism of bone destruction is not known. The X-ray appearance can vary from rarefaction to thickening and sclerosis resembling a bone tumor. The mandible, ribs, and spine are the bones most frequently involved but infections of the humerus, phalanx, knee, maxilla, mastoid, cranium, and others have been described (21, 70, 80). Cope (14) gives a good review indicating that sixty-six cases of bone involvement have been described in the literature through 1951.

Central Nervous System Actinomycosis: An excellent review (24) indicates that there are over one hundred reports of actinomycosis of the brain and spinal cord but of these only twenty were verified by cultures. Involvement of the CNS usually results from direct extension of cervicofacial actinomycosis or from a hematogenous spread of a thoracic or abdominal locus. Either of the latter two may extend directly into the spinal canal (6, 91) or the spinal column is directly involved (14). The predominant symptoms are usually directed toward the primary site of infection but the patient may complain of headache, show evidence of increased intracranial pressure or symptoms of focal seizures, hemiparesis, aphasia, ataxia or abnormal reflexes.

Skin and Wound Actinomycosis: Primary infections of the skin (74) usually have a history of trauma resulting from a human bite, fistfight or barbed wire although in some there is no obtainable history of injury or even evidence of an endogenous source. The infections usually develop slowly and may eventually involve the subcutaneous tissue, muscle and even bone with diagnosis dependent upon the presence of sulfur granules, filaments in gram strains or positive cultures. Treatment is usually successful with surgical drainage and/or antibiotics. The antibiotic of choice and in all forms of actinomycosis is penicillin.

ETIOLOGY

In 1877 Harz (5) microscopically examined pus from a case of bovine actinomycosis and observed the ray-like appearance of the sulfur granules and from this applied the name *Actinomyces bovis* to the causative bacterium. It was not until 1940 (20) that the human and bovine species were differentiated although the primary human species had been referred to as the Wolff-Israel type since the work of Wolff and Israel (117) in 1891 and that of Wright (118) in 1905. The name *Actinomyces israelii* was established in 1898 (59). The other species have been described more recently. *A. naeslundii* in 1951 (112); *A. odontolyticus* in 1958 (2); *A. viscosus* in 1965 (50); but renamed in 1969 (32); *A. eriksonii* in 1965 (33) although some authors indicate this species should be in *Bifidobacterium*.

Arachina propionica was originally described as an actinomycete but was reclassified in 1969 because it produces propionic acid from glucose and has diaminopimelic acid in the cell wall (87, 102).

A. bovis, as it is now defined and identified, has not been isolated from human infections. However, all the other species have been isolated from infections in man and have been shown to produce experimental infections in animals (10, 86). *A. israelii* is most frequently involved causing classical actinomycosis with sulfur granules although the other species may cause clinically similar infections. Also, infections of the various organs and tissues without sulfur granules have been reported and overall may be more numerous than classical actinomycosis. Certain of these species may be directly or indirectly involved in the development of caries and periodontal disease in man (108).

Holm (47, 48) initiated the concept that human actinomycotic diseases are multiple or combined infections which arise through synergism between anaerobic actinomycetes and certain other microbes including *Actinobacillus actinomycetemcomitans, Bacteroides,* anaerobic streptococci and others. This thesis is supported by workers in Germany (66) and Norway (45). There is little question that in many cases, particularly cervicofacial, that other organisms are introduced into the tissue along with the *Actinomyces* and certainly add to the pathological process. In addition, these organisms may well complicate the treatment in being resistant to antibiotics. However, there is no doubt that when one has actinomycosis an *Actinomyces* is present and that the disease with sulfur granules can be produced in experimental animals (10, 31); thus, these oragnisms are the etiological agents of actinomycosis.

SOURCE OF INFECTION

Over the past sixty years or more there has accumulated an impressive amount of experimental evidence that supports the concept that the oral cavity consistently harbors the various species of *Actinomyces* and thus is the source of these organisms when they cause infections in man.

This began when Israel (54) in 1879 described a case of pulmonary actinomycosis and postulated that the tonsils could harbor the organisms and then in 1887 (55) he described another case with a piece of tooth embedded in the pulmonary lesion and from this concluded that diseased teeth act as a depot for the organisms. Filamentous bacteria were demonstrated on the surface of teeth and it was postulated that they played a role in the development of caries in 1907 (3). Then in 1910 material from carious teeth and tonsils was injected intraperitoneally into guinea pigs and the majority of the animals developed peritoneal abscesses containing gram-positive filaments and in some cases typical sulfur granules (67, 68). In 1938 Emmons (17) isolated anaerobic actinomycetes from 11 percent of two hundred pairs of tonsils; this was confirmed by Slack (101) in 1942 and more recently demonstrated using the fluorescent antibody technique (4, 49). Histological studies demonstrating clumps or masses of *Actinomyces* in tonsillar crypts from persons without actinomycosis have been reported by several authors (37, 39, 116). Although previously filamentous bacteria had been associated with teeth (3, 67, 68), the anaerobic actinomycetes were not isolated from the oral cavity until 1925 (79). Since then a number of authors have reported the presence of various species of *Actinomyces* in both plaque and calculus (19, 111). Recently in our own laboratory (104), using the fluorescent antibody technique, we have demonstrated that four species (*A. israelii, A. naeslundii, A. odontolyticus* and *A. viscosus*) are consistently present in plaque and calculus and that in many specimens all four species were present. Their presence in appreciable numbers indicates that *Actinomyces* play a significant role in the development of plaque and calculus and that they also play a role in caries and periodontal disease (107).

With these organisms in the oral cavity it is understandable how they can invade areas of the face and neck or be carried into the lungs via the tracheobronchial tree. However, the source of the organisms in abdominal actinomycosis is more difficult to explain. These organisms have not been reported to be normal inhabitants of the intestinal tract, thus they must be transient occupants gaining entrance into adjacent tissue through an ulcerative or perforative gastrointestinal disease or through trauma. It is, of course, always possible that they are carried by the blood stream and lodge in an injured or thrombosed site.

It now seems appropriate to state three truisms about these organisms and the disease in man and thus hopefully putting the contrasting myths to rest.

1. The *Actinomyces* are bacteria, they are not fungi.
2. The source of the organisms is the oral cavity of man, not grasses or grains.
3. Actinomycosis is just as likely to occur in urban as in rural inhabitants, the disease is not primarily associated with cattle or agriculture.

GEOGRAPHIC DISTRIBUTION OF ACTINOMYCOSIS

United States: In 1885 the first two cases of cervicofacial actinomycosis were reported to the Chicago Medical Society (77) and three more were added in 1891 (78). This was followed by seventy-two cases in 1899 (95) plus thirty-one in 1902 (22) giving a total of 103 recorded cases through 1902. The majority of these were reported from New York, Minnesota, Illinois, and Massachusetts.

The most extensive survey in this country was conducted by Sanford (97, 98) in which he not only reviewed the literature but canvassed health officers, medical schools, hospitals, and physicians collecting 575 cases (334 had not been published or reported) which gave a total of 678 cases in the U. S. through 1923. The patients ranged in age from twenty-eight days to eighty-two years with the median falling between twenty and thirty years. Nearly 80 percent of the cases were males. Over one-half of the patients were urban dwellers having no contact with cattle indicating the disease is not related to occupation although many cases were related to injury. The anatomical distribution approximated 60 percent cervicofacial, 18 percent abdominal and 14 percent thoracic but practically every part of the body was reported to be infected. Geographic location of these cases on a regional basis included New England—86; North Atlantic Coast—138; South Atlantic Coast—16; East

Central—52; Mississippi Valley—191; Northwest Central—95; Southern—35; Plateau—37; and Pacific Coast—28. Kolouch and Peltier (58) extend the literature review of cases through 1945 and added thirty-eight new cases which plus the above gives a total of 879 cases of actinomycosis reported in the literature through 1945 (Table 2-I). From 1945 on, it becomes difficult to separate cases included in the above total and those reported by the various authors, thus a listing of papers will be given in which a number of cases are given but no attempt will be made to give overall totals (Tables 2-IV, 2-V).

TABLE 2-I

NUMBER OF REPORTED CASES OF ACTINOMYCOSIS IN THE UNITED STATES, 1885 TO 1945

		Clinical Distribution				
Date	*Number Cases*	*Cervico-facial*	*Thoracic*	*Abdominal*	*Other*	*Ref.*
1885	2	2				77
1891	3	2		1		78
1899-1900	67	33	14	16	4	95, 96
1902	31	19	6	6		22
1923-1925	575	346	80	104	45	98
1946	201	90	40	71		58
	879	492	140	198	49	

Table 2-II presents the crude death rates reported to the Bureau of Vital Statistics during the years of 1949 through 1969 with an average of twenty-five deaths per year. The Spearman Rank correlation of —.605 has a probability value of $p<.01$ which indicates a statistically significant downward trend. However, it should be noted that the years 1962, 1957, and 1954 are low crude death years thus there is considerable yearly fluctuation. Unfortunately this data does not extend to the preantibiotic era to allow a comparison of crude death rates between these two periods as one would expect a very significant drop beginning in the latter 1940's.

TABLE 2-II

ACTINOMYCOSIS—REPORTED MORTALITY FROM VITAL STATISTICS OF U. S. CRUDE DEATH RATE, 1949 TO 1969

Year	*Year Rank*	*Deaths*	*United States Resident Population* x 1,000*	*Reported Crude Death Rate Per 100 Million*	*Crude Death Rate Rank*	*d*	*d^2*
1969	21	15	201,385	7.45	1	20	400
1968	20	16	199,399	8.02	2	18	324
1967	19	28	197,457	14.18	11	8	64
1966	18	21	195,576	10.74	6	12	144
1965	17	26	193,526	13.43	9	8	64
1964	16	31	191,141	16.22	16	0	0
1963	15	35	188,483	18.57	17	-2	4
1962	14	17	185,771	9.15	4	10	100
1961	13	21	182,992	11.48	7	6	36
1960	12	28	179,979	15.56	14	-2	4
1959	11	27	177,135	15.24	13	-2	4
1958	10	21	174,149	12.06	8	2	4
1957	9	15	171,187	8.76	3	6	36
1956	8	24	168,088	14.28	12	-4	16
1955	7	23	165,069	13.93	10	-3	9
1954	6	17	161,884	10.50	5	1	1
1953	5	30	158,956	18.87	18	-13	169
1952	4	25	156,393	15.99	15	-11	121
1951	3	37	153,982	24.03	21	-18	324
1950	2	36	151,868	23.70	20	-18	324
1949	1	32	149,304	21.43	19	-18	324
							2472

Correlation, Mortality vs. Year.

$$\text{Spearman's } r = 1 - \frac{6 \Sigma d^2}{n(n^2-1)} = 1-6(2472) = 1-1.605 = -.605$$

*Statistical Abstract of the U. S. 1972, Table No. 2, P. 5, 93ed, U. S. Commerce Dept. Government Printing Office, Washington, D. C.

Table 2-III gives the number of cases of actinomycosis reported to the Center for Disease Control (CDC) in Atlanta, Georgia, with a list of the states from which the cases were reported. The states reporting ten cases or more in descending frequency are Minnesota, Iowa, Illinois, Louisiana, Connecticut, Maine, Mississippi, Arizona and Arkansas. One must question whether or not this information really correlates with incidence, particularly when a populous state like California has not reported a case in some twenty years. Also Sanford (97) more than doubled the number of cases he collected by making direct inquiries to physicians and hospitals. This data lends itself to the same type of analysis as presented in Table 2-II with a correlation of –.654 and a probability value of $p<.01$ indicating a downward trend of incidence. The reported incidence varies from three to eleven per 100 million persons. However, as there

TABLE 2-III

NUMBER OF CASES OF ACTINOMYCOSIS REPORTED IN THE UNITED STATES, 1950 TO 1971

Year	*Number Cases*	*States Reporting*
1971	6	Ar., 2; Ct., 1; Il., 1; La., 1; Mn., 1
1970	7	Fl., 2; Il., 1; Ia., 1; Ma., 1; Mi., 1; Ms., 1
1969	13	Ct., 2; Fl., 1; Il., 1; In., 1; La., 3; Ma., 1; Mn., 2; Mt., 1; Va., 1
1968	9	Ct., 1; Il., 2; Ia., 2; La., 3; Mn., 1
1967	10	Il., 3; In., 2; Ia., 1; La., 3; Ms., 1
1966	11	Ar., 1; Fl., 2; Il. 1; Ia., 4; La., 1; Ma., 1; Mn., 1
1965	10	Al., 1; Ct., 1; Ia., 1; Ks., 1; Ma., 1; Mn., 2; N.H., 1; Pa., 2
1964	8	Ct., 1; Ia., 2; La., 1; Mi., 1; Mn., 2; Pa., 1
1963	8	Ar., 1; Ct., 1; Fl., 1; Ia., 1; La., 1; Ma., 2; R.I., 1
1962	15	Me., 1; R.I., 1; Ct., 1; Pa., 3; Oh., 1; Ia., 1; De., 1; Ms., 2; Ar., 1; La., 2; Az., 1
1961	8	Al., 1; Az., 1; Ct., 1; In., 1; Ia., 3; Mi., 1
1960	6	Ar., 1; In., 1; La., 1; Me., 1; Mi., 1; Mt., 1
1959	18	Az., 1; Fl., 1; Il., 3; Ia., 1; Ma., 1; Mi., 5; Mn., 2; Ut., 1; Va., 1; Wi., 1; Wy., 1
1958	14	Al., 1; Az., 1; Il., 1; Ia., 1; Ks., 5; La., 1; Mi., 1; Or., 1; Pa., 1; Wy., 1
1957	11	Ct., 1; Il., 3; Mn., 2; Mo., 1; Oh., 1; Ut., 1; Wi., 2
1956	11	Az., 1; Il., 2; Ia., 1; Ma., 3; Mn., 2; Mo., 1; Wi., 1
1955	18	Az., 5; Ar., 2; Ct., 2; Ga., 1; Il., 1; In., 2; Ia., 1; Mn., 1; Tn., 1; Wi., 2
1954	16	Az., 1; Co., 1; Il., 2; Ma., 1; Mi., 1; Mn., 5; S.D., 1; Tn., 3; Va., 1
1953	11	Az., 1; Co., 2; In., 1; Ma., 1; Mi., 1; Mn., 1; Oh., 1; S.D., 1; Tn., 1; Wa., 1

*Table from CDC Morbidity and Mortality Reports, Atlanta, Ga. The years 1951 and 1952 are not included as optionally reported diseases were not recorded for these two years.

are fewer cases reported each year than there are deaths recorded and as the literature reports do not correlate with either deaths or incidence it is doubtful that any statistical analysis would be valid or lend itself to a meaningful interpretation.

Table 2-IV gives a list of those authors reporting on ten or more cases and Table 2-V is a rather detailed review of case reports for the years 1966 through 1972. These serve the purpose of emphasizing that actinomycosis occurs in the United States and will provide a good reference source for anyone interested in particular kinds of cases or desiring to do a more complete literature review.

TABLE 2-IV

LITERATURE REPORTS OF 10 CASES OR MORE OF ACTINOMYCOSIS IN THE UNITED STATES, 1942 TO 1972*

		Clinical Distribution				
Year	*Total Cases*	*Cervico-facial*	*Thoracic*	*Abdominal*	*Other*	*Ref.*
1946	19	1	13	5		88
1947	65		65			57
1947	15	15				61
1948	110				110, CNS	56
1948	46	26	.9	11		83
1949	21	4	5	12		115
1950	122			122		92
1957	37	9	5	23		44
1962	10	6	2	2		51
1966	13				13, brain	73
1968	86				86, cardiac	15
1968	28	13	9	5	1, brain	71
1969	30		30			40
1969	10		2	7	1, CNS	34
1970	15		15			25
1971	18		18			26
1972	24	5	15	4		16
1972	9	2	5	2		113
1972	11	2	1	4	4, eye, finger	7†

*There is duplication between some of the cases in these reports and those listed in Table 2-I. The year of publication does not necessarily indicate when the case(s) occurred.

†Cases caused by *Arachia propionica* are included here although published in early 1973.

TABLE 2-V

CASES OF ACTINOMYCOSIS IN THE UNITED STATES REPORTED IN THE LITERATURE FOR THE YEARS, 1966 TO 1972*

		Clinical Designation			
Journal	*Date*	*Cervico-facial*	*Tho-racic*	*Ab-dominal*	*Other*
Amer. J. Med. Sci. *263*:369	1972	1	1		
†Amer. J. Surg. *124*:46	1972	2	5	2	
Ann. Intern. Med. *77*:629	1972			1	
J. Amer. Med. Ass. *221*:1052	1972		1		
J. Oral Surg. *30*:362	1972	1			
Lancet *1*:641	1972		1		
Oral Surg. Oral Med. Oral Path. *34*:199	1972	1			
S. Dak. J. Med. *25*:15	1972	1	1		
N. Y. State J. Med. *72*:2797	1972	1			
South. Med. J. *65*:762	1972			1	
South. Med. J. *65*:839	1972	5	15	4	
Virginia Med. Mon. *99*:142	1972		1		
Amer. J. Surg. *122*:414	1971			1	
J. Oral Surg. *29*:440	1971	1			
†Minn. Med. *54*:593	1971		18		
N. Y. State J. Med. *71*:364	1971		1		
South. Med. J. *64*:987	1971	1			
Oral Surg. Oral Med. Oral Path. *32*:276	1971	4			
†Amer. J. Roentgenol. *110*:707	1970		15		
Ann. Thor. Surg. *9*:307	1970		12		
Arch. Otolaryngol. *92*:468	1970	3			
Arch. Surg. *101*:258	1970			2	
J. Amer. Med. Ass. *212*:2260	1970	2	2		
J. Neurosurg. *33*:347	1970	1			
J. Urol. *103*:126	1970			1	
New Engl. J. Med. *282*:614	1970			1	
N. Y. State Med. *70*:2833	1970		1		
Oral Surg. Oral Med. Oral Path. *29*:138	1970	3			
Postgrad. Med. *48*:59	1970		1		
†Amer. J. Clin. Path. *52*:445	1969		2	7	1
Amer. J. Obstet. Gynecol. *103*:908	1969			1	
Arch. Intern. Med. *123*:430	1969		7		
Del. Med. J. *41*:297	1969		1		
†Dis. Chest. *55*:119	1969		2		
J. Amer. Med. Ass. *210*:552	1969			1	
J. Maine Med. Ass. *60*:159	1969		1		
J. Pediat. *74*:763	1969			1	
Med. Ann. D. C. *38*:197	1969			1	
Mil. Med. *134*:281	1969			1	

TABLE 2-V—Continued

CASES OF ACTINOMYCOSIS IN THE UNITED STATES REPORTED IN THE LITERATURE FOR THE YEARS, 1966 TO 1972*

		Clinical Designation			
Journal	*Date*	*Cervico-facial*	*Tho-racic*	*Ab-dominal*	*Other*
Nebraska Med. J. *54*:317	1969			1	
Postgrad. Med. *46*:73	1969		2		
S. C. Dent. J. *27*:5	1969	1			
Surg. Gynecol. Obstet. *128*:259	1969		1		
Arch. Surg. *96*:58	1968				1
Dis. Chest. *54*:463	1968				1
J. Thor. Cardiov. Surg. *55*:193	1968		2		
Oral Surg. Oral Med. Oral Path. *26*:374	1968	1			
South. Med. J. *61*:849	1968	3			
†Surgery *64*:905	1968	13	9	5	1
Arch. Surg. *94*:292	1967			1	
Arch. Surg. *94*:344	1967			1	
Cutis *3*:739	1967	1			
Clin. Pediat. *6*:221	1967		1		
J. Amer. Med. Ass. *199*:1002	1967	1			
J. Amer. Med. Ass. *200*:156	1967		1		
New Engl. J. Med. *276*:515	1967	1			
Postgrad. Med. *42*:288	1967	1			
Obstet. Gynecol. *29*:71	1967			1	
Radiology *88*:9	1967			1	
Radiology *88*:536	1967				1
Surgery *62*:431	1967			8	
Advan. Cardiopul. Dis. *3*:123	1966		3		
Amer. J. Surg. *111*:678	1966			1	
Dis. Chest. *50*:211	1966		1		
Ill. Med. J. *130*:665	1966			1	
J. Kans. Med. Soc. *67*:471	1966				
†N. Y. State J. Med. *66*:2155	1966				1
South. Med. J. *59*:613	1966				1

*The date of publication does not necessarily indicate when the case actually occurred. As there may be duplication of cases in these reports and those listed in Tables 2-I and 2-IV there is no attempt to determine the total number of cases. No doubt there are additional reports in the literature although this will serve as a good beginning for one interested in doing a literature review. Most of the cases listed represent new cases.

†Reports also listed in Table 2-IV.

The previous tables show conclusively that actinomycosis occurs throughout the United States and that cases are reported by one means or another every year. It is, however, impossible to arrive at any meaningful figure as to incidence, except to indicate that it is neither a rare nor common disease in the United States. This shortcoming in our Vital Statistics could well be remedied if it was mandatory to provide morbidity and mortality reports on all infectious diseases.

CANADA: The first case was recorded by Bell in 1900 (*Montreal Med. J.*, *34*:81, 1905) followed by reports of forty in Montreal (76), fifty in Edmonton (41) and fourteen in the Vancouver area (109). There are a number of single cases in the literature with two very interesting ones being that of a primary breast infection (114) and a thyroiditis caused by *A. naeslundii* (63).

SOUTH AMERICA, CENTRAL AMERICA, MEXICO, AND PUERTO RICO: In Argentina, Negroni (81, 82) indicates that the first case was reported in 1903 and that over one hundred cases have been observed in Buenos Aires. He also gives references to cases in Brazil, Chile, Peru, and Uruguay.

Actinomycosis is either not common or seldom reported in the literature from these countries as recent reviews either list only a very few cases or none at all. These include *Brazil—Thorax 17*:224, 1968; *Oral Surg, Oral Med., Oral Path. 24*:817, 1967; *Colombia—Am. J. Clin. Path. 51*:470, 1969; *47*:505, 1967; and *Venezuela—Thorax 16*:135, 1967; *Acta Odont. Venez. 1*:3, 1967. In Mexico, Macotela-Ruiz reports from the National Medical Center in Mexico City (Int. Symp. Mycoses, 1970, WHO pub. 205) that from 1,000 confirmed cases of mycotic infections eighty-seven were deep seated with eight being actinomycosis. In Panama, Calero et al. (*Am. J. Trop. Med. Hyg. 10*:877, 1961) reported the first case from this country. Nadal and Munoz (*Bol. Assoc. Med. P.R. 57*:225, 1965) of *Puerto Rico* described a case of abdominal actinomycosis and indicated that the disease was first described by Carrion (*P.R.J. Pub. Hlth.*

Trop. Med. 13:367, 1938). An incidental problem in these and other countries where mycetomas are prevalent is the indiscriminate use of the terms actinomycosis or actinomycotic for infections due to *Actinomyces, Nocardia* or *Streptomyces.* It would be most helpful if authors would extend the practice of naming the disease after the etiological agent which in these cases would then be actinomycosis, nocardiosis and streptomycosis.

ENGLAND: V. Z. Cope (12, 13, 14) has provided a great deal of information on the incidence of actinomycoses in England and throughout the world. In his book (14) he gives excellent clinical descriptions of the various types of actinomycosis and compiles a total of 1,330 cases from the world literature (750 cervicofacial, 199 thoractic, 296 abdominal and 79 other types). This information is supplemented by a recent book from Germany (8) which emphasizes case reports and clinical descriptions.

The first case in England was reported by Acland in 1884 (*Trans Path Soc London, 37*:546, 1866) and later he compiled 109 cases with forty cervicofacial, twenty thoracic, forty-two abdominal and seven other types. Then Foulerton (27) discusses seventy-eight cases he observed in a London hospital over a thirteen-year period and appends a list of seventy additional cases from other hospitals. Cope (13) tabulates 182 cases from thirteen hospitals through 1935 and indicates that these had not been previously reported, these were classified as eighty cervicofacial, twenty-eight thoracic, sixty-two abdominal and twelve other types. This gives a total of at least 439 cases recorded in England by 1935. However, this does not accurately portray the incidence as 902 mortalities from actinomycosis were recorded for 1916 through 1935 (13). Since then there does not seem to be a comprehensive compilation of cases but numerous authors have reported on a number of cases, usually of a particular type. These are listed in Table 2-VI. There are at least twenty individual cases reported in the literature through 1972. Two of particular interest are a sinus infection (110) and an infection of the head following a fist fight (72).

TABLE 2-VI

REPORTS OF FIVE OR MORE CASES OF ACTINOMYCOSIS IN ENGLAND, 1952 TO 1973

			Clinical Distribution			
Journal	*Year*	*Total Cases*	*Cervico-facial*	*Tho-racic*	*Ab-dominal*	*Other*
Tubercle, *33*:258	1952	47		47		
Proc. Roy. Soc. Med. *46*:209	1953	15				15, eye
Brit. J. Surg. *42*:77	1954	9			9	
Thorax. *12*:99	1957	85		85		
Brit. Dent. J. *104*:314	1958	12	12			
Brit. Dent. J. *109*:235	1960	11	11			
Brit. J. Surg. *49*:266	1961	14			14	
Brit. J. Surg. *51*:345	1964	6			6	
Brit. J. Dermatol. *76*:421	1964	5	5			
Brit. Dent. J. *120*:423	1966	46	46			
Brit. Dent. J. *121*:23	1966	5	5			
Oral Surg. Oral Med. Oral Path. *29*:735	1970	7	7			
Thorax. *28*:73	1973	7		7		

Slade et al. (106) state that the number of cases reported to the Public Health Service is as follows:

	1966	1967	1968	1969	1970
No. cases	25	27	21	60	36—Total 169

This is considerably above the fifty reported in the U. S. (Table 2-III) during this period and probably reflects a greater sense of responsibility in reporting diseases in England.

Scotland and Ireland: Porter (89) collected a total of ninety-eight cases occurring in Scotland from 1936 through 1948 or 7.5 per year with a clinical distribution of seventy-two cervicofacial, six thoracic, fourteen abdominal and three other types with twelve deaths recorded during this same period. In Ireland, MacCarthy in 1955 (69) reported a case involving the uterus and in a review of the literature indicated that ten other cases had been recorded in Great Britain with a total of 157 reported in the world literature. Three additional cases have been reported from Ireland but information on incidence is difficult to obtain as actinomycosis is not a reportable disease.

AUSTRALIA: The first case was reported by McInerney in 1894 (*Aust. Med. J. 16*:39, 1894). Gardiner in a series of papers with extensive literature reviews (28, 29, 30) describes thirty cases, mostly cervicofacial, occurring in the Newcastle region. A review of cases from 1946 through 1956 lists four individual cases but indicates that fourteen occurred in Sydney in 1949 and that the average annual rate was ten (*Mycopath. Mycol. Appl. 9*:80, 1958). A second report for the years 1956 to 1969 adds six more cases (*Med. J. Aust. 2*:1117, 1970). Studies from the Institute of Dental Research in Sydney report on the culturing of exudate from 192 patients with oral swellings and diagnosing sixteen as actinomycosis (*Oral Surg. Oral Med. Oral Path. 8*:877, 1955; *Aust. Dent. J. 2*:259, 1957). Actinomycosis is reported in the aborigenes (*Med. J. Aust. 1*:184, 1965). Roveda (93) reports on two cases involving salivary glands and states that from 1965 through 1971 he observed fourteen additional cases of cervicofacial actinomycosis.

NEW ZEALAND: Two cases of cervicofacial actinomycosis have been reported (*N.Z. Dent. J. 64*:111, 1968; *62*:216, 1966).

DENMARK: The first case was reported by Bang in 1883 (*Hospitals.* Tidende, p. 673). Beginning with Orskov in 1923 (84) most of the studies on actinomycosis have been done at the State Serum Institute in Copenhagen where Holm (46, 47, 48) reports studying 801 patients and from this developed his thesis that actinomycotic diseases are a multiple or combined infection. Glahn (*Acta. Chir. Scand. 99*:537, 1950; *108*:183, 1954) indicated that ninety-one cases of cervicofacial actinomycosis were observed in Copenhagen. Then Rud in 1967 (94) reported that 224 cases were diagnosed from 1945 through 1950 with 90 percent being cervicofacial and indicated ten more were observed from 1954 through 1967.

NORWAY: In 1911 Harbitz and Grondahl (42) collected a series of eighty-seven cases (39 cervicofacial, 20 thoracic, 26 abdominal and 2 skin) in which over half gave positive cultures. They indicate the first case was described in Norway in 1887. Svane (*Acta Chir. Scand. 131*:160, 1966) indicates that eleven cases (5 cervicofacial, 1 thoracic and 5 abdominal) have been diagnosed and treated during the years 1941 through 1950.

SWEDEN: Hertz (*J. Int. Coll. Surg. 34*:148, 1960; *Sven Tandlak Tidskr 65*:129, 1971) tabulated seventy-five cases occurring from 1956 through 1969 followed by a description of eleven cases, six of which are described as being atypical because the facial swelling attached to the bone without fistulas. One additional case is reported in a review of pulmonary mycoses. (*Scand. J. Resp. Dis. 47*:1, 1966).

FRANCE: No articles were found which comprehensively reviewed the incidence of actinomycosis in France and one gains the impression that it is relatively rare. Segretain et al. (100) in a rather extensive article indicates actinomycosis is universal and sufficiently frequent but cites no actual cases. Lamarque et al. (60) discuss the radiological aspects of four cases of pulmonary actinomycosis but fewer than fifteen additional cases have been reported in the literature.

GERMANY: Illich (52) in 1892 compiled 492 cases (234 cervicofacial, 58 thoracic, 89 abdominal and 11 other) occurring in Germany. In recent years Lentze (64, 65, 66) at the Institute for Hygiene in Cologne has been a major contributor to the identification of the organism and in recognition of the disease. He gives statistics on 1,002 cases of bacteriologically and clinically proven actinomycosis which were distributed as follows: 929 cervicofacial, forty-three thoracic, twenty abdominal and ten of the tongue. The overwhelming number of cervicofacial cases is due to the cooperative efforts between the Institute and Department of Maxillosurgery in Cologne. Buchs (9) compiled data on fifty cervicofacial cases successfully treated with a heterovaccine and Freitag et al. (*Dent. ZaKnart, Z. 25*:333, 1035, 1970) report on fifty-two cervicofacial cases observed over an eight-year period. There are a number of single cases reported in the literature.

Czechoslovakia and Poland: Bronner and Bronner (8) relate personal communications from Warsaw and report at some length on sixty-nine cervicofacial cases observed during the years of 1952 through 1969. This is followed by a report from Poznan of 264 cervicofacial cases observed and treated during the years 1952 through 1970. Sazama (99) indicated that forty-five cervicofacial cases were treated at a clinic in Hradec Kralove, Czechoslovakia during the years of 1946 through 1962 and five cases of parotitis are described in detail.

Greece: Gogas et al. (*Int. Surg. 57*:664, 1966) describe two cases of actinomycosis of the breast responding to surgery. Sechas et al. (*Dis. Colon, Rectum 15*:366, 1972) reported on two additional cases simulating neoplasms.

Spain: An unusual case involving the liver and pancreas is reported (*Digestion, 2*:262, 1969) as well as a brain abscess which responded to surgery (*Rev. Clin. Esp. 87*:144, 1962).

Israel, Iraq, Iran: In Israel (*Isr. J. Med. Sci. 8*:148, 1972) sixteen cases (8 cervicofacial, 5 thoracic and 3 abdominal) have been treated over a fifteen-year period. An abdominal case is reported from Iraq (*Dis. Colon, Rectum 12*:30, 1969) and two cases of actinomycosis of the tongue are described from Iran (*Laryngoscope, 82*:2149, 1972).

Japan, India, Hawaii: Tokiwa et al. (*Bull. Tokyo Med. Dent. Univ. 6*:135, 1959) indicate that 283 cases were treated between the years 1951 to 1959. Takohashi (*Mycopath. Mycol. Appl. 19*:105, 1963) in a survey states that actinomycosis is quite common throughout Japan and lists seventy cervicofacial, three thoracic and fifteen abdominal cases. More recently Yamada et al. (*Am. J. Surg. 121*:341, 1971) in a detailed article describes a case involving the liver.

In India three cases of abdominal actinomycosis are described (*J. Ind. Med. Ass. 58*:426, 1972). Payner (*Hawaii Med. J. 13*:189, 1954) indicates that from 1940 through 1954 a total of thirty cases (10 cervicofacial, 14 thoracic, 4 abdominal and 2 other) had been observed in Hawaii and then Ajello (*Mycoph. Mycol.*

Appl. 46:87, 1972) indicates cases have been reported in Hawaii and in Fiji.

RUSSIA: No reports of the overall incidence of actinomycosis in Russia were found but Minsker and colleagues at the Institute of Parasitology and Tropical Medicine in Moscow report on treating over four hundred cases most of which were cervicofacial and they indicate the use of skin tests and the complement fixation tests as aids to diagnosis (*Vest. Derm. Veneroi, S.S.S.R.* 7:59, 1968; *Klin. Med. S.S.S.R.* 12:107, 1968). Pinzur et al. (*Sovetsk. Med.* 6:89, 1968) report ninety cases involving the perirectal region and the buttocks and Pliner (*Stomatol Mosk.* 50:84, 1971) reports on fifteen cases of actinomycosis of the tongue.

SUMMARY

1. Actinomycosis in man is most frequently caused by *Actinomyces israelii* although *A. naeslundii, A. odontolyticus, A. viscosus, A. eriksonii* or *Arachnia propionica* can cause the same disease with the same symptoms.
2. The disease is usually divided into cervicofacial (most common), thoracic and abdominal actinomycosis but any area of the body such as the brain, bone or skin may be involved.
3. These organisms may play a role in the development of caries and periodontal disease in man. This potential has been established by producing such lesions in experimental animals.
4. Actinomycosis occurs throughout the world without relation to race, seasons or occupation. It is not an opportunistic disease.
5. Males develop actinomycoses more frequently than females. Reported ratios vary from two to four males per female.
6. The disease occurs in all age groups being reported in infants as well as adults in their eighties. Overall, the greatest number of cases have been reported in persons between the ages of fifteen to thirty-five.

7. In relation to mortality rates, Cope (13) states that in Germany there were thirty-one deaths per year from 1914 to 1924 and that in England the average was forty-eight per year from 1916 through 1935. In Scotland (89) twelve fatalities were recorded for the year 1936 to 1948. In the United States an average of twenty-five deaths per year have been reported (Bureau of Vital Statistics) for the years 1949 through 1969 but a statistical analysis of the data (Table 2-II) indicates a downward trend in mortalities.
8. From the information presently available it is not possible to establish a meaningful case rate (the U. S. reported incidence varies from 3 to 11 cases per 100 million population) nor to pinpoint particular areas of incidence. The only conclusion is that "Actinomycosis occurs through the world and it is neither a rare nor a common disease."

REFERENCES

1. Adar, R., Antebi, R., David, R., Mozes, M.: Abdominal actinomycosis. *Isr J Med Sci, 8*:148, 1972.
2. Batty, I.: *Actinomyces odontolyticus*, a new species of actinomycete regularly isolated from deep carious dentine. *J Pathol Bact,* 75:455, 1958.
3. Bergey, D. H.: Aktinomyces der mundhole. *Zentralb Bakteriol Parastenk Infektionskr Abt I Ref, 40*:361, 1907.
4. Blank, C. H., Georg, L. K.: The use of fluorescent antibody methods for the detection and identification of *Actinomyces* species in clinical material. *J Lab Clin Med,* 71:283, 1968.
5. Bollinger, O.: Ueber eine neu pilzkrankheit beim rinde. *Zentralb Med Wiss, 15*:481, 1877.
6. Bolton, C. F., Ashenhurst, E. M.: Actinomycosis of the brain: Case report and review of literature. *Can Med Assoc J, 90*:922, 1964.
7. Brock, D. W., Georg, L. K. Brown, J. M., Hicklin, M. D.: Actinomycosis caused by *Arachnia propionica. J Clin Pathol, 59*:66, 1973.
8. Bronner, M., Bronner, M.: *Actinomycosis* (ed. 2). Bristol: John Wright and Sons, 1971.
9. Buchs, H.: Zur klinik und therapie der cervicofaciaten aktinomykose. *Deut Zahnaerztl Z, 18*:1060, 1963.
10. Coleman, R. M., Georg, L. K.: Comparative pathogenicity of *Actinomyces naeslundii* and *Actinomyces israelii. Appl Microbiol, 18*:427, 1969.

11. Coodley, E. L.: Actinomycosis: Clinical diagnosis and management. *Postgrad Med, 46*:73, 1969.
12. Cope, V. Z.: A clinical study of actinomycosis with illustrative cases. *Br J Surg, 3*:55, 1915.
13. Cope, V. Z.: *Actinomycosis.* Oxford University Press, London, 1938.
14. Cope, V. Z.: Actinomycosis of bone with special reference to infection of vertebral column. *J Bone Joint Surg, 33-B*:205, 1951.
15. Dutton, W. P., Inclan, A. P.: Cardiac actinomycosis. *Dis Chest, 54*:463, 1968.
16. Eastridge, C. E., Prather, J. R., Hughes, F. A., Young, J. M., McCaughan, J. J.: Actinomycosis: A twenty-four year experience. *S Med J, 65*:839, 1972.
17. Emmons, C. W.: The isolation of *Actinomyces bovis* from tonsillar granules. *Pub Hlth Rep,* 1, 1938.
18. Emmons, C. W., Binford, C. H., Utz, J. P.: *Medical Mycol.* Philadelphia: Lea and Febiger, 1963.
19. Ennever, J., Robinson, H. B. G., Kitchen, P. C.: *Actinomyces* and the dentobacterial plaque. *J Dent Res, 30*:88, 1951.
20. Erikson, D.: Pathogenic anaerobic organisms of the *Actinomyces* group. London: His Majesty's Stationery Office. *Med Res Council Spec Rep No. 240*:1, 1940.
21. Ernst, J., Ratjen, E.: Actinomycosis of the spine. *Acta Orthop Scand, 42*:35, 1971.
22. Erving, W. G.: Actinomycosis hominis in America, with report of six cases. *Bull Johns Hopkins Hosp, 13*:261, 1902.
23. Everts, E. C.: Cervicofacial actinomycosis. *Arch Otolar, 92*:468, 1970.
24. Fetter, B. F., Klintworth, G. K., Hendry, W. S.: *Mycoses of the Central Nervous System.* Baltimore: Williams Wilkins Co., 1967.
25. Flynn, M. W., Felson, B.: The roentgen manifestations of thoracic actinomycosis. *Am J Roent Radium Ther Nuclel Med, 110*:707, 1970.
26. Foley, T. F., Dines, D. E., Dolan, C. T.: Pulmonary actinomycosis. *Minn Med, 54*:593, 1971.
27. Foulerton, A. G. R.: Some observations on a series of 78 cases of streptothrix infections. *Proc Roy Soc Med, 6*:132, 1913.
28. Gardiner, S. S.: Actinomycosis of the fallopian tubes with report of a case. *Aust N Z J Surg, 4*:279, 1935.
29. Gardiner, S. S.: Actinomycosis of the head and neck. *Aust N Z J Surg, 6*:186, 1936.
30. Gardiner, S. S.: Actinomycosis of the urinary system. *Aust N Z J Surg, 12*:210, 1943.
31. Georg, L. K., Coleman, R. M.: Comparative pathogenicity of various *Actinomyces* species. The *Actinomycelates. Jena Int Symp Taxon, 1*:35, 1970.

32. Georg, L. K., Pine, L., Gerencser, M. A.: *Actinomyces viscosus* comb. nov., A catalase positive, facultative member of the genus *Actinomyces. Int J Syst Bact, 19*:291, 1969.
33. Georg, L. K., Robertstad, G. W., Brinkman, S. A., Hicklin, M. D.: A new pathogenic anaerobic *Actinomyces* species. *J Infect Dis, 115*:88, 1965.
34. Gerszten, E., Allison, M. J., Dalton, H. P.: A ten-year study of mycotic infections in a Virginia general hospital. *Am J Clin Pathol, 52*:445, 1969.
35. Goldstein, B. H., Sciubba, J. J., Laskin, D. M.: Actinomycosis of the maxilla; Review of literature and report of case. *J Oral Surg, 30*:362, 1972.
36. Graybill, J. R., Silverman, B. D.: Sulfur granules, second thoughts. *Arch Intern Med, 123*:430, 1969.
37. Gruner, O. P. N.: *Actinomyces* in tonsillar tissue. *Acta Pathol Microbiol Scand, 79*:77, 1971.
38. Guidry, D. J.: *Actinomycosis in Human Infection with Fungi, Actinomycetes and Algae,* Baker, R. D. (ed.), N. Y.: Springer-Verlag, 1971.
39. Hall, W. E. B.: *Actinomyces* in the tonsils. *Am J Clin Pathol, 14*:215, 1944.
40. Halseth, W. L., Reich, M. R.: Pulmonary actinomycosis treated by lung resection. *Dis Chest, 55*:119, 1969.
41. Hamilton, W. S.: A review of actinomycosis. *J Can Dent Assoc, 8*:427, 1942.
42. Harbitz, F., Grondahl, N. B.: Actinomycosis in Norway: Studies on the etiology, mode of infection and treatment. *Am J Med Sci, 142*:386, 1911.
43. Harley, J. H., Schatten, W. E.: Cervicofacial actinomycosis. *Plast Reconstr Surg, 51*:44, 1973.
44. Harvey, J. C., Cantrell, J. R., Fisher, A. M.: Actinomycosis: Its recognition and treatment. *Ann Int Med, 46*:868, 1957.
45. Hertz, J.: Actinomycosis. Borderline cases. *J Int Coll Surg, 34*:148, 1960.
46. Holm, P.: Comparative studies on pathogenic anaerobic *Actinomyces. Acta Pathol Microbiol Scand Suppl, 3*:151, 1930.
47. Holm, P.: Studies on the aetology of human actinomycosis. I. The "Other Microbes" of actinomycosis and their importance. *Acta Pathol Microbiol Scand, 27*:736, 1950.
48. Holm, P.: Studies on the aetiology of human actinomycosis. II. Do the "Other Microbes" of actinomycosis possess virulence? *Acta Pathol Microbiol Scand, 28*:391, 1951.
49. Hotchi, M., Schwarz, J.: Characterization of actinomycotic granules by architecture and staining methods. *Arch Pathol, 93*:392, 1972.

50. Howell, A., Jordon, H. V., Georg, L. K., Pine, L.: *Odontomyces viscosus,* Gen. Nov., Spec. Nov., A filamentous microorganism isolated from periodontal plaque in hamsters. *Sabouraudia, 4*:65, 1965.
51. Hutter, R. V. P., Collins, H. S.: The occurrence of opportunistic fungus infections in a cancer hospital. *Lab Invest, 11*:1035, 1962.
52. Illich, A.: Beitrag zur klinic der akinomycose. *J Safir,* Wien (quoted by Cope, 1938).
53. Israel, J.: Neue beobachtungen auf dem gebiete der mykosen des menschen. *Arch Pathol Anat Phys Klin Med, 74*:15, 1878.
54. Israel, J.: Neue beitrage zu den mykotischen erkrankungen des menschen. *Arch Pathol Anat Phys Klin Med, 78*:421, 1879.
55. Israel, J.: Ein beitrag zur pathogenese der lungenaktinomykose. *Arch Klin Chir, 34*:160, 1887.
56. Jacobson, R. J., Cloward, R. B.: Actinomycosis of the central nervous system. *JAMA, 137*:769, 1948.
57. Kay, E. B.: Bronchopulmonary actinomycosis. *Ann Int Med, 26*:581, 1947.
58. Kolouch, F., Peltier, L. F.: Actinomycosis. *Surgery, 20*:401, 1946.
59. Lachner-Sandoval, V.: Ueber Strahlenpilze. Inaugural-Dissertation Strassburg. Universitats Buchdruckerei Von Carl Georgi, Bonn, 1898.
60. Lamarque, J. L., Combes, C., Senac, J. P., Ampelas, S.: Aspects radiologiques de l'actinomycose pulmonaire. *J Radiol Electrol Med Nucl, 53*:5, 1972.
61. Lamb, J. H., Lain, E. S., Jones, P. E., Actinomycosis of the face and neck. *JAMA, 134*:351, 1947.
62. Lambert, F. W., Brown, J. M., Georg, L. K.: Identification of *Actinomyces israelii* and *Actinomyces naeslundii* by fluorescent antibody and agar-gel diffusion techniques. *J Bact, 94*:1287, 1967.
63. Leers, W. D., Dussault, J., Mullens, J. E., Volpe, R.: Suppurative thyroiditis: An unusual case caused by *Actinomyces naeslundii. Can Med Assoc J, 101*:715, 1969.
64. Lentze, F. A.: Zur bakteriologie und vakzinetherapie der aktinomykose. *Zentral Bakteriol Abt 1, Orig, 141*:21, 1938.
65. Lentze, F. A.: Die Aktinomykose des Menschen. *Lehrbuch der medizinische Mikrobiologie und Infektions Krankheiten.* Fisher, Stuttgart, 1961.
66. Lentze, F. A.: Die Aktinomykose und die Nocardiosen. *Die Infektionskrankheiten des Menschen und ihre Erregen.* A. Bumgach ed. George Thieme, Stuttgart, 1969.
67. Lord, F. T.: The etiology of actinomycosis. *JAMA, 55*:1261, 1910.
68. Lord, F. T.: A contribution to the etiology of actinomycosis. The experimental production of actinomycosis in guinea pigs inoculated

with the contents of carious teeth. *Boston Med Surg J, 163*:82, 1910.
69. MacCarthy, J.: Actinomycosis of the female pelvic organs with envolvement of the endometrium. *J Pathol Bact, 69*:175, 1955.
70. Main, J. H. P., MacPhee, I. T.: Actinomycosis of the maxilla in relation to a periodontal abscess. *Oral Surg Oral Med Oral Pathol, 17*:299, 1964.
71. McQuarrie, D. G., Hall, W. H.: Actinomycosis of the lung and chest wall. *Surgery, 64*:905, 1968.
72. Mendelsohn, B. G.: Actinomycosis of a metacarpal bone. *J Bone Joint Surg, 47B*:739, 1965.
73. Mincy, J. E., Peck, F. C.: Actinomycotic subdural empyema. *N Y State J Med, 66*:2155, 1966.
74. Montgomery, R. M., Welton, W. A.: Primary actinomycosis of the upper extremity. *Arch Dermatol, 79*:578, 1959.
75. Moore, W. R., Scannell, J. G.: Pulmonary actinomycosis simulating cancer of the lung. *J Thorac Cardiov Surg, 55*:193, 1968.
76. Morton, H. S.: Actinomycosis. *Can Med Assoc J, 42*:231, 1940.
77. Murphy, J. B.: Actinomycosis in the human subject. *N Y Med J, 41*:17, 1885.
78. Murphy, J. B.: Actinomycosis hominis, with report of five cases. *Practitioner, 3*:593, 1891.
79. Naeslund, C.: Studies of *Actinomyces* from the oral cavity. *Acta Pathol Microbiol Scand, 2*:110, 1925.
80. Nathan, M. H., Radman, W. P., Barton, H. L.: Osseous actinomycosis of the head and neck. *Am J Roentg Radium Ther Nucl Med, 87*:1048, 1962.
81. Negroni, P.: Micosis Profundas. Los Micetomas, Vol. 1, El Ateneo, Buenos Aires, 1954.
82. Negroni, P., Bonfiglioli, H.: Morphology and biology of *Actinomyces israelii. J Trop Med Hyg, 40*:226, 240, 1937.
83. Nichols, D. R., Herrell, W. E.: Penicillin in the treatment of actinomycosis. *J Lab Clin Med, 33*:521, 1948.
84. Orskov, J.: *Investigations into the Morphology of the Ray Fungi.* Levin and Munksgaard, Copenhagen, 1923.
85. Pheils, M. T., Reid, D. J., Ross, C. F.: Abdominal actinomycosis. *Br J Surg, 51*:345, 1964.
86. Pine, L., Howell, A., Watson, S. J.: Studies of the morphological, physiological and biochemical characters of *Actinomyces bovis. J Gen Microbiol, 23*:403, 1960.
87. Pine, L., Georg, L. K.: Reclassification of *Actinomyces propionicus. Int Bull Bact Nomencl Taxon, 15*:143, 1969.
88. Poppe, J. K.: Treatment of pulmonary actinomycosis with a report of seven arrested cases. *J Thorac Surg, 15*:118, 1946.

89. Porter, I. A.: Actinomycosis in northeast Scotland. *Br Med J, 1*:1360, 1951.
90. Prather, J. R., Eastridge, C. E., Hughes, F. A., McCaughan, J. J.: Actinomycosis of the thorax. *Ann Thorac Surg, 9*:307, 1970.
91. Prolo, D. J., Hanbery, J. W.: Secondary actinomycotic brain abscess. *Arch Surg, 96*:58, 1968.
92. Putman, H. C., Dockerty, M. C., Waugh, J. M.: Abdominal actinomycosis: An analysis of 122 cases. *Surgery, 28*:781, 1950.
93. Roveda, S. I. L.: Cervicofacial actinomycosis. Report of two cases involving major salivary glands. *Aust Dent J, 18*:7, 1973.
94. Rud, J.: Cervicofacial actinomycosis. *J Oral Surg, 25*:229, 1967.
95. Ruhrah, J.: Actinomycosis in man, with special reference to cases which have been observed in America. *Ann Surg, 30*:417, 605, 722, 1899.
96. Ruhrah, J.: Actinomycosis in man with special reference to cases which have been observed in America. *Ann Surg, 31*:235, 1900.
97. Sanford, A. H.: Distribution of actinomycosis in the United States. *JAMA, 81*:655, 1923.
98. Sanford, A. H., Voelker, M.: Actinomycosis in the United States. *Arch Surg, 11*:809, 1925.
99. Sazma, L.: Actinomycosis of the parotid gland. *Oral Med Oral Surg Oral Pathol, 19*:197, 1965.
100. Segretain, G., Drouhet, E., Mariat, F.: Classification des mycoses, mycoses rares in France, actinomycosis. *Rev Praticien, 18*:2843, 1968.
101. Slack, J.: The source of infection in actinomycosis. *J Bact, 43*:193, 1942.
102. Slack, J. M.: Genus *Actinomyces. Bergey's Manual for Determinative Bacteriology*, 8th ed. Baltimore, William Wilkins, 1974.
103. Slack, J. M., Gerencser, M. A.: *Actionmyces, Filamentous Bacteria: Biology and Pathogenicity*. Minneapolis, Burgess, 1975.
104. Slack, J. M., Landfried, S., Gerencser, M. A.: Identification of *Actinomyces* and related bacteria in dental calculus by the fluorescent antibody technique. *J Dent Res, 50*:78, 1971.
105. Slack, J. M., Moore, D. W., Gerencser, M. A.: Use of the fluorescent antibody technique in the diagnosis of actinomycosis. *W Va Med J, 62*:228, 1966.
106. Slade, P. R., Slesser, B. V., Southgate, J.: Thoracic actinomycosis. *Thorax, 28*:73, 1973.
107. Socransky, S. S., Manganiello, S. D.: The oral microbiota of man from birth to senility. *J Periodontol, 42*:485, 1971.
108. Socransky, S. S., Hubersak, C., Propas, D.: Induction of periodontal destruction in gnotobiotic rats by a human oral strain of *Actinomyces naeslundii. Arch Oral Biol, 15*:993, 1970.

109. Spilsbury, B. W., Johnstone, F. R. C.: The clinical course of actinomycotic infections. *Can J Surg, 5*:33, 1962.
110. Stanton, M. B., Actinomycosis of the maxillary sinus. *J Laryng Otol, 80*:168, 1966.
111. Sullivan, H. R., Goldsworthy, N. E.: A comparative study of anaerobic strains of *Actinomyces* from clinically normal mouths and from actinomycotic lesions. *J Pathol Bact, 51*:253, 1940.
112. Thompson, L., Lovestedt, S. A.: An Actinomyces-like organism obtained from the human mouth. *Proc Staff Meet Mayo Clin, 26*: 169, 1951.
113. Tomm, K. E.: Raleigh, J. W., Guinn, G. A.: Thoracic actinomycosis. *Am J Surg, 124*:46, 1972.
114. Trempe, F.: Actinomycose mammaire-primitive. *Can J Surg, 1*:210, 1958.
115. Weed, L. A., Baggenstoss, A. H.: Actinomycosis, A pathologic and bacteriologic study of twenty-one fatal cases. *Am J Clin Pathol, 19*:201, 1949.
116. Wilkinson, H. F.: Pathologic changes in tonsils. *Arch Otolaryng, 10*: 127, 1929.
117. Wolff, M., Israel, J.: Ueber reincultur des Actinomyces und seine uebertragbarkeit auf thiere. *Arch Pathol Anat Phys Klin Med, 126*:11, 1891.
118. Wright, J. H.: The biology of the microorganism of actinomycosis. *J Med Res, 8*:349, 1905.
119. Yamada, T., Sakai, A., Tonouchi, S., Kawashina, K.: Actinomycosis of the liver. *Am J Surg., 121*:341, 1971.

Chapter 3

THE EPIDEMIOLOGY OF NOCARDIOSIS

Norman L. Goodman

Unfortunately, human nocardiosis cannot be discussed in classical epidemiological terms because of the paucity of information on the disease and the lack of tools and expertise in identifying infections. Thus, there are no data on the incidence of nocardiosis in any given human population. Therefore, we are obliged to resort to the study of existing case study data and thereby draw conclusions, as best as possible on the nature of this disease in the population.

Nocardiosis is a generalized infection in man and animal which is characteristically pulmonary in origin. The infection may be subclinical, acute or chronic in nature and frequently spreads hematogenously to other organs of the body.

Nocardiosis had its origin, as a clinical entity in man, in 1890, when Eppinger described the disease in a fifty-two-year-old male glassblower (11). The disease in the first reported human case involved the lungs, pleura, peribronchial lymph nodes, meninges and brain.

Subsequent to Eppinger's case, additional cases were reported infrequently and diagnosis were almost invariably made at autopsy. Also, the reported cases were frequently confusing in that a clear distinction between nocardiosis and actinomycosis was often not made and many cases were not verified by culture, but only by visual observations of clinical specimens. In 1957 Ballenger and Goldring (5) reviewed the literature and reported ninety-five cases as authentic nocardiosis. Reports in the literature since that time have had better mycological and pathological documentations, and thus provide a more firm basis for clinical and mycological evaluations (1, 10, 19, 24).

NOCARDIA ASTEROIDES

Systemic nocardiosis is caused by *Nocardia asteroides,* a gram-positive, aerobic, actinomycete having branching hyphae of approximately one micron in diameter. The soil is the natural habitat of this organism and it has been isolated from various types of soil throughout the world (16, 22, 31). Presumably, the organism is inhaled in aerosolized dust and thus infects the human; of which the more susceptible host progress to various states of disease. Communicability from human to human, human to animal, or animal to animal has not been reported.

Nocardiosis has been reported in a wide variety of animals throughout the world, with the largest number of infections being in dairy herds in California and Hawaii (3, 13).

Nocardiosis in man was once considered a rare and fatal disease, as indeed the literature indicates; however, with improved microbiological methods and an increased awareness of fungal infections, this disease is now being recognized more frequently in nonfatal infections (6, 25).

Opportunism

The ability of *N. asteroides* to invade and cause pulmonary disease in a healthy individual has been questioned, thus many consider it an opportunist, causing secondary disease concomitant with a primary disease. There is convincing evidence that this organism is indeed commonly associated with secondary infections of individuals with chronic debilitating diseases, and diseases requiring immunosuppressive drugs of radiation therapy. Young, et al. (37) reported twenty-two cases of nocardiosis concomitant with and complicating neoplastic disease. Others have reported fewer similar cases. This disease has also been associated with other underlying conditions such as: dysproteinemia, disseminated lupus erythematous, immunosuppression after organ transplantation, pulmonary alevolar proteinosis, ulcerative colitis, intestinal lipodystrophy, sarcoidosis, and Cushings disease. It is becoming clear that this is not a rarely encountered disease, but one that may be easily overlooked with subsequent high mortality.

Occurrence and Distribution

Nocardiosis has been reported as a disease of males, primarily with occupations associated with farming or other jobs which bring the individuals close to the soil. A review of the case histories to 1973, fails to substantiate this, however this is primarily because of the lack of occupation histories.

A search of the literature provided 267 cases of culturally proven cases of nocardiosis (1, 19, 20, 24). Table 3-I shows the distribution of nocardiosis by sex, with 61 percent of the cases being male, 27 percent female and 12 percent with sex not reported, thus a ratio of over 2 to 1, males to females, with nocardiosis.

When these cases are categorized by the organ(s) involved, the largest number, 130 (4%) have lung involvement only, with the next largest category being the disseminated form with seventy-seven cases, or 29 percent (Table 3-II). The percentages drop precipitously to the next category of brain involvement only, extra pulmonary, etc. Thus, nocardiosis is primarily a pulmonary disease which frequently becomes disseminated (4, 12, 14, 18, 23, 27, 28). The organism is reported to have a predilection for brain, although this is not reflected in the case studies where 46 of 267 (17%) cases had brain involvement, sixteen (6%) of which had brain infection only. This indicates a prevalence of 17 percent brain involvement with 6 percent of the cases having brain involvement only (Table 3-II).

TABLE 3-I

DISTRIBUTION OF HUMAN NOCARDIOSIS BY SEX

Sex	*No.*	*Percent*
Male	164	61
Female	73	27
Sex Not Reported	30	12

TABLE 3-II

DISTRIBUTION OF HUMAN NOCARDIOSIS BY CLINICAL DIAGNOSIS

Type Disease	*Number*	*Percent*
Lung only	130	47
Lung and Brain	15	6
Brain only	16	7
Disseminated (lung and/or brain and other internal organs)	77	29
Extra Pulmonary (internal organs exclusive of lung and brain)	15	6
Subcutaneous	14	5

TABLE 3-III

DISTRIBUTION OF PULMONARY NOCARDIOSIS BY AGE

Age (yr.)	*No.*	*Percent*
0-1	5	2
2-10	16	7
11-20	21	8
21-30	29	11
31-40	53	20
41-50	45	18
51-60	37	13
61-70	31	11
71-80	1	0.3
81+	3	1
Age Not Reported	26	9

In the early literature, nocardiosis was considered a dread disease with grave prognosis. This was indeed the case, as there was a 72 percent mortality rate in cases reported to 1950 (9). The mortality rate of nocardiosis still remains high, with 139 deaths in 267 cases reported; a 52 percent mortality rate. This high mortality rate is undoubtedly a partial result of the lack of good diagnostic procedures for diagnosing the disease. This is borne out by the fact that 20 percent of the reported cases were diagnosed post mortem; a real challenge to the clinical microbiologist.

Age

Nocardiosis has been diagnosed in individuals of ages ranging from six months to eighty-two years (5, 10, 34, 36). As indicated in Table 3-III, the age distribution is relatively even from ages eleven through seventy. However, 50 percent of the cases reported were in individuals of ages thirty-one through sixty-nine. Thirty-six percent of the cases were in the thirty-one through fifty age group, possibly indicating a higher risk of nocardiosis or higher risk of exposure in the middle aged indivdual.

Types of Infection

Pulmonary involvement in nocardiosis is one of the most stable features of the disease, although there are many extrapulmonary manifestations. In the group of 267 cases studied, 84 percent showed pulmonary involvement, with and without extrapulmonary manifestations (2, 7, 14, 26). Of the 267 cases, 130 or 47 percent had pulmonary disease only. This comprised the largest component of the group studied. A closer look at these cases of pulmonary nocardiosis without dissemination showed that 60 percent were male, 24 percent female and 16 percent of the cases had no sex reported (Table 3-IV). This is approximately the same ratio for all forms of nocardiosis.

TABLE 3-IV

DISTRIBUTION OF PULMONARY NOCARDIOSIS BY SEX

Sex	*No.*	*Percent*
Male	78	60
Female	31	24
Sex Not Reported	21	16
Total	130	100

The age distribution of pulmonary nocardiosis indicates that no particular age group was more susceptible than another. Tables 3-V and 3-VI show the age distribution of males and females with pulmonary nocardiosis only. Approximately 50 percent of the male cases were in the thirty-one through seventy age group while 50 percent of the female cases were in the twenty-one through forty age group, thus the male distribution is more even from age one through seventy. Also approximately 12 percent of the male cases were ten years of age or less. This represents nine males in that age group, while only one female of this age group was reported.

TABLE 3-V

AGE DISTRIBUTION OF MALES WITH PULMONARY NOCARDIOSIS ONLY

Age (yr.)	*No.*	*Percent*
0-1	4	5.1
2-10	5	6.4
11-20	10	12.8
21-30	6	7.6
31-40	15	19.2
41-50	12	16.3
51-60	10	12.8
61-70	14	17.8
71-80	0	0
81+	2	2.5
Total	78	100.0

TABLE 3-VI

AGE DISTRIBUTION OF FEMALES WITH PULMONARY NOCARDIOSIS ONLY

Age (yr.)	*No.*	*Percent*
0-1	0	0.0
2-10	1	3.2
11-20	4	12.9
21-30	8	25.8
31-40	8	25.8
41-50	3	9.7
51-60	4	12.9
61-70	3	9.7
71-80	0	0.0
81+	0	0.0
Total	31	100.0

The overall mortality rate for reported cases of pulmonary nocardiosis is 43 percent with a 51 percent mortality rate for males and 36 percent for females. The age distribution relative to the mortality in pulmonary nocardiosis is shown in Tables 3-VII and 3-VIII. There is no particular age group of males with a higher mortality, however, the mortality in females apparently increases with age.

TABLE 3-VII

AGE SPECIFIC MORTALITY RATE OF PULMONARY NOCARDIOSIS IN MALES

Age	*Total No.*	*Deaths*	*Percent Mortality*
0-1	4	2	50
2-10	5	3	60
11-20	10	7	70
21-30	6	1	16
31-40	15	11	73
41-50	12	5	42
51-60	10	5	50
61-70	14	6	43
71-80	0	0	0
81+	2	0	0

TABLE 3-VIII

AGE SPECIFIC MORTALITY RATE OF PULMONARY NOCARDIOSIS IN FEMALES

Age	*Total No.*	*Deaths*	*Percent Mortality*
0-1	0	0	0
2-10	1	0	0
11-20	4	1	25
21-30	8	3	38
31-40	8	3	38
41-50	3	0	0
51-60	4	2	50
61-70	3	2	66
71-80	0	0	0
81+	0	0	0

Pulmonary nocardiosis may be summarized as 1) being more prevalent in males than females, 2) having no increased prevalence in any particular age group, 3) having an increased mortality rate with increasing age in females and a more evenly distributed mortality rate in males relative to age.

Disseminated nocardiosis occurs as a result of hematogenous spread from a primary focus of infection, usually the lungs. Disseminated disease was diagnosed in 77 of 267 cases of nocardiosis (29%) of the seventy-seven cases, 57 or 74 percent were in males (4, 12, 21).

The majority of cases of disseminated nocardiosis appears to occur in the middle age group of males and females. However, this is also true of nocardiosis in general. Of fifty-seven cases of disseminated nocardiosis in males, thirty-one cases, or 54 percent occurred in the thirty-one through sixty age group (Table 3-IX). The same distribution is found in females, with thirteen of twenty cases, or 65 percent in the thirty-one through sixty age group (Table 3-X). It should be noted that of the five cases of nocardiosis reported in infants, three were disseminated.

TABLE 3-IX

AGE SPECIFIC DISSEMINATION RATE OF NOCARDIOSIS IN MALES

Age	*No.*	*Percent*
0-1	3	5.2
2-10	1	1.7
11-20	3	5.2
21-30	7	12.2
31-40	10	17.5
41-50	9	15.7
51-60	12	21.0
61-70	7	12.2
71-80	0	0
81+	0	0
Unknown	5	8.7
Total	57	100.0

TABLE 3-X

AGE SPECIFIC DISSEMINATION RATE OF NOCARDIOSIS IN FEMALES

Age	*No.*	*Percent*
0-1	0	0
2-10	2	10
11-20	1	5
21-30	2	10
31-40	3	15
41-50	7	35
51-60	3	15
61-70	2	10
71-80	0	0
81+	0	0
Total	20	100

3. Ayers, K. M., Garner, F. M., Griner, L. A.: Disseminated nacardiosis in a North African antelope. *JAVMA, 159*:5, 1971.
4. Baikie, A. G., MacDonald, C. B., Mundy, G. R.: Systemic nocardiosis treated with trimethoprim and sulphamethoxazole. *Lancet, 2*:261, 1970.
5. Ballenger, C., Goldring, D.: Nocardiosis in childhood. *J Pediatr, 50,* 1957.
6. Brine, J. A. S.: Human nocardiosis: A developing clinical picture. *Med J Aust, 1*:339, 1965.
7. Burbank, B., Morrione, T. G., Cutler, S. S.: Pulmonary alveolar proteinosis and nocardiosis. *Am J Med, 28*:1002, 1960.
8. Carlsen, E. T., Hill, Jr., R. B., Rowlands, Jr., D. T.: Nocardiosis and pulmonary alveolar proteinosis. *Ann Int Med, 60*:2, 1964.
9. Conant, N. F., Smith, D. T., Baker, R. D., Callaway, J. L.: *Manual of Clinical Mycology.* Saunders, Philadelphia, ed. 3, 1971.
10. Dolan, Jr., T. F., McCullough, N. B., Gibson, L. E.: Nocardiosis, report of two cases in children. *Am J Dis Child, 99*:234, 1960.
11. Eppinger, H.: Ueber Eine Neue Pathogene Cladothrix Und Eine Durch Sie Hervorgerufene Pseudotuberculosis. *Wien Klin Wchnschr, 3*:321, 1890.
12. Failes, D.: Systemic nocardiosis presenting as a breast abscess. *Med J Aust, 1*, 1965.
13. Fawi, M. T., Tag El Din, M. H., El Sanousi, S. M.: Canine distemper as a predisposing factor for Nocardia asteriodes infection in the dog. *Vet Record, 88*, 1971.
14. Freese, J. M., Young, Jr., W. G., Sealy, W. C., Conant, N. F.: Pulmonary infection by *Nocardia asteriodes. J Thorac Cardiovas Surg, 46*:4, 1963.
15. Goodman, J. S., Koenig, M. G.: Nocardia infections in a general hospital. *Ann N Y Acad Sci, 174*:2, 1970.
16. Gordon, R. E., Hagan, W. A.: A study of some acid-fast actinomycetes from soil with special reference to pathogenicity for animals. *J Infect Dis, 59*:200, 1936.
17. Gydell, K., Juhlin, I., Ljunggren, H., Norden, J. G., Fors, B.: Nocardiosis During Steroid Treatment of Auto-immune Haemylytic Anaemia. *Acta Medica Scand, 178*:2, 1965.
18. Hall, G. V.: A case of pulmonary nocardiosis with apparent cure with sulphadiazine. *Med J Aust, 1*:455, 1964.
19. Hathaway, B. M., Mason, K. N.: Nocardiosis, study of fourteen cases. *Am J Med, 32*:903, 1962.
20. Hoeprich, P. D., Brandt, D., Parker, R. H.: Nocardial brain abscess cured with cycloserine and sulfonamides. *Am J Med Sci, 255*:208, 1968.

21. Iyer, P. K. R., Rao, A. T., Acharjyo, L. N., Sahu, S., Mishra, S. K.: Systemic nocardiosis in a hill mynah (Gracula Religiosa), A pathological study. *Mycopath Mycol Appl, 48*:2-3, 1972.
22. Kishimoto, R. A., Baker, G. E.: Pathogenic and potentially pathogenic fungi isolated from beach sands and selected soils of Oahu, Hawaii. *Mycologia, 61*:537, 1969.
23. Langevin, R. W., Sol, Katz: Fulminating pulmonary nocardiosis. *Dis Chest, 46*:3, 1964.
24. Larsen, M. C., Diamond, H. D., Collins, H. S.: *Nocardia asteriodes* infection: A report of seven cases. *Arch Intern Med, 103*:712, 1959.
25. Murray, J. F., Finegold, S. M., Froman, S., Will, D. W.: The changing spectrum of nocardiosis. *Am Rev Respir Dis, 83*:3, 1961.
26. Neu, H. C., Silva, M., Hazen, E., Rosenheim, S. H.: Necrotizing nocardial pneumonitis. *Ann Intern Med, 66*:274, 1966.
27. Pinkerton, J. A., Lawler, M. R., Foster, J. H.: Pulmonary nocardiosis. *Am Surgeon, 37*:729, 1971.
28. Pinkhas, J., Oliver, I., De Vries, Andre, Spitzer, S. A., Henig, E.: Pulmonary nocardiosis complicating malignant lymphoma successfully treated with chemotherapy. *Chest, 63*:3, 1973.
29. Raich, R. A., Casey, F., Hall, W. H.: Pulmonary and Cutaneous Nocardiosis. *Am Rev Resp Dis, 83*:505, 1961.
30. Rifkind, D., Marchioro, T. L., Schneck, S. A., Hill, Jr., R. B.: Systemic fungal infections complicating renal transplantation and immunosuppressive therapy. *Am J Med, 43*:28, 1967.
31. Rodda, G. M. J.: *Nocardia* strains in the environment. *Med J Aust, 1*:13, 1964.
32. Rouge-Mont, M. J., Mlle. Battesti, Manuel, Y., Goutelle, A.: Abcès du cervelet par *Nocardia asteriodes. J Med Lyon*, 605, 1963.
33. Saltzman, H. A., Chick, E. W., Conant, N. F.: Nocardiosis as a complication of other diseases. *Lab Invest, 11*:2, 1962.
34. Stites, D. P., Glezen, W. P.: Pulmonary nocardiosis in childhood. *Am J Dis Child, 114*:101, 1967.
35. Taleghani-Far, M., Barber, J. B., Sampson, C., Harden, K. A.: *Cerebral Nocardiosis and Alveolar Proteinosis.* Howard Univ. Col. Med., Washington, D. C., 1963.
36. Webster, B. H.: Pulmonary nocardiosis simulating pulmonary tuberculosis in the aged. *Am J Geriat, 10*:192, 1962.
37. Young, L. S., et al.: *Nocardia asteroides* infection complicating neoplastic disease. *Am J Med, 50*:356, 1971.

Chapter 4

THE EPIDEMIOLOGY OF HISTOPLASMOSIS

Howard W. Larsh

The subject of this chapter has been explored rather extensively since Darling discovered the disease in 1905. Many excellent papers have been written in which each investigator's viewpoints have been presented, but not to the satisfaction of all epidemiologists. Furcolow's review in the treatise on histoplasmosis constitutes the most comprehensive coverage up to 1960 (16). Since this publication several national and international symposia have included discussions dealing with various aspects of the epidemiology of this mycotic infection.

In view of the completeness and expertise of the authors on the overall subject of the epidemiology of histoplasmosis, the scope of this chapter will be limited. Review of recent research and an emphasis on basic concepts of the biology of *Histoplasma capsulatum* are necessary to understand fundamental factors affecting the epidemiology of histoplasmosis.

GROWTH AND DISSEMINATION OF HISTOPLASMA

It is essential at the outset to know the source of the etiological agent in nature. The role of environmental factors on the growth and development of *H. capsulatum* must be examined and well understood. Two parameters, moisture and temperature, have been associated with the growth of the fungus in the laboratory and in experiments in nature. Many earlier studies have revealed that *H. capsulatum*, like other fungi, shows a preference for moderate temperatures and moist environments. These observations have been corroborated under natural as well as experimental conditions. The growth and development of *H. capsulatum* are affected by certain temperature and humidity ranges. Under experimental laboratory conditions, sterile soil cultures of *H. capsulatum* show no detectable growth in less than 100 percent relative humidity and only in the temperature range 68 to 86 degrees F. Goodman and Larsh (19), in comparative studies, have shown that *H. capsulatum* will survive best in moist soils at temperatures below 0 degrees C and up to 37 degrees C. However, in dry soil the mycelium rapidly dehydrates and lysis occurs. Nevertheless, microaleuriospores and macroaleuriospores remain morphologically unchanged and viable. The lysis and eventual destruction of the mycelium and long exposure to dry conditions results in the loss of viability of these infectious units. Microaleuriospores likewise are destroyed when subjected to excessive exposure to dry conditions as well as to very low and high temperatures. Only the macroaleuriospore can survive the extremes of temperature and moisture ranges for this organism. There is a rapid death of the fungus in moist soil at 40 degrees C, which is most likely due to inactivation of enzymes at this temperature. Earlier laboratory experiments, which have been confirmed by recent studies of natural soils, show a rather sharp line of heat tolerance between 37 degrees and 40 degrees C.

The author has always considered *H. capsulatum* to be a rather common soil microorganism and that man and other animals are fortuitously susceptible to it. Unfortunately, many soil samples collected from areas in which positive histoplasmosis cases occurred failed to yield the fungus when inoculated onto artificial media and into experimental laboratory animals. The failure to recover the fungus from such soil specimens in environments in which optimal humidity and temperature requirements were present does not necessarily preclude that it was not present. There are several reasons that could be cited for such failures. In many instances only a very small sample was actually processed. Also, a limited number of infectious units may have been present and these may have been in competition with other microorganisms that contaminated the artificial media or destroyed the experimental animals. It is also true that soil from one small area will be positive, whereas a specimen only a few inches away will not yield the fungus. These common findings introduce an obvious question, "Are there other environmental factors playing a role in the ecology of *H. capsulatum* in nature?" Emmons (13) first isolated the fungus in 1949 from soil collected from a rodent burrow under a chicken coop. Zeidberg (34) and his coworkers first reported the frequency of isolation of *H. capsulatum* from soil in chicken yards and houses in comparison to isolations from other areas on farms. Stimulated by the reports of these and other investigators, a search for other factors which may be necessary for the growth and maintenance of *H. capsulatum* in the environment began.

Routine chemical analyses to establish the composition of soil specimens did not completely resolve the problem, but they did lead to laboratory studies suggesting that certain chemicals were essential for growth and development of the fungus in nature. In our laboratory it was established that certain additives, which were constituents of soil from which the fungus was isolated, enhanced its growth on artificial media. Smith (30) has presented a more sophisticated study showing that specific chemical substances may play a significant role in the ecology of the fungus in nature.

It has been evident since 1949 that soils contaminated by animal droppings enrich the environment and play a major role in the ecology of *H. capsulatum*. Bats, starlings, blackbirds, chickens, and other avian species are especially associated with this relationship.

Due to the early suggestions that chicken droppings may play a significant role on the biology of *H. capsulatum*, an attempt was made to determine the effect of chicken excrement on the growth of this fungus. The rationale was to study specific chemical constituents in chicken excrement as environmental factors possibly associated with humidity and temperature in maintaining *H. capsulatum* in the environment. In view of this hypothesis, a water extract of chicken droppings was produced for laboratory studies and designated as "chimanex" (24, 30). This was added in varying amcunts to sterilized soil, natural soil, and Sabouraud's dextrose agar medium. A definitive inoculum was added to each experimental medium and incubated at 25 degrees C for thirty days. After incubation quantitative counts were made from each soil and artificial culture medium to determine the number of infectious units per milliliter of sample. A stimulatory effect was observed at lower levels and a deleterious effect at higher levels. Luxuriant mycelial growth and sporulation occurred at the 2.5 and 5.0 percent additive levels, whereas the fungus was destroyed at 25 percent. The preliminary chemical analysis of chimanex showed it to contain 1.20 mg/ml total nitrogen by Kjedahl method and 0.21 mg/ml nonprotein nitrogen. A later more comprehensive analysis of chimanex established that carbohydrates, nitrogen, phosphate, and cationic salts very similar to those reported by Smith were present, as were other chemical elements. From these results information was obtained for a plausible explanation of the existence of the fungus in places where the excrement has aged, but not where it is fresh. The relatively high concentration of certain chemicals in fresh excrement, especially ammonium and ammonium compounds proved detrimental to the fungus.

Presence of the etiological agent in nature is not the sole prerequisite for infection in human and other animal species. In recent years it has been clearly established that active disturbance of the environment may be necessary for the dissemination of the infectious particles. The outbreak of histoplasmosis in Delaware, Ohio, in 1970 is a classical example which shows that activity within the environment may lead to infection by *H. capsulatum.* This small epidemic resulted in the publication of two papers which are descriptive and relevant to the epidemiology of histoplasmosis. The subjects of these papers are, "Caution: Ecology Can Be Hazardous to Your Health" (14) and "Earth Day Histoplasmosis: A New Type of Urban Pollution" (15). It is obvious from this and many other "epidemics" of histoplasmosis that if the environment, especially soil, is disturbed, dissemination of the fungus occurs within the immediate vicinity.

The dissemination of *H. capsulatum* within the environment is dependent on many factors, including the growth status of the fungus, disturbance of the immediate area in which the fungus is present, velocity of the wind currents, etc. As stated above, there are many basic environmental factors which must be available in nature for active growth of the fungus. However, if the humidity remains high, although reproductive bodies are produced, they will not be easily detached from the mycelium. The micro- and macroaleuriospores do not become separated from the mycelium until there is dehydration. Laboratory experiments have shown that extremely high wind velocities did not cause a release of these spores until the cultures showed signs of active dehydration. It can be extrapolated that similar activities are necessary in nature. The basic question is whether man and other animals become infected following dissemination of the fungus in air by prevailing winds. Reports in the literature have increased over the past decade, indicating that disturbance of areas in which excrement from bats and birds have contaminated the soil results in infections. Thus, under certain conditions and in many areas throughout the world, *H. capsulatum* has joined the list of pollutants in man's environment.

The size of the infectious particles is of consequence in an infection. In most descriptive discussions of histoplasmosis, the characteristic and diagnostic spore is the macroaleuriospore. The size of this spore ranges from 8 to 15 μ and is the most difficult to disengage from the mycelium. It is difficult to imagine that the macroaleuriospore is the principal infectious unit in histoplasmosis. The size and other morphological characteristics preclude that it can enter deeply into the respiratory tract. Brown et al. (5) have shown that particles of 5 μ or greater are usually filtered out of the air prior to reaching the larger bronchi. Sufficient evidence has been presented that in most artificial cultures of *H. capsulatum* microaleurospores and mycelial fragments greatly outnumber the macroaleuriospores. The latter spores in reality constitute only a small portion of the total number of infectious units in an *H. capsulatum* culture. The most abundant spore is the microaleuriospore, which ranges in size from 1 to 5 μ. Also mycelial fragments can be of such size that they too can be potentially infectious. In laboratory experiments in which the various environmental factors were investigated, it was learned that predominant infectious units produced were the microaleuriospore and mycelial fragments. From these results and those from animal experimentation, it is clearly evident that infectious particles of the size capable of penetrating into the alveoli of the lungs are produced by *H. capsulatum.* Although all of particles produced by this fungus: macroaleuriospore, microaleuriospore, and mycelial elements are viable and potentially infectious, the microaleuriospore would appear to be the most dangerous.

METHODS OF DETECTING MAN'S INVOLVEMENT WITH THE FUNGUS

The distribution and significance of histoplasmosis throughout the world are questions that remain unclear and debatable. Skin-test surveys reveal that the prevalence of histoplasmin sensitivity is highest in the United States. This information on the epidemiology of histoplasmosis has come from skin-test studies that have led to predictions that over 40 million individuals are infected by *H. capsulatum* in the United States alone. In addition, there is an annual increase in skin sensitivity of 500,000 individuals to the antigen histoplasmin. These present concepts on the epidemiology of histoplasmosis have resulted almost entirely from studies of "epidemics" among small groups of persons. One interesting finding from these studies has been the determination of the source of the inoculum in nature and its association with bird or bat feces.

Edwards and Billings (10) summarizes in a comprehensive fashion the data regarding skin-test sensitivity to histoplasmin throughout the world. Ajello (1) has updated the distribution of *H. capsulatum* in the United States as of 1971 and emphasized the tendency of investigators to overlook the fact that the organism is indigenous to areas outside of the east central endemic region. These publications extend the endemic areas but corroborate that the organism is commonly found in tropical and subtropical zones and that several large endemic areas are located in temperate regions. It is apparent from studying the maps of the endemic areas, as well as the actual skin-test results, that infection rates may vary widely over relatively short distances.

This fact, along with the consistent observation that only a small number of the millions of suspected infected persons develop clinical diseases, is a disturbing problem to the epidemiologist. One suggestion often used to explain this situation is that very large doses of inoculum are required to produce clinical disease. In experimental animals, however, this has not proved to be the case. Relatively small numbers of infectious units have caused overt disease in guinea pigs, dogs, and rhesus monkeys. Earlier experiments in our laboratory have shown mice and guinea pigs become infected with as few as ten spores by the inhalation route and these animals regularly showed lesions and clinical disease (23). Bauman and Chick (3) have infected rhesus monkeys by installation of the yeast phase directly into the lung by the intrathecal route. Graded doses of *H. capsulatum* yeast showed that cavitation can result from these experimental procedures. Therefore, it is plausible that man's susceptibility to infections by *H. capsulatum* may not be entirely dependent on unusually large doses of the organism. It is true nevertheless, that most of our knowledge of the epidemiology of histoplasmosis has come from investigations of the epidemic type of infection. Exposure of individuals to dusty environments in which the soil contained excrement from birds and bats produced miliary lung lesions. This type of lung involvement would suggest that large numbers of infectious particles were inhaled, but individuals from the same environment often present only a few pneumonic lesions. These localized epidemics produce only a fraction of the number of suspected clinical cases of histoplasmosis throughout the world. It is this aspect of skin-test survey which is the most difficult to rationalize, because only a very limited number of the 40 million infected persons develop clinical disease.

It is obvious that skin-test surveys of human and other animal populations have contributed significantly to the understanding of this fungus infection. Positive histoplasmin reactors suggest that the fungus is present in the environment and that individuals are being exposed to sources of the fungus in nature. The frequency of positive reactors in the endemic areas provides evidence of the growth, development, and dissemination of the infectious agent within the environment. Likewise, extensive surveys with histoplasmin have revealed that some lifelong residents in endemic areas fail to become infected, but in other areas nearly everyone is a positive reactor and clinical disease is fairly common. However, as stated by Edwards and Billings (10), "Even though information is fragmentary or entirely lacking for vast areas, data from many areas are sufficient to depict the geographical distribution and prevalence of histoplasmal infection in man."

Although histoplasmin skin testing is an excellent epidemiological tool, there remain many pitfalls that limit its efficiency. There is the old dilemma of cross-reactions with antigens from other systemic mycotic agents. It remains necessary to speculate or to extrapolate in determining the specific causal agent in patients in which cross-reactions occur. The procedure of diluting the various antigens to ascertain which antigen is the cause of the reaction is still followed. Usually the homologous antigen will produce the larger reaction in an infected host. Statistically this may be true, but on the other hand, no hard and fast rule can be followed. For this reason, mycologists must continue sophisticated chemical purification and characterization of fungal antigens. Through modern physical-chemical procedures, better antigens are becoming available for clinical trials. Standardization of and the use of such antigens must be followed if skin testing is to remain a useful procedure in determining the true distribution of histoplasmosis.

The interpretation of the skin-test reaction to histoplasmin needs further study. The size of the reaction, along with cross-reactions should be reevaluated in light of the reports by Edwards and Palmer (9), and Goodman (18). There is an excellent possibility that fungi other than those associated with the common systemic fungi may cause antigenic response in patients with histoplasmosis. Such an association was reported by Asgari and Conant (2) from studies conducted in Iran. Two strains of *Chrysosporium* species were isolated from soil collected around the homes of four persons presenting positive histoplasmin reactions. Guinea pigs infected with either *Chrysosporium* species or *H. capsulatum* reacted with antigens produced from each genus and showed cross-reactions with both types of antigens. The

Chrysosporium isolates inoculated into experimental animals resulted in generalized dissemination with development of nodular infiltrates in various organs. Larsh and Goodman (25) found similar results from fungi isolated from sputum specimens in patients in two chest hospitals. Certain fungi proved mildly pathogenic and cross-reactions occurred in experimental animals infected with *H. capsulatum* and other specific fungi. Antigens prepared from these isolates, as well as with histoplasmin, showed cross-reactions when tested on homologous and heterologous infected animals. There is at least more than a remote possibility that man might contract a subclinical infection to these "potential pathogens," thus resulting in cross-reactions when skin tested with histoplasmin.

Another area that should be considered in detecting man's possible involvement with the fungus lies within serological tests and their interpretation. It is not at all uncommon to find patients with clinical symptoms compatible with histoplasmosis only to find their skin-test reaction negative. An unequivocal diagnosis of histoplasmosis is based on the isolation of *H. capsulatum* from clinical specimens. Success is not always obtained and many failures result when clinical or soil specimens are cultured for pathogenic fungi. These circumstances make diagnosis on presumptive evidence necessary and immunologic procedures often provide the first evidence of the existence of clinical infections by these agents.

The skin-test reaction is useful in defining endemic areas of histoplasmosis; however, it has limited value as an epidemiologic or diagnostic tool since it does not distinguish between previous or present infections. A single histoplasmin skin test may increase the level of complement-fixing antibodies, precipitins, and agglutinins to *H. capsulatum* antigens. These reactions should be circumvented by drawing blood previous to applying the skin-test antigen. Kaufman's (20) studies show that increased antibody responses were detected in serum specimens drawn fifteen days after skin testing. He, too, suggests that blood samples should be drawn for serological studies before skin testing. However, the patient can be bled within two or three days after the skin test without induced antibodies being detected in the serum. There has been no evidence that a single histoplasmin skin test can produce serological responses in nonsensitized individuals.

Carefully planned serological surveys have produced incriminating evidence for late definitive or retrospective diagnosis of histoplasmosis. These findings have stimulated active epidemiological studies which resulted in a specific diagnosis instead of earlier reports of unusual forms of pneumonia.

Since antibody responses differ in nature and serological tests usually become positive within a month after infection and remain positive for varying intervals of time, a battery of tests should be employed. The complement-fixation, immunodiffusion, and latex agglutination tests should be performed alone or in combinations. The most widely used test is complement-fixation, either as a tube or microtitration procedure. Information obtained by these techniques, if performed correctly, can be of value in diagnostic as well as epidemiological studies. It is essential that the specificity and the sensitivity of the antibody response be interpreted correctly. The antigenic responses to most mycotic agents are relatively low and are significant between the range of 1 to 8 and 1 to 16. The specificity of the reactions are best judged with a battery of serological tests, using homologous and heterologous antigens. At the CDC (Center for Disease Control) laboratory "a presumptive diagnosis of histoplasmosis is reported on those sera which exhibit only *H. capsulatum* reactions regardless of the test used and on those showing homologous and heterologous CF antibodies but no precipitins for blastomycin and coccidioidin" (20).

The use of data from skin-test as well as serological surveys enhances our chances of becoming more knowledgeable on the role *H. capsulatum* plays in man's natural environment.

THE ROLE OF ANIMALS IN THE EPIDEMIOLOGY OF HISTOPLASMOSIS

In 1938 DeMonbruen (7) isolated *H. capsulatum* from a dog experimentally infected with active histoplasmosis. Since this early report, histoplasmosis has been found by many investigators to occur in several domestic and wild animals. Menges et al. (26) and Menges (27), presented the clinical features of the disease in domestic, captive, and wild animals. However, in these reports the infection in dog is the only one adequately described, due to so few cases documented in other animals.

The important finding in animal studies is that histoplasmosis is not a communicable disease, but each individual contracts the infection from its environment. Therefore, lower animals, as is man, are exposed to the fungus through the disturbance of the environment and its dissemination as a pollutant. It is not plausible to state unequivocally that animals do not have a direct effect of seeding *H. capsulatum* in nature. The rate of active, naturally acquired histoplasmosis, particularly in dogs, in certain areas of the United States is well known. Many of these animals succumbed to histoplasmosis, and with the decomposition of their bodies the fungus may be introduced into specific foci in nature. Whether or not the organism can withstand the chemical and biological activities associated with decomposition is questionable. Nevertheless, it is well known that if experimentally infected animals are not cultured soon after death, *H. capsulatum* is seldom recovered from the tissue.

From all indications, this possible seeding of the organism in nature is not the apparent role animals play in the biology of *H. capsulatum*. On the other hand, an indirect relationship can be a major contribution to the growth and development of the fungus in nature which may eventually influence the epidemiology of histoplasmosis.

Emmons' earlier investigations directed attention to the possibility that the growth of *H. capsulatum* was enhanced in soil contaminated with chicken excrement. Another era of exploration in the epidemiology and ecology of *Histoplasma* occurred when Emmons (12) in 1958 reported the possible relationship of house-dwelling bats to histoplasmosis. He was successful in recovering the fungus from soil collected adjacent to a bat-infested house in Maryland. Later reports confirmed his findings when bat guano was found harboring the fungus in Trinidad and Panama (11, 22). These data proved that sources of infecting inoculum other than bird droppings in soil and similar natural materials may be of consequence to the epidemiology of histoplasmosis.

There also have been several authenticated cases of histoplasmosis reported in individuals visiting or exploring caves, as well as among professional spelunkers. Gonzales-Ochoa (17) in his review of the relationship between bat habitats and histoplasmosis cites an early description by Mexicans of an acute, febrile, respiratory disease among employees of bat guano mines. This syndrome has been commonly described as *cave disease.* Public health records of 1895 and later in 1930 describe very well, and contain accurate descriptions of this bat-human association.

More recently, Shacklette, Diercks, and Gale (29) reported the recovery of *H. capsulatum* from bat tissue. The significance of the fungus in caves was elucidated by the report of Klite and Diercks (21). These researchers clearly showed the fungus was present in fecal contents and organs of bats in the Canal Zone.

Di Salvo (8) has thoroughly reviewed the role bats play in the ecology of *H. capsulatum*. In addition he has presented the history and the pertinent literature of *Chiroptera* and the association of the fungus in guano and tissue of these mammals. Evidence has been accumulated on the isolation of *H. capsulatum* from bat guano throughout the world and at least twenty-five chiropteran species have been incriminated as harboring this mycotic agent.

The question that still exists, however, is can the bat be an important factor in the dissemination of the fungus or is this mammal an incidental or fortuitous host? Although it is most difficult to answer this question, the fact that the same species of bat can be positive in one area of the world and negative in another would support an hypothesis that specific caves may be the source of the infective agent. If this is true, then guano, like soil, contaminated with excrement of avian species would provide the growth factors for the saprophytic existence of the organism.

The bat cave associated histoplasmosis as described above can be adequately illustrated by the report in the CDC, Morbidity and Mortality Weekly Report ending April 14, 1973 (28). This is a classical example of an epidemiological investigation and illustrates an important basic fact that *H. capsulatum* can be a common air pollutant in specific disturbed areas.

On February 10, 1973, a healthy 18-year-old girl from North Central Florida was admitted to the University of Florida Medical

Center in severe respiratory distress. Therapy with supplemental oxygen, systemic corticosteroids, and ventilatory assistance was initiated for presumed influenza pneumonia. On the third hospital day, the patient's mother related the occurrence of a respiratory illness in several of her daughter's friends, three of whom had been recently hospitalized elsewhere. Subsequently, *Histoplasma capsulatum* was cultured from a bone marrow aspirate.

On further questioning, it was learned that between January 1 and 21, 1973, the patient and 28 members of a church-sponsored youth group, 21 males and 8 females, had explored a bat-infested limestone cave in Suwanne County, Florida. They had entered the cave on one or two occasions for approximately 30 minutes attempting to encourage the bats to fly. The youths had thrown soil from the cave floor at them. Upon experiencing mild shortness of breath in the dusty atmosphere they left the cave.

Twenty-three of the 29 spelunkers were subsequently identified as infected (28).

Through many similar epidemic studies it has been learned that bats, chickens, starlings, blackbirds, and other avian species have a profound indirect effect on the epidemiology of histoplasmosis. Like the patients in the Florida bat epidemic, individuals in most of the other epidemics had positive skin and serological reactions, whereas individuals not closely associated with the disturbed environments were nonreactors.

The features of urban histoplasmosis have usually been associated with demolition of old buildings contaminated with bird or bat excrement. A great number of small epidemics have been related to such activities as early as 1938. These associations tend to support earlier suggestions, particularly in areas of low skin-test sensitivity, that the fungus has an extremely limited existence in nature. This localized association in contrast to generalized distribution of the organism resulted in the *point source* theory of infection. Accordingly, individuals became exposed and infected by visiting these specific habitats of the fungus. However, as emphasized by many students of the epidemiology of histoplasmosis, it is most difficult to account for the large numbers of infections in man, solely through contact with the fungus in localized areas of proliferation.

In recent years exposure to *H. capsulatum* in open urban areas has come into prominence. Rapid urbanization has resulted in the disruption of virgin areas and the removal of trees and other structures that were previously bird habitations. Such activities have increased the number of disturbed foci of the fungus in nature which in turn caused a greater number of active cases of histoplasmosis. Urbanization also has resulted in the addition of geographical areas in which the disease has not been reported previously.

Campbell (6) recently stated in her summary of *the Need for an Improved Serological Test for Histoplasmosis,* that "*H. capsulatum* is far more important as an air pollutant in this contemporary era of massive upheaval of soil and increasingly dense aggregated human populations and probably accounts for an infinitely greater number of cases than all those traceable to direct exposure to microfoci in nature combined."

The emerging patterns of urban histoplasmosis are of interest, since the disease has previously been considered to have almost an exclusive rural distribution. A more plausible explanation of the high rates of skin-test sensitivity in some areas of the world can be made, based on *H. capsulatum* more as an urban pollutant than by the *point source* exposure to infection. Therefore, it is more realistic to accept that millions of humans and lower animals reacting to histoplasmin obtained their delayed sensitivity from a pollutant of the air than merely from exposure to the fungus in microenvironments. The number of active cases of histoplasmosis admitted to the Missouri State Chest Hospital since January 1, 1973, with no evidence of a microenvironment exposure, further substantiates that the fungus may be an important air pollutant following disturbances within man's environment. It is obvious, however, that these limited observations will not be accepted as prima facie evidence of no association with point sources of the fungus. This is particularly true, since the patients in Missouri were from a small west central community and many epidemiologists would consider this entire area rural. However, critical and thorough clinical histories of the patients failed to uncover any evidence of limited exposure of possible point sources or the organism. Nevertheless, the occupations of all but one, a fourteen-year-old student, were such that they were exposed to massive clouds of dust as a result of their job activities. It is more remarkable that these infections occurred in an area in which rainfall during the latter part of 1972 and in 1973 through the month of May was many inches above normal. Soil samples collected from an urban site in this area which was being prepared for a building project yielded positive isolations from three of the six samples. One positive isolation was from soil collected below trees, which had a history of being a starling roost. The other two positive isolations were from samples collected from virgin soil in which no trees were present.

The increasing number of bona fide urban sources of exposure, in which the fungus has been isolated from areas within cities lends more credence to the hypothesis that *H. capsulatum* is an autochthonous soil organism; also, that under disturbances of its environment the fungus becomes airborne and constitutes a hazard to the health of man and other animals.

DISTRIBUTION OF HISTOPLASMOSIS THROUGHOUT THE WORLD

An appreciation of the epidemiology of histoplasmosis requires knowledge of the incidence, geographical distribution, sources of the infectious inoculum, and the types of infections.

Although acute, chronic, and disseminated histoplasmosis has been well documented in many areas of the world, the knowledge of the overall distribution of this mycotic disease is based very little on clinical information. It is imperative, however, that the relationship of the various factors which may determine or influence the frequencies and distribution of histoplasmosis in the human population be understood. Clinical and pathological studies have clearly established that this fungus disease occurs in all age groups. It is true that certain types may be found more frequently in particular age groups. For example, the incidence of extrapulmonary fatal histoplasmosis is highest in infants, with almost equal frequency among the aged. This is clearly evident if the patient does not receive prompt and adequate therapy. Studies of histoplasmosis in children under ten years of age showed that there is no definite prediction in favor of either sex. However, among adult patients, the male predominates, and this is usually believed to be associated with exposure risk. Many investigators have reported that there are no significant differences in racial susceptibility. Nevertheless, in our chest hospital, disseminated histoplasmosis followed the well-recognized pattern of pulmonary disease in that it predominantly affected the white male. The ratio of white over black patients was 24 to 1 and the infection was found very infrequently in our female patients. In our investigations we have observed *Histoplasma* as the primary organism and as a concomitant organism. Frequently, histoplasmosis has been regarded as a disease only in individuals who have some impairment of their immune mechanism or who suffer from debilitation. The infection has been found associated with such syndromes as sarcoidosis, leukemia, diabetes, tuberculosis, Hodgkin's disease, and others. These observations may be extremely useful in determining the actual distribution and significance of histoplasmosis throughout the world.

Information obtained from clinical ecological, epidemiological, and immunological studies has proved advantageous in determining world areas of *H. capsulatum* endemicity. Histoplasmin skin testing has been in use since 1945 and this antigen has permitted the accumulation of a vast amount of knowledge as to the distribution and significance of histoplasmosis. A positive reaction to histoplasmin theoretically indicates that the individual has had or is presently infected with the etiological agent, whereas, a nonreactor has not been infected. Within a strict interpretation there may be difficulty, since known infected individuals may not react to the histoplasmin skin test. In addition, it has not been possible to perform extensive surveys, or in some areas of the world no survey has been done or at least information is not available from these areas. In spite of these apparent pitfalls, sufficient numbers of individuals have been observed to permit more than speculation by epidemiologists as to the distribution of histoplasmosis among the world's population. Also, through these studies it is now clear that most epidemic foci are located in the tropical and subtropical zones of the world. Nevertheless, there are significant foci in temperate regions and perhaps the largest or at least the most publicized one is within the continental United States.

Literature reviews such as those of Ajello (1), and Edwards

and Billings (10) on the occurrence of histoplasmosis in the United States and other regions of the world are monumental contributions. These investigators have collected all available data on the distribution of this infection and have concisely mapped the areas of endemicity as known up to 1971. Information obtained from cultural studies of human and animal cases as well as soil isolations clearly demonstrates that *H. capsulatum* is endemic in thirty-one of the forty-eight contiguous states. Even a casual study of these data suggests that the size of the endemic areas in addition to the intensity of colonization of the fungus obviously varies within specific states and especially from state to state. It is also clear that to illustrate distribution of a fungus solely by isobars on a map does not present the true picture.

Epidemiological and ecological investigations show that Arkansas, Kentucky, Missouri, and Tennessee have the greatest densities of the fungus. It is not at all uncommon to find nearly 100 percent skin-test reactors in the young adult population in these central states. Thirty-one of the forty-eight continental states have been proved as endemic areas of this pathogen, although soil isolations have not been obtained from specimens from twenty states. However, naval recruits tested from eight of the states with negative soil cultures were positive to the histoplasmin skin test. This latter information, along with additional circumstantial evidence, is encouraging and allows speculation that eventually the fungus may be isolated from specific habitats in most of the states.

Outside the United States, histoplasmosis is endemic throughout most of Central and South America. Although it appears to be uncommon in lifelong residents in Europe and adjacent areas, the recent two reports of small localized foci in Italy has stimulated medical mycological activity in the Mediterranean region. Endemic areas have been reported in Africa and Asia, but it is in these parts of the world that extensive studies of lifelong residents are badly needed. Further observations by Bezjak and Farsley (4) in East Africa suggest that histoplasmosis is more common than previously reported. However, the diagnosed cases to date are too few to positively indicate the incidence and geographical pattern of the disease. The southeastern region of Asia and the western tropical areas of Africa have shown the highest skin-test reactivity but documentation of the actual involvement of histoplasmosis in Africa and Asia will have to await more thorough coverage of these continents.

There have been very few additional reports of skin-test reactors and active disease since Edwards and Billings published their comprehensive data in Table 1 of "*Skin Sensitivity in Histoplasmosis.*" There were a number of papers read at the Eighth International Congresses for Tropical Medicine and Malaria, September, 1968, Teheran (Iran) on histoplasmosis in countries throughout the world. These were published as a monograph in *Mycopathologia et Mycologia Applicata,* Vol. 40, 1970, and should be consulted for further information.

There are two publications worthy of mention, since they represent welcome news of interest in medical mycology. Stepanishtcheva et al. (31) have reported twenty-seven patients with histoplasmosis that have been registered in Russia. These results were from a two-year investigation by members of the newly formed Department of Deep Mycoses at the Martzinovsky Institute of Medical Parasitology and Tropical Medicine in Moscow, USSR. In Greece sensitivity to the histoplasmin skin test was documented in 1952 among school children but the first active case of histoplasomosis was recently reported (33).

Until clinicians throughout the world show a greater interest in and a concern for the infectious potential of mycotic organisms our knowledge of the distribution and significance of histoplasmosis will remain incomplete and fragmentary. There must be a universal adoption of world-wide reporting and surveillance of the mycoses before these infections can be relegated to minor importance and of little significance to the public health of the world.

AFRICAN HISTOPLASMOSIS (*HISTOPLASMA DUBOISII*)

African histoplasmosis occurs more frequently as an involvement of mucocutaneous tissues than as the pulmonary type that is generally associated with *H. capsulatum.* In this disseminated mycosis there is often generalized enlargement of the lymphatic system. Death usually occurs in a few weeks, especially in patients with pronounced liver or spleen symptomatology. The origin of the infection in man is not unequivocally established, but indications are that the portal of entry is the respiratory route, after which dissemination occurs. However, the skin has also been suggested as a route of infection.

The epidemiology of African histoplasmosis is not well understood, although skin-test surveys have been done in several regions throughout Africa. There are complications in determining the distribution and significance of *H. duboisii* in this continent. This is particularly true in East Africa, where individuals may contract histoplasmosis from either *H. capsulatum* or *H. duboisii*. Cases of African histoplasmosis have been reported in several patients in the region of Uganda, whereas in Kenya and Tanzania this form of histoplasmosis is rarely diagnosed. To further complicate the problem of differentiation of the histoplasmas in Africa, *Blastomyces dermatitidis* has been isolated from patients with a life-long history of residency in Africa. There is sufficient resemblance in signs and symptoms of these mycotic diseases that cultures of clinical specimens are essential in making a diagnosis of African histoplasmosis. The mycelial cultures of the three organisms have many similarities and it may be necessary to convert the isolated fungus to the yeast phase for a positive identification.

Unfortunately, skin-test surveys have not proved fruitful in distinguishing the reactions due to *H. capsulatum* from patients previously infected with *H. duboisii*. Current information suggests that histoplasmin testing is not reliable, since a substantial percentage of patients with African histoplasmosis are not sensitive to the available histoplasmins. Antigen differences between *H. duboissii* and most of the *H. capsulatum* isolates have been documented; nevertheless, standardized *H. duboisii* histoplasmins have not been employed in human skin testing. There have been only a limited number of histoplasmins from *H. duboisii* critically evaluated, even in animals experimentally infected with isolates of this mycotic agent.

In view of the sparcity of information on the epidemiology of African histoplasmosis, there should be a concentrated effort to utilize all the known clinical ecological, and immunological information to further our knowledge. Although there is a close antigenicity between *H. capsulatum* and *H. duboisii,* there are sufficient differences which warrant skin testing in native African populations with partially purified and separated antigens from culture filtrates of the mycelial phase of *H. duboisii.*

It also is of interest that Vanbrueseghem (32) has stated that the known African endemic areas of *H. duboisii* have high average rainfall and humidity levels, with very slight differences in night and day temperature. These climatic factors, controlled under laboratory conditions, and the fungus inoculated into sterile soil cultures resulted in luxuriant growth and development of the mycelial phase. The knowledge that the African histoplasmosis agent is an autochthonous soil microorganism whose ecology may be determined by specific factors similar to those necessary for the colonization of *H. capsulatum* in nature is most encouraging to epidemiologists.

Development of more sophisticated skin-test antigens and the recognition that factors do exist which influence the growth of *H. duboisii* in Africa are suggestive that eventually the epidemiology of African histoplasmosis will be better understood.

REFERENCES

1. Ajello, L.: Distribution of *Histoplasma capsulatum* in the United States. *Proc. 2nd Nat. Con. on histoplasmosis,* 1971.
2. Asgari, M., Conant, N. F.: A preliminary note on interreaction of skin-test sensitivity between histoplasmin and chrysosporin in experimental animals. *Mycopath Mycol Appl,* 23:321, 1964.
3. Bauman, D. S., Chick, E. W.: Serologic response to *Histoplasma capsulatum* in *Maccaca mulatta. Bact Proc, 119,* 1971.
4. Bezjak, V., Farsley, S. J.: Prevalence of skin sensitivity to histoplasmin and coccidioidin in various Ugandan populations. *J Trop Med Hyg, 19*:664, 1970.
5. Brown, J. H., Cook, K. M., Ney, F. G., Hatch, T.: Influence of particle size upon the retention of particle matter in the human lung. *Am J Pub Hlth, 40*:450, 1950.
6. Campbell, C. C.: The need for an improved serologic test for histoplasmosis. *Proc. 2nd Nat. Conf. on histoplasmosis,* 1971.
7. Demonbreun, W. A.: The dog as a natural host for *Histoplasma capsulatum. Am J Trop Med, 19*:565, 1939.
8. DiSalvo, A. F.: The role of bats in the ecology of *Histoplasma capsulatum. Proc. 2nd Nat. Conf. on histoplasmosis,* 1971.

9. Edwards, P. Q., Palmer, C. E.: Nationwide histoplasmin sensitivity and histoplasmal infection. *U S Pub Hlth Rep, 78*:241, 1963.
10. Edwards, P. Q., Billings, E. L.: Worldwide pattern of skin sensitivity to histoplasmin. *J Trop Med Hyg, 20*:288, 1970.
11. Emmons, C. W., Greenhall, A. M.: *Histoplasma capsulatum* and house bats in Trinidad, W. I. *Sabouraudia, 2*:18, 1962.
12. Emmons, C. W.: Association of bats with histoplasmosis. *Pub Hlth Rep, 73*:590, 1958.
13. Emmons, C. W.: Isolation of *Histoplasma capsulatum* from soil. *Pub Hlth Rep, 64*:892, 1949.
14. Faigel, H. C.: Caution: ecology can be hazardous to your health. *Clin Pediatr*, 245, 1971.
15. Fass, R. J., Saslaw, S.: Earth day histoplasmosis. A new type of urban pollution. *Arch Intern Med, 128*:588, 1971.
16. Furcolow, M. L.: Epidemiology of histoplasmosis. *Histoplasmosis.* Springfield, Thomas, 1960.
17. Gonzalez-Ochoa, A.: Relaciones entre el habitat del murcielago y el *Histoplasma capsulatum. Rev Ins Salubr Enferm Trop, 23*:81, 1963.
18. Goodman, N. L.: Cross reactivity to histoplasmin skin testing. *Proc. 2nd Nat. Conf. on histoplasmosis*, 1971.
19. Goodman, N. L., Larsh, H. W.: Environmental factors and growth of *Histoplasma capsulatum* in soil. *Mycopath Mycol Appl, 33*:145, 1967.
20. Kaufman, L.: Serological tests for histoplasmosis: their use and interpretation. *Proc. 2nd Nat. Conf. on histoplasmosis*, 1971.
21. Klite, P. D., Diercks, F. H.: *Histoplasma capsulatum* in fecal contents and organs of bats in the Canal Zone. *Am J Trop Med, 14*:433, 1934.
22. Klite, P. D.: The focal occurrence of histoplasmosis in house-dwelling bats on the Isthmus of Panama. *Sabouraudia, 4*:158, 1965.
23. Larsh, H. W.: Natural and experimental epidemiology of histoplasmosis. *Ann N Y Acad Sci, 89*:78, 1960.
24. Larsh, H. W.: Ecology and epidemiology of histoplasmosis. *Proc Intern Sym on mycoses*, 1970.
25. Larsh, H. W., Goodman, N. L.: Sputum mycology. *Sputum.* Springfield, Thomas, 1972.
26. Menges, R. W., Habermann, R. T., Selby, L. A., Ellis, H. R., Behlow, R. F., Smith, C. D.: A review and recent findings on histoplasmosis in animals. *Vet Med, 58*:331, 1963.
27. Menges, R. W.: Clinical manifestations of animal histoplasmosis. *Proc 2nd Natl Conf on histoplasmosis*, 1971.
28. *Morbidity and Mortality. 22*:125, 1973.
29. Shacklette, M. H., Diercks, F. H., Gale, N. B.: *Histoplasma capsulatum* recovered from bat tissue. *Science, 135*:1135, 1962.

30. Smith, C. D.: The role of birds in the ecology of *Histoplasma capsulatum. Proc 2nd Natl Conf on histoplasmosis,* 1971.
31. Stepanishtcheva, Z. G., Arievitch, A. M., Minsker, O. B., Sooteyeva, T. B.: Investigation of deep mycosis in the USSR. *Intern J Dermatol, 11*:181, 1971.
32. Vanbreuseghem, R.: Essai de Mise au Paint Sur l'Histoplasmose Africaine. *Bull Acad Roy Med Belg, 23*:686, 1958.
33. Vlachos, J. D.: First case of histoplasmosis in Greece. *Pathol Europaea,* 7:289, 1972.
34. Zeidberg, L. D., Ajello, L., Dillon, A., Runyon, L. C.: Isolation of *Histoplasma capsulatum* from soil. *Am J Pub Hlth, 42*:930, 1952.

Chapter 5

THE EPIDEMIOLOGY OF COCCIDIOIDOMYCOSIS

FRANK E. SWATEK

COCCIDIOIDOMYCOSIS IS AN exogenously acquired infection, the result of a single etiologic agent, *Coccidioides immitis.* Three basic types of infection are known: 1) primary pulmonary coccidioidomycosis (valley fever, San Joaquin Valley fever) which is an acute self-limiting disease with an annual incidence in endemic areas of approximately 80,000 cases; 2) disseminated coccidioidomycosis (coccidiodal granuloma), a chronic malignant disease, beginning with a pulmonary episode, but disseminating into the viscera, bones, meninges, subcutaneous and cutaneous tissues. This form of the disease has a low incidence, showing racial preference for the subspecies of man, with a higher incidence among the darker skinned races; and 3) primary cutaneous coccidioidomycosis which is very rare, with less than a dozen authenticated cases being presented in the literature.

Coccidioidomycosis is known to occur in infants from three months of age to seventy-year-old adults in the endemic regions. There also seems to be a greater frequency of males than females acquiring the infection as a primary pulmonary syndrome. Before the age of puberty both the male and female patients respond in approximately the same manner to the primary pulmonary infection. After the age of puberty there is a tendency for females to show the allergic manifestation of erythema nodosum in about

25 percent of the cases, while this allergic syndrome is seen in only about 5 percent of the teenage males. It also has been observed that males tend to disseminate more frequently than do females.

The disease produces a granuloma whether in the lungs or disseminated throughout the body, with changes in hematological and serological values. For example, there is a slight leukocytosis or even a mild leukopenia associated with the disease. The leukocyte population remains unchanged, while the sedimentation rate continues to be elevated during the course of the disease. There is also a hypochromic type of anemia which can be detected in the majority of cases. In the study of the primary pulmonary infection, specimens can be secured from the sputum; after dissemination, biopsy material or excised pustular material from cutaneous lesions and spinal fluid are also suitable materials for laboratory study. Serologically, the disease can be followed by the use of complement-fixation, precipitin, and gel-diffusion, as well as skin testing. This battery of serological tests enables the physician to detect infections and follow the disease with some accuracy as to the type of host response that is occurring. The incubation period of the disease is from ten to fourteen days. The following time schedule should be kept in mind in the utilization of these serological tests. The skin test becomes positive by the second week after the onset of symptoms, which means that the test should be performed after the first month of infection. Precipitin antibodies can be detected in ten to fourteen days after the onset of symptoms, and these antibodies disappear by the end of the first month. Therefore, the precipitin test must be performed early in the course of the disease. Complement fixation antibodies form after the second or third month of infection, and as implied, a rise in titer generally is indicative of dissemination. Gel-diffusion antibodies are also detected after the second month from the onset of symptoms, and carry the same connotation of dissemination as the complement-fixation antibodies. Indeed, the gel-diffusion and complement-fixation tests show good correlation so that one or the other test could be performed. In this disease it has been shown that individuals who disseminate will have a rise in their complement-fixation titer and that as the disease progresses to the terminal stages, their skin-test reaction will convert from a positive to a negative.

Mycology

Coccidioides immitis is a diphasic organism, living in nature as a septate mycelial forming fungus. The description of isolates of *C. immitis* from human material shows the growth of a scant woolly off-white colony with tendency to form pseudocoremia and to have a neutral or sometimes slightly darkened reverse, and producing chlamydospores, vesicles, racquet hyphae, right angle branching and arthroaleuriospores characterized as having a "dead" space between them. Huppert et al. (28) have reported on variation in some seventy odd cultures markedly different from those which would be called textbook types (described above). Huppert et al, in their discusson of these atypical colonial types, make a very valid observation that in the isolation of these organisms back from test animals in the proof of Koch's postulates, the colonial morphology is maintained, and there is no apparent shift to that of a so-called typical *C. immitis* colony. In the course of one epidemic studied by the author and co-workers this phenomenon of the appearance of cultural variation was very useful as an epidemiological marker in showing organisms isolated from the soil and patients from one site were different from a more typical strain isolated a few hundred yards away which also was the cause of infection (32). In the author's experience, *C. immitis* isolated from naturally infected animals culturally appears like that predominantly isolated from man.

Coccidioides immitis grows *in vivo* by the swelling of the arthroaleuriospores into spherules. The cytoplasm of the spherules undergoes cleavage either with or without central vacuolations of the cytoplasm to produce endospores. This is followed by the rupture of the spherule's wall, presumably through enzymatic activity, to free the endospores. The endospores which are not identical in size or shape at the time of release, to be uninuclear in nature, have the capability of rounding up to form a new parasitic spherule. The parasitic phase in man, animal or test tube is seen in this form of metamorphosis from either the arthroaleuriospore or vegetative mycelial cell to the large rounded up spherules. In Figure 5-1 the life cycle of *C. immitis* is diagrammatically presented.

Epidemiological Studies of *C. Immitis* in the World

Data to establish the distribution of *C. immitis* in the world has been derived through three main sources: 1) recognition of proven cases; 2) use of skin tests as an epidemiological tool in delineating those areas in which the nonmobile population or domestic animals show a high incidence of reactivity; and 3) ecological studies in those regions in which "epidemics" have occurred or have a high skin-test reactivity. The precise site of growth of *C. immitis* in the soil is sought in this last type study. Although this report is not one to contain the veterinary side of coccidioidomycosis, it is noteworthy to mention that *C. immitis* is a pathogenic organism with a wide host range. It is known to produce infections experimentally in all warm-blooded animals that have been challenged. It also has produced experimental infections in cold-blooded vertebrates such as lizards and has been shown to produce the mycelial form of growth with great enzymatic activity in crustaceans (64).

The first case of coccidioidomycosis was reported by Posadas in 1892 in the Argentine (48). The second case was recognized in 1894 in the United States, and for more than a score of years these reports delineated the distribution of *C. immitis* (54). By 1912 only nineteen cases of coccidioidal granuloma were reported in the literature. In 1916 the first case was seen east of the Mississippi, thus establishing an awareness in the medical world of this granulomatous disease in areas other than the strict endemic region which at that time was defined as the San Joaquin Valley in California and the Chaco region of the Argentine (34). In 1923 a case report was presented in Chicago (26). By the mid-1920's serological studies, especially the development of skin-testing procedures, became an important adjunct to the study of this disease, providing both prognostic as well as epidemiological tools. In 1928 Jacobson presented the theory of the allergic reaction of the skin, thus establishing our understanding of erythema nodosum (29). In 1931 the first epidemiology paper

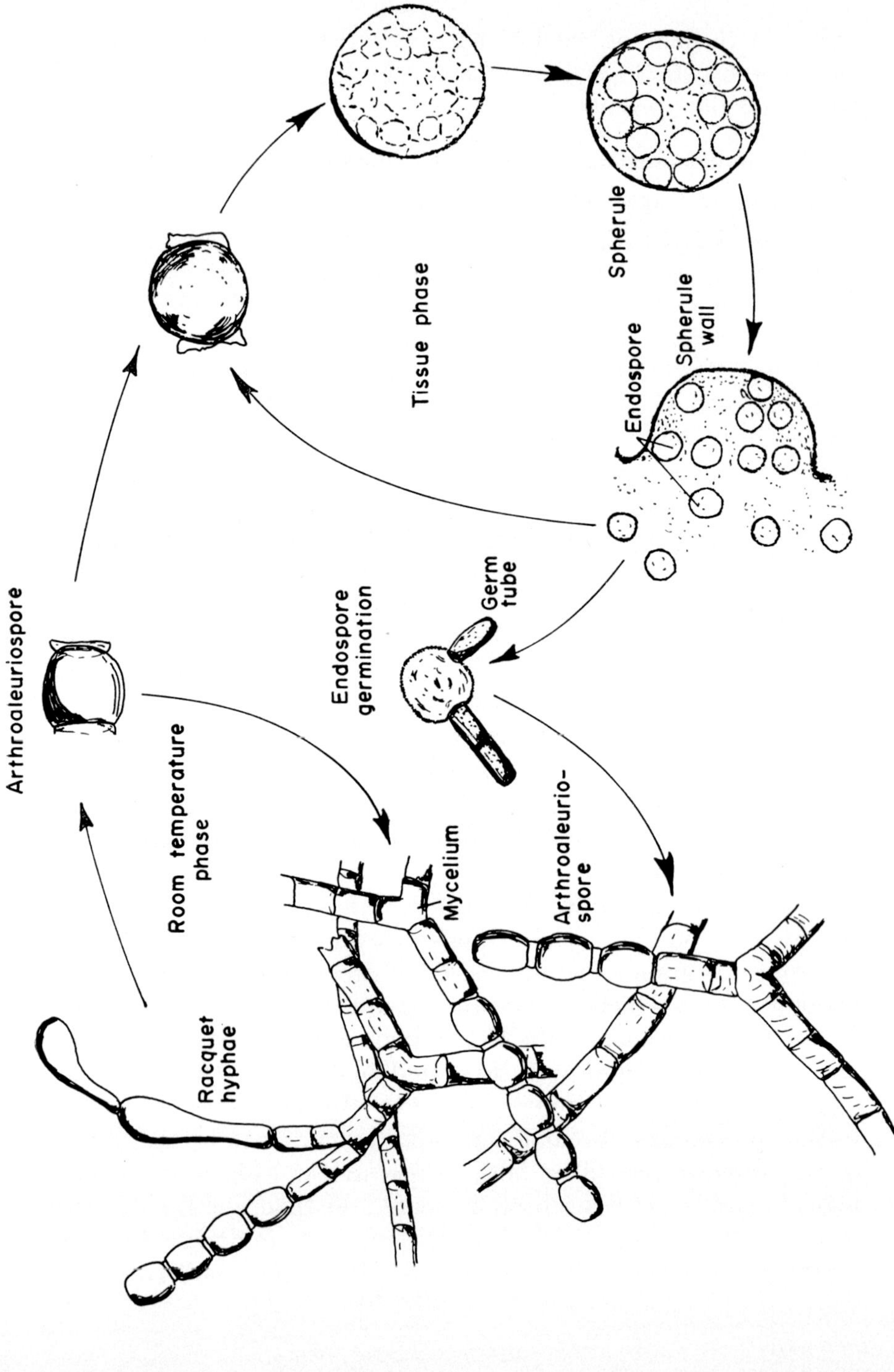

Figure 5-1. Diagrammatic scheme for growth of *Coccidioides immitis*.

as such was presented by Beck in California discussing the many aspects of coccidioidal disease and its interrelationship with the population of the San Joaquin Valley (3). By 1932 Texas was reporting cases of coccidioidomycosis in which the origin of the disease was believed to be Texas, not California, thus expanding the endemic region for this infectious agent (4). Also Moore classified *C. immitis* for the first time in 1932 as a mycological agent in relationship to other fungi (44). In this same year Stewart and Meyer made the first isolation from nature of this fungus (62) followed by the report of the first case in 1934 from Hawaii (20, 49).

A turning point in the study of coccidioidomycosis occurred with the work of Gifford and Dickson in the years of 1936 to 1937 in which the disease was shown to be a self-limiting primary pulmonary type of infection, and that coccidioidal granuloma was a much more rare complication from the primary pulmonary portal of entry (12, 13, 21). In 1942 an extensive survey had been completed by Emmons and his co-workers showing that rodents were naturally infected also in endemic regions of Arizona (18, 19). In 1942 Emmons' group made the second isolation of *C. immitis* from the soil in Arizona (18). In 1942, prompted by the events of World War II, a survey was conducted at Fort Roberts on the occurrence of coccidioidomycosis among the trainees (57). The 1942 reports of Emmons and co-workers on the presence of *C. immitis* in wild rodents had grown into a theory by 1943 postulating the possible reservoir of *C. immitis* in these animals, however, this theory was shown by further investigations to be erroneous.

Seven of fourteen students became infected in 1942 after trying to dig a rattlesnake out of a squirrel hole in the Panoche Valley in San Benito County, California. This epidemic site was confirmed by soil isolation of *C. immitis* (11). Another epidemic was recorded in the Western Flying Training Command, and this represented the first of a number of epidemics which have since been reported in the literature in which *C. immitis* is seen as a natural agent occurring in military training facilities or in areas in which maneuvers are conducted by service personnel (33). Recognition of this problem for the military brought forth in 1946 a recommendation by C. E. Smith to control the dust in the endemic areas with anticipation of the environmental seasonal effects on the growth of the fungus (60). By 1950, Gomez published on the endemicity of coccidioidomycosis in the Chaco region (23), while Hoekenga presented the results of skin tests of three hundred men (27). Further, a case of coccidioidomycosis believed acquired in Los Angeles, which is out of the San Joaquin Valley, was put forward (31). The endemic regions in the Argentine and in the state of Sonora were also presented in the year 1950, a most productive year in the study of distribution and ecology of *C. immitis* (42).

In this chronological review it can be seen that coccidioidomycosis was recognized mainly on an individual patient basis and only a few "epidemics" had been reported. Thus the epidemiological study of this disease had its major turning point in the 1950's as reports began to appear on the acquisition of coccidioidomycosis by students, especially anthropologists and archeologists in universities.

The Era of Epidemics

In 1950 case reports extended by skin-testing procedures provided the early detection of the endemicity of *C. immitis* in Los Angeles County with the publication of Kritzer et al. of a group of sixty-one boys in a forestry camp near Saugus, California (31). This site is just north of the San Fernando Valley. Twenty positive skin tests were detected in the group, with only a few showing histories of ever being in a known endemic region in California. Soil and dung samples were collected and processed from the area; no positives were recovered. Three years later the author began a two-year study of this area, processing soil samples and trapping rodents in the search for the endemic site. More than five square miles were studied in the investigation, but all efforts were negative after collecting 1,109 rodents and 469 soil samples. To this day, this elusive site in the Saugus region remains to be found.

In 1957 Plunkett and Swatek reported on the first anthropological epidemic at an old Indian campsite near Inyokern, California, in Kern County (47). This campsite was believed to be close to 2,000 years old and had been used up to within 200 years from the time of infection and subsequent sampling. About two weeks after a field trip four students became ill, and a fifth who had been only cleaning the artifacts brought back to the laboratory developed primary pulmonary coccidioidomycosis. This is one of the most extensively studied known *C. immitis* sites in California, in which the organism resides in the soil throughout the year in a space eight by ten feet.

In 1960 Joffe reported an epidemic of thirty-three cases of coccidioidomycosis at Edwards Air Force Base, which is situated very near the city of Mojave in Kern County, California, and about fifty miles from the Inyokern site (30). This epidemic was correlated with bulldozing activity in preparation for a building project. Before this epidemic, only one case of coccidioidomycosis had been reported at the air base. Attempts to isolate *C. immitis* from the air were all negative. In 1961, for the first time, Walch et al. reported an epidemic of *C. immitis* from San Diego County in the southeastern border of the city of Lakeside (66). This epidemic was brought to the attention of investigators after topsoil had been carried into the city to be used to upgrade the fertility of the soil at a residence. This soil had been taken at the site of an old Indian campground. In the course of this very thorough study a total of twenty-four cases of coccidioidomycosis were brought to light over a period of several years. This site has proven to be a resident year round site for *C. immitis,* with isolations having been made over a ten-year period at the same small patch of soil. In 1963 Winn et al. reported an epidemic of ten children who acquired coccidioidomycosis while playing in the confines of their dusty back yard (69). The soil was dry, contaminated by bird droppings and denude of grass or small plants. This epidemic, like that of Walch, was confirmed by soil isolations of *C. immitis* from the site at the time of the epidemic. In 1964 Eckmann and his co-workers reported on an epidemic among six individuals from bedside interhuman transmission of *C. immitis* which had grown on the removed cast material from an individual with a broken leg (14).

From the 1960's to the present, epidemics have been reported with greater frequency in relationship to group activity in which soil had been disturbed. Thus in 1965 Cowper reported on an outbreak of coccidioidomycosis in Canoga Park in the San Fernando Valley, California, in the County of Los Angeles (10). Roberts in 1967 reported on an epidemic in El Paso, Texas, where ten children contracted *C. immitis* from the soil of an upgraded field near their housing development (55). Soil isolations were made and a very small endemic site was identified. Two years later Loofbourow reported on an epidemic among ten college students in the Capay Valley of Yolo County, California (35), where they acquired their infection from digging for Indian artifacts. In 1970 Ramras et al. reported on an epidemic among eight young boys who had been playing on a sandy cleared off hill in the Pacific Beach area of San Diego County near the city of San Diego, California (50). This site, in view of Mission Bay and 2.5 miles from the Pacific Ocean, was shown to be positive for *C. immitis* by soil isolation. In the same year a localized outbreak of coccidioidomycosis in southern Texas was reported (65). In 1971 Lacy filmed an anthropology field trip in Madera County, California, in an Indian site which was believed to be negative for *C. immitis.* Twenty-eight of the thirty students became ill, with one developing meningitis (32). Soil isolates confirmed this epidemic. Rao, in 1972, was able to establish the endemic foci of *C. immitis* in Los Angeles County near the city of Los Angeles (51). Also in 1972 Werner reported on an epidemic among college students frequenting Indian mounds in the northern part of California (67). So it is at the time of this writing that there have been limited true epidemics of coccidioidomycosis brought to medical attention, for which only some have been verified as to the source of the epidemic by culture of the organism in a specific locale. Indeed, *C. immitis* in its endemic area remains a puzzle in that its plasticity of metabolic enzymes enables it to grow in many varied conditions on laboratory media and in the soil, yet in nature it seeks out and grows only in very restricted areas to command larger areas as a wind-borne spore.

Distribution of Coccidioidomycosis

The endemicity of coccidioidomycosis has been much more widely published upon than the true epidemiology of epidemics.

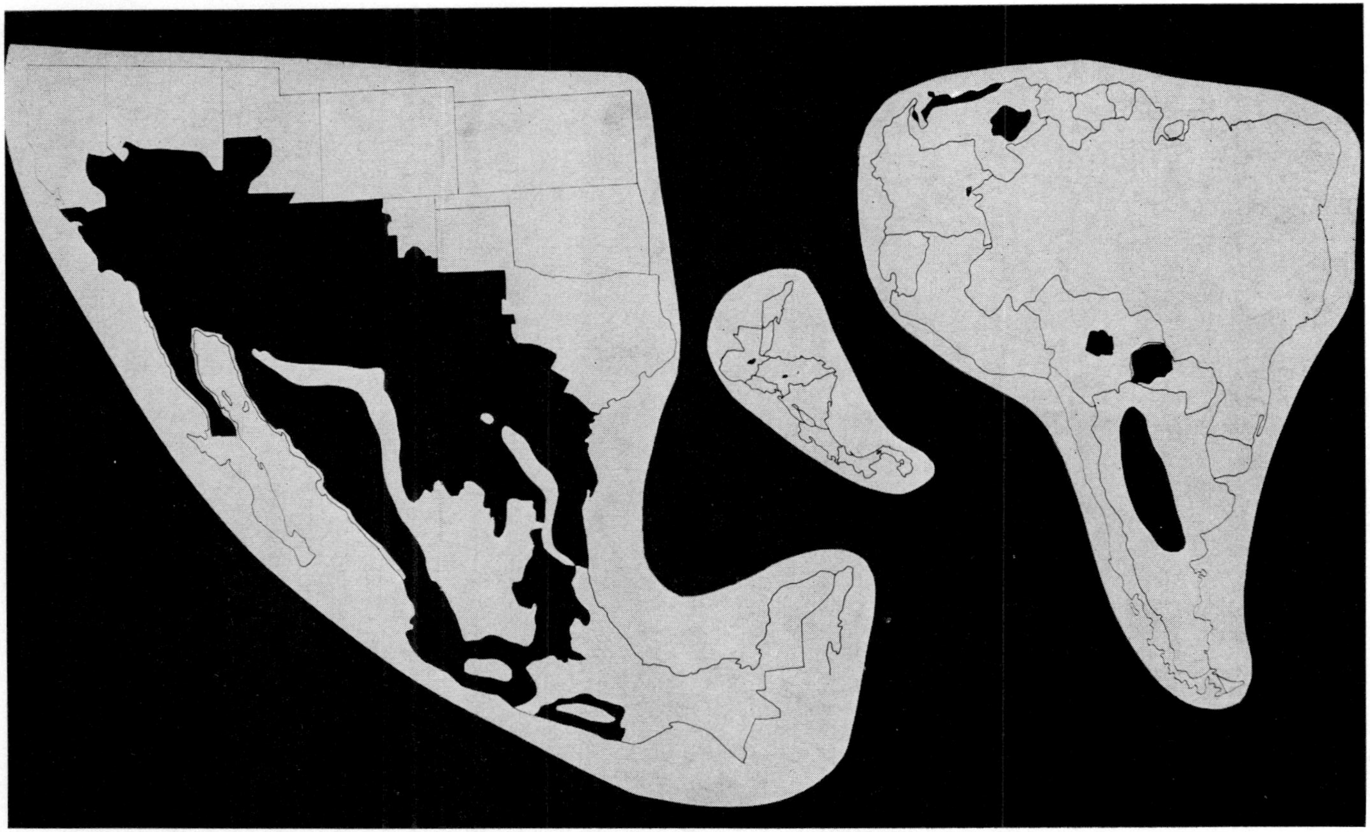

Figure 5-2. Endemic regions of *Coccodioides immitis* in the Americas as determined by skin testing (from data compiled from the literature).

Thus in the year 1973 a number of regions in North, Central and South America have been identified by use of skin testing procedures on the populace of these areas (Figure 5-2). In many instances, however, the infectious agent has not yet been recovered from the soil or any other natural source. Much of what is known about the ecology of *C. immitis* has relied upon investigations which have been most extensive in California and Arizona.

NORTH AMERICA

Six states in the United States of America show regions in which skin testing indicates the presence of *C. immitis* in varying amounts, namely, Arizona, California, Nevada, Texas, New Mexico and Utah. The same skin-test surveys indicate that Arizona, California and Texas have the largest areas and the most extensive ecological studies being conducted on this disease. The report of Edwards and Palmer in 1957 (15) provided an overview and has been since regionally reinforced by later skin testing (Figure 5-3). In Table 5-I the known sites where *C. immitis* has been isolated from nature are shown. It should also be pointed out that in the United States of America there has been a Veterans' Administration and Armed Forces Coccidioidomycosis Cooperative Study going on for a number of years. This cooperative study has brought together annually investigators with different research approaches, clinical and surgical, as well as epidemiological-ecological interests. The cooperative study has attempted to systematically guide the investigations and share the results from one area of medicine and science to another.

Arizona

The first case of coccidioidomycosis was presented in 1938 by Woolley in Arizona (70). The early case reports that followed established the presence of *C. immitis* in the Tucson and Phoenix areas. Aronson et al. in 1942 skin tested Indians on the reservations in Arizona, finding a high percent of reactivity among certain tribes (2). In 1964 Sievers et al. again skin tested Indians in the age group of five to fourteen years in this endemic area and reported results which were at slight variance with those of Aronson (58). Most recently, in 1973, Geller et al. reported

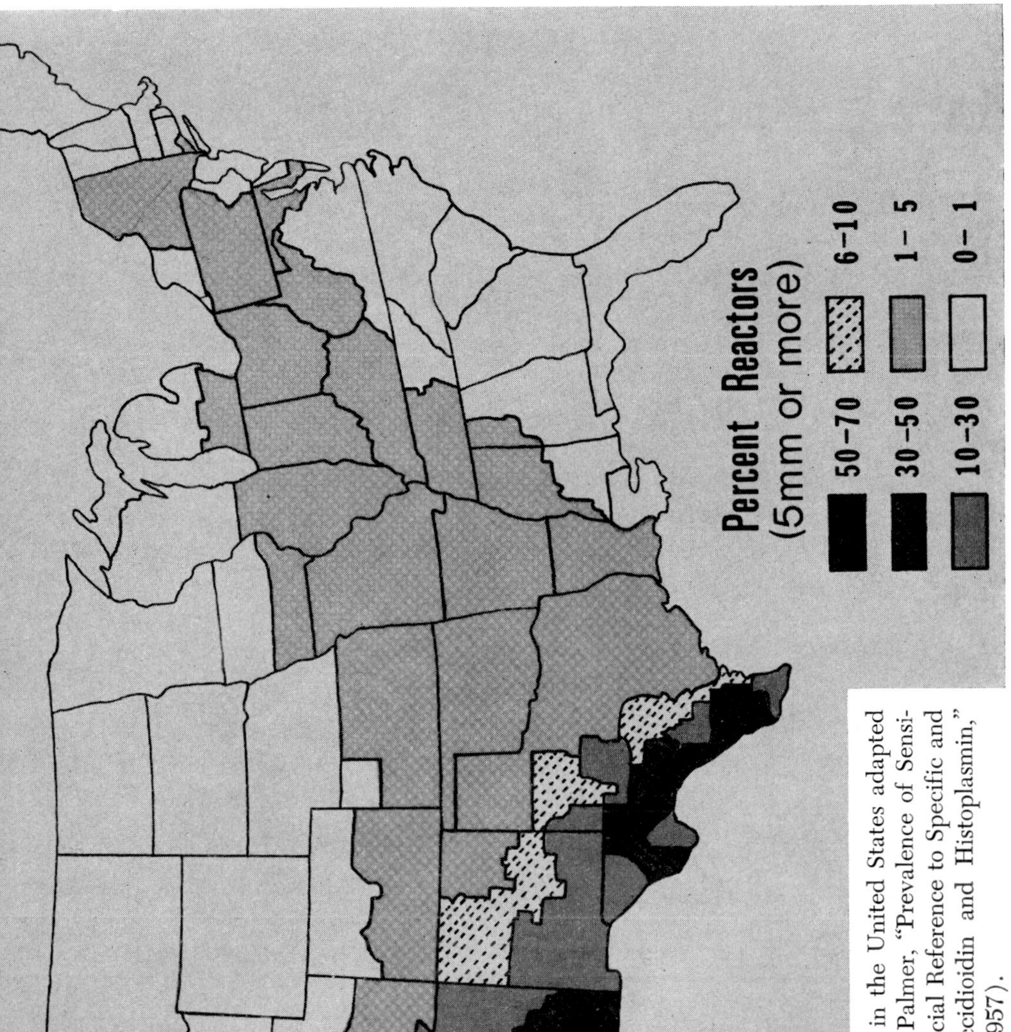

Figure 5-3. Skin-test sensitivity in the United States adapted from P. Q. Edwards and C. E. Palmer, "Prevalence of Sensitivity of Coccodioidin, with Special Reference to Specific and Non-Specific Reactions to Coccidioidin and Histoplasmin," *Diseases of the Chest, 31*:35 (1957).

TABLE 5-I

ISOLATION SITES OF *COCCIDIOIDES IMMITIS* FROM THE SOIL

Site	*Worker(s)*	*Year*
Delano, Kern County, Calif.	Stewart & Meyer	1932
Panoche Valley, San Benito County, Calif.	Davis et al.	1942
San Carlos, Gila County, Ariz.	Emmons	1942
Oildale, Kern County, Calif.	Plunkett et al.	1953
Buttonwillow & McKittrick, Kern County, Calif.	Egeberg & Ely	1956
Newman, Stanislaus County, Calif.	Plunkett & Swatek	1956
Panoche Valley, San Benito County, Calif.	Plunkett & Swatek	1956
Bakersfield, Kern County, Calif.	Plunkett & Swatek	1956
Maricopa, Kern County, Calif.	Plunkett & Swatek	1956
Blythe, Riverside County, Calif.	Swatek & Plunkett	1956
Palo Verde, Riverside County, Calif.	Swatek & Plunkett	1956
Inyokern, Kern County, Calif.	Plunkett & Swatek	1957
Cactus, Maricopa County, Ariz.	Maddy	1959
Hermosillo, Sonora, Mex.	Sotomayor et al.	1960
Lakeside, San Diego County, Calif.	Walch & Pribnow	1961
Los Banos, Merced County, Calif.	Plunkett et al.	1963
Woodville, Tulare County, Calif.	Levine & Winn	1964
Tucson, Pima County, Ariz.	Converse & Reed	1966
Sharktooth Hill, Oildale, Kern County, Calif.	Swatek et al.	1967
Lakeside, San Diego County, Calif.	Swatek et al.	1967
Santee, San Diego County, Calif.	Swatek et al.	1967
Capay Valley, Yolo County, Calif.	Pappagianis	1967
Maricopa, Kern County, Calif.	Schmidt & Howard	1968
Pacific Beach Area, San Diego, San Diego County, Calif.	Ramras et al.	1969
Reedley, Fresno County, Calif.	Sorensen	1970
Panoche, San Benito County, Calif.	Sorensen	1970
El Paso, Tex.	Teel	1970
El Tocuyo, Lara, Venezuela	Campins	1970
Richardson Springs, Butte County, Calif.	Ramsdell & Kellog	1970
Coalinga, Fresno County, Calif.	Sorensen	1971
Amerindian Village, Kern County, Calif.	Lacy & Swatek	1974
Amerindian Village, Madera County, Calif.	Lacy & Swatek	1974

on a much lower rate of skin-test reactivity among certain of the basic groups of Indians in this area (22). The earliest to the latest skin tests all support the concept of the regional presence of *C. immitis* in Arizona and the need for a continuous supply of susceptible individuals. The regional presence of *C. immitis* in Arizona has also been well established by Emmons and co-workers who reported on natural infections of *C. immitis* in rodents trapped on the Indian reservations both in the northern and southern parts of Arizona (18, 19). Maddy has shown natural infections of coccidioidomycosis among cattle and dogs in Arizona (37, 38). Thus by using the skin-testing data gathered both for man and animal it would appear that the Phoenix and Tucson areas still rank as the high endemic areas of coccidioidomycosis in this state. Phoenix, Scottsdale and Paradise Valley seem to have especially high endemic foci for this organism, yet in those areas in which skin testing for both animals and man has shown high infectivity, only a small percentage of soil samples have proven to be positive. One exception to this was the report made by Maddy in 1967 of the recovery of *C. immitis* from around burial sites of dogs that had expired of coccidioidomycosis in the Paradise Valley region (41). These findings would support the idea that if contaminated material were placed in a suitable climatic environment *C. immitis* would be able to establish within the soil and maintain itself. The parameters that are needed for the establishment of *C. immitis* within the soil in Arizona, or indeed in any other part of the world, are not known with any exactness, therefore the reporting of these infectious sites, if recovery is replicated year after year, will strongly indicate a possible means of distribution of this agent into new endemic areas. Another observation made in Arizona by Maddy was the direct growth of the mycelial phase of *C. immitis* in the soil (40). In his microscopic observation of this growth of *C. immitis* he did not report on any special nutritional prerequisite in the environment for growth, therefore we are left with the conclusion that *C. immitis* must be growing upon diffuse materials that have been rendered to the molecular level through enzymatic activities of the soil. Arizona soils have also been used to expose animals to endemic sites of *C. immitis* in nature. These field studies have been conducted with both monkeys and dogs. In comparing the results of the monkey and dog it appears that the monkey is much more susceptible to an extensive infection than is the dog (9).

It is also through the studies of Maddy in Arizona that the relationship of the general distribution of *C. immitis* in North and Central America has been shown to coincide with Merrian's definition of the Lower Sonoran Life of plant life (Fig. 5-4)(39). The Lower Sonoran Life Zone overlaps the greatest part of the known *C. immitis* endemic regions, unconscious of the geographic boundaries which man has placed upon countries, states or counties. Climatic changes have taken place with the result that certain of the margins of the Lower Sonoran Life Zone as projected by Merrian must be adjusted. The recognized climatic and soil conditions required by the types of plant found in the Merrian Lower Sonoran Life Zone seem to be, but not exclusively so, the types of environments in which *C. immitis* has come to colonize throughout these two continents. The recognition by Ochoa Gonzalez in Mexico of *C. immitis* in two endemic sites in the tropical rain forest, the recognition of the site by Walch and co-workers in Pacific Beach, California, along the ocean, by Lacy et al. in the mediterranean woodland regions of the upper part of California, give us ample reason to use the generalities put forward by Maddy as a rule of thumb, but to be cautious of the exceptions which nature seems to be providing for this generalization. It also seems significant to mention at this point the relationship of *C. immitis* distribution in nature and the creosote bush (*Larrea tridentata*). A great deal has been written about the overlapping of these two forms of biological life. Indeed, the creosote bush is one of the prime types of vegetation to be found in the Lower Sonoran Life Zone, therefore one would not be surprised to find it there, and if *C. immitis* is also present, that it too would be in the area. But the relationship here appears to be a superficial one. For, of the millions of creosote bushes existing in the Lower Sonoran Life Zone, which extends over thousands of square miles, the absence of *C. immitis* is better known than its presence. Indeed, these bushes do not seem to provide any unique or special place for the growth of this organism in nature, but only chance colonization in the mounds beneath these particular types of shrubs. The work of Riker has been substantiated by others to show that the creosote bush is inhibitory to the growth of *C. immitis* (53). This is not the only type of vegetation in the Lower Sonoran Life Zone that showed marked inhibitory action on the growth of *C. immitis*. The majority of reported soil isolations of *C. immitis* in Arizona have been

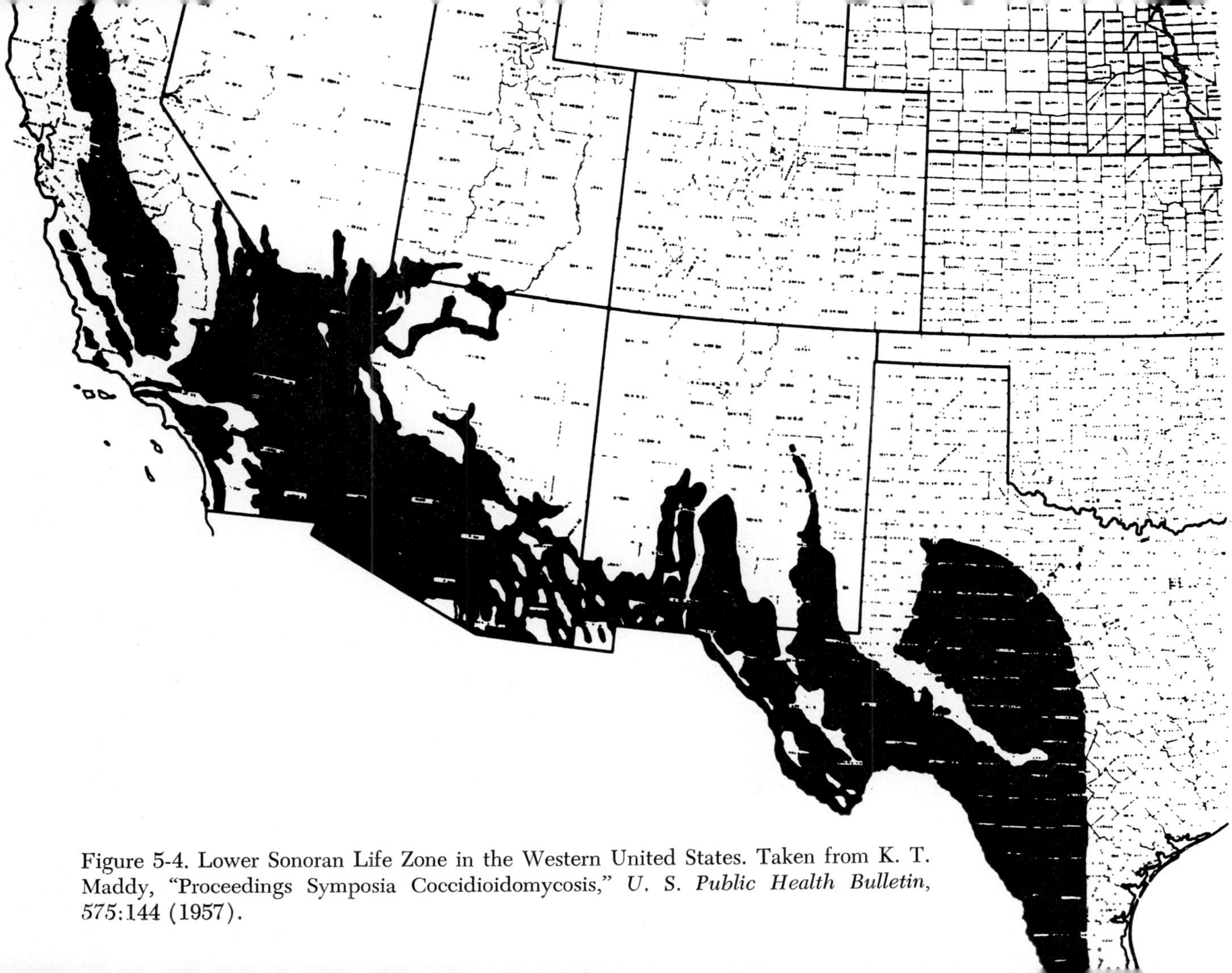

Figure 5-4. Lower Sonoran Life Zone in the Western United States. Taken from K. T. Maddy, "Proceedings Symposia Coccidioidomycosis," *U. S. Public Health Bulletin*, 575:144 (1957).

from rodent holes or a creosote bush mound. However, these ecological niches have not been the sole sources in other endemic area where this fungus has been demonstrated to have long term residence.

California

Rixford reported the first case of coccidioidomycosis in California in 1894. Since this early report the geographic distribution of *C. immitis* in California has been established both by skin testing and ecological studies. By far the greatest number of infections in California seem to have occurred in the southwestern part of the San Joaquin Valley, with Kern and Tulare counties probably being the most heavily endemic of any in the state. Infections, even soil isolations, are known in counties outside of the San Joaquin Valley, especially Yuba, Inyokern, San Bernardino, Riverside, Los Angeles and San Diego counties. These latter named counties are geographically removed from the San Joaquin Valley by a substantial range of mountains and constitute geographic and biologic isolation from the San Joaquin Valley per se. In California the endemic zone takes on different geographical appearances. Much of what is known about the distribution of *C. immitis* in California falls within the Lower Sonoran Life Zone. However, a variety of exceptions do exist, for isolations have occurred at sea level and at elevations of more than 3,200 feet. The majority of isolations have occurred in areas in which the extremes of weather are mild, others where the winter is hard every few years, complete with snow and freezing of the surface soil. Most of the endemic sites in California have been recognized as a direct result of either institutional field trips, wartime installation activities, or amateur museum archeological and anthropological groups seeking artifacts in the desert from either Indian habitats or marine fossil remains. Even the first epidemic, already mentioned of a group of graduate students in 1942 seeking out a rattlesnake in a ground squirrel hole, was an institutional field trip for the collection of biological specimens.

The exact sites in endemic regions in California are being carefully delineated by the use of soil isolation procedures repeated for years, not months, to identify the resident natural infective site. Isolations of *C. immitis* have been made from Indian burial grounds in San Diego County in the south, Inyokern to the mid northeast, Madera and Yuba in the central and northern part of the state. In these counties sites are known in which *C. immitis* is found as a resident autochthonous part of the normal flora of the soil, following a seasonal growth pattern from the surface to the deeper parts of the soil as the water table rises and falls and the heat and cold of the seasons incubate the soil. Like the situation with the creosote bush in Arizona, hundreds of samples have been processed by different investigators, but only an occasional creosote bush has been the site for the isolation of *C. immitis.* In the experience in California, these are not resident sites, but only seasonal sites at which the wind-borne, water or animal transported spores have been collected at random along with other sample material and rarely yield repeatable isolation from the mounds. Likewise, not all Indian burial sites investigated in California have been productive. In one study, Lacy et al. worked with eleven midden sites for a total of 178 samples tested, in which 8.5 percent of the soil samples were found to be positive for *C. immitis.* Sixty-seven adjacent nonmidden samples were cultured, and none were found to be positive. Of the eleven midden sites sampled, six were found to be positive for *C. immitis.* Extensive investigations of the soil and other ecological factors of these midden sites and the adjacent nonmidden soil have yielded a collection of ideas and potential theories but no single cardinal characteristic to differentiate them and identify a uniformly positive characteristic for the growth of *C. immitis* in such soils (32). Egeberg and co-workers (17), Sorensen and others (61) have studied the soil salt composition in the endemic regions. *C. immitis* has been demonstrated to have a tolerance for high salt concentrations and a greater tolerance for sodium borate than that of isolated antagonist organisms, yet no single chemical factor has been detected in these studies to explain the presence of or exclusion from the soil of *C. immitis* in endemic regions.

Ecological studies of the physical environment such as temperature have shown that in nature the surface soil down to 2.0

cm experiences temperatures which our laboratory data would imply to be lethal for *C. immitis* within an hour or so, and yet these temperatures are reached day after day for many months. The pH of the soil ranges from 7 to 10, but again does not give us a definitive clue as to the selective needs of *C. immitis* in nature. Solar radiation, especially ultraviolet radiation, has been studied in a number of sites in California, however these studies have not provided any special survival clues for soil colonization. Biological antagonists of the soil have also been pursued, especially the work of Egeberg and co-workers (16) in trying to find some biological inhibition as a controlling mechanism in nature. These studies are still too preliminary to give us a satisfactory answer for the controlling mechanism of the distribution of *C. immitis* in nature in California soil.

Besides the midden soils being a potential source of contamination of *C. immitis* in the endemic regions, the marine deposit sites such as Shark's Tooth Hill (63) just outside of Oildale near Bakersfield in the southeastern part of the San Joaquin Valley present an unusual ecological situation in that the range of hills known as Shark's Tooth Hill extends for a little better than three miles and rises from the basement of the plains near the Kern River to about 2,000 feet elevation. About a third of the way down from this range of mountains on a southwest exposure there is a single site that has been identified in which *C. immitis* has been repeatedly isolated from the soil. Extensive sampling of these three miles of mountain has been performed. This area is subject to violent cloudbursts with little ground cover to retain the water which rushes with great force down the hills, through the ravines and onto the plain below. At the base of an old sycamore tree is one of the favorite campsites in this area for dove hunters and overnight fishermen. This site has been found to be randomly positive for *C. immitis* intermittently over a period of almost twenty years. Being exposed and frequented it is subject to extensive abuse by the campers, and as a result many times the experimental stakes are lost at this site, thus exact replicate samples have not always been possible. It has always been a puzzle to the author as to whether the old sycamore site is contaminated by the wind eddies that come down through the canyon from the known *C. immitis* site or whether it is via the water that washes down through the canyon in the form of mud slurrys. The same question can be posed for the animal burrows that have been dug up repeatedly throughout the canyons leading up to Shark's Tooth Hill which yield random positives but for which repeated isolation has failed to materialize at these sites.

It is possible to generalize from the data that has been collected in California by saying that *C. immitis* is in limited pockets within the endemic regions, and that the chemistry of these sites does not appear to be significantly different, nor the physical basic soil structure. Although, it cannot be denied, that in the Indian middens there is a large amount of charcoal and a heavier residue of organic material than in some of the surrounding non-midden areas, while in the marine fossil deposit areas the calcium sulfate predominates along with diatomaceous earth being present as a substantial component of the soil complex. A sandy soil, occasionally silty, and even more rarely a clay soil, can be the home of *C. immitis* as seen at this time in California. From field work completed by our laboratory it would appear that coccidioidal blooms in the soil need 56 to 90 percent humidity for several weeks. This provides sufficient available water for growth of the organism in these naturally infected soils (32). In field studies where testing of the basic humidity, beneath the surface of the earth was conducted, a comparison between the humidity of animal burrows as well as test holes showed no appreciable difference. Therefore, no apparent environmental microniche seems to be provided *C. immitis* in a rodent hole over its natural resident sites. Studies in which infected soils have been transported *in toto* from one site to a negative site a few hundred yards away have become negative within a few months to a year of continuous study. Thus the establishment of *C. immitis*, even when transported with a large amount of its basal supportive soil, does not insure long-term establishment in the soil for this organism in areas that do not provide the total needs of the organism.

A great deal of work still needs to be carried out in order to understand *C. immitis* in California soils.

New Mexico

In 1927 the first case of coccidioidal granuloma was reported in New Mexico by Riesman et al. (52). This case was reported from the southern part of the state near the Texas-Arizona border. The opposite northeastern quarter of the state is apparently free of coccidioidal infection, falling out of the skin-test sensitivity pattern of Edwards and Palmer. It is worth noting that *Histoplasma capsulatum* invades the state of New Mexico, as does *C. immitis,* and that these two fungal agents have been reported as close as fifteen miles from each other's endemic zones. Soil isolations and ecological studies are still wanting in the state of New Mexico.

Texas

The first reported case of coccidioidomycosis infection in Texas was established by MacNeal in 1913 (36), with five cases known by 1932. The use of the skin-testing procedures show the fungus to be endemic along the entire Rio Grande Valley, with epidemics being reported in the city of El Paso, Texas. In the 1950's the military began to investigate the incidence of *C. immitis* at air force bases. Air force bases at Big Springs, San Angelo and Laredo, Texas, were surveyed and compared with the air base at Chandler, Arizona. It was observed that there was about a 2.5, 2.3 and 4.3 percent conversion each year of susceptible individuals at Big Springs, San Angelo and Laredo, respectively. These low percentages were compared to that of 31 percent at Chandler, Arizona, a recognized high endemic area (68). Data such as this again reinforces our concept of need to identify the precise geographic site of *C. immitis* in nature, and infections which occur within endemic areas may be correlated back to exceedingly small foci within the environment.

Nevada and Utah

Skin-testing surveys indicate the presence of small pockets of endemic coccidioidomycosis in Utah and Nevada. No sites, however, have been detected from direct isolation of this organism from the soil. The trapping of rodents has yielded *C. immitis* indicating the distinct regional presence of this organism within limited geographical range of the rodents collected (59). Soil ecological studies are wanting for this organism in these two states.

Republic of Mexico

The first case of coccidioidomycosis was reported in the Republic of Mexico in 1932 by Cicero et al. (8) followed by Madrid reporting a case in the State of Sonora in 1948 (42). Through the epidemiological skin-testing work of Gonzalez-Ochoa involving nearly a million subjects three endemic regions have been laid out geographically (24). The northern zone, bordering the United States, has a skin-test incidence which parallels that found in the United States. It is noteworthy that the skin-testing sensitivity moves from a 50 percent incidence in the west down to about a 10 percent incidence in the east. The second, or Pacific littoral, zone shows a high skin-test sensitivity in the north, and decreases toward the equator. In the third, or central zone, most reactors are found in the northwest with a general decrease toward the southeast. Two isolated tropical regions have been detected by skin testing and case reports in Mexico. Indeed, coccidioidal granuloma has been diagnosed among children who have never left these tropical regions. The highest skin-test sensitivity in these two tropical zones is seen in Colima and Michoacan where 10 to 29 percent positive reactors have been detected. A lower rate of 5 to 9 percent has been reported in Guerrero. These regions are not well delineated at this time, but are well out of the Lower Sonoran and creosote bush growth zones. The three other zones recognized in Mexico are within the basic projections of the Merrian Lower Sonoran Life Zone or Garcia's projection of the distribution of the creosote bush, *Larrea tridentata*, in Mexico (Fig. 5-4).

Coccidioidomycosis is being studied at a national level in Mexico with a great deal of interest. The total number of published cases are few, and many more cases are recognized than reported, strewing the true incidence of this disease at this time. The future should produce interesting data on the exact distribution of *C. immitis* through ecological studies and more complete case reporting.

CENTRAL AMERICA

The reported cases of coccidioidomycosis are only now beginning to appear in the literature. The first case was published in 1951 in the Camayaga Valley of Honduras by Castro and Trejos (7). Through skin-testing survey Mayorga (43) has identified two endemic sites in the Camayaga Valley, Zacapa and Gualan. The skin-testing survey of 1,104 individuals from these two endemic areas showed 25.5 percent positive reactors. Skin tests of 341 individuals in Escuintla, a nonendemic site showed only 2.6 percent positive reactors. This skin-testing evidence accentuates the spotty, limited geographic distribution of *C. immitis* in its environment. The skin-testing survey of Guzman (25) in 1968 of 19,846 Hondurans showed a very low accumulative overall reactor (0.2%). The isolation of *C. immitis* from nature has not been successful, however with its success an explanation of some of the skin-testing variation may come to light.

Guatemala to the north of Honduras reported coccidioidomycosis for the first time in 1960 (46). To date four human cases and seven veterinary have been reported. The skin-test studies of Andrade (1) in 1945 on 1,200 residents in the capital of Guatemala did not shed much light on the endemicity of *C. immitis* in this country, since these results show an overall 0.5 percent positive reaction. Suspicion is shed at this time on the Motagua Valley as a possible endemic site, though empirical data is wanting. No cases of coccidioidomycosis have been reported from Costa Rica, Nicaragua or Panama. There has been one veterinary report from Nicaragua in a dog (45) and two human cases from Colombia (56). Skin-testing data showed a positive coccidioidin reactor of 3.3 percent in the north and 6.3 percent in the north central region of Colombia.

SOUTH AMERICA

Venezuela

Campins et al. (6) diagnosed the first case of coccidioidomycosis in Barquisimeto, Venezuela in 1948. The endemic regions recognized today are the result of skin testing and case reports in the states of Lara, Falcan and Zulia. A total of thirty-five cases have been diagnosed from these states. Attempts have been made to isolate *C. immitis* from the soil at suspected sites but to date all results have been negative. Skin-sensitivity surveys have by far been the most productive, yielding positive reactors ranging from 0.74 to 46.4 percent (5).

Argentina

It was in Buenos Aires, Argentina, in 1892 that Alejandro Posadas presented the first case of coccidioidomycosis. It was not until 1929 that Mazza et al. saw the second case, although the fungus was misidentified, and it was not until 1932 that Almeida properly recognized the infection. Up to this point twenty-seven cases of coccidioidomysis have been reported from the Argentine, a shockingly small number compared to those in the other endemic regions found in the northern hemisphere. Skin-testing surveys conducted at different times reveal skin reactors among primary school children to range from 7.5 to 19.8 percent. Eight cases are recognized to have come from the endemic zone Santiago del Estero, four from Cordoba, three from the arid zone of the Chaco, two from the Rio Nigro, two from Mendoza, and one each from Tucuman Catamarca, San Luis and Buenos Aires. No soil sampling or ecological work has been conducted which would shed light on the distribution of this organism in nature.

Summary

The disease coccidioidomycosis has since its beginning puzzled man as to its nature, its appearance at first believed to be protozoan instead of its true fungous nature, and the fact that it existed in a mild form for many years before being detected and considered as part of a cycle preceding the granulomatous stage. In the study of coccidioidomycosis we have a true granuloma, a powerful antigen capable of stimulating a number of different kinds of antibodies within the human body, but within some, a small percent of the human population, the protective antibody and proper overall body response does not occur to contain *C. immitis* in a self-limiting form. These people, as J. Walter Wilson has identified them, are "immunologically deficient." This is a disease that imparts with its strong antigenic properties a strong immunity against reinfection. The pathogenic and virulence range of this organism make it a formidable adversary and one in which epidemics will surely continue to be recognized as man continues to disturb the face of the earth and uncover those special locales in which for whatever reasons *C. immitis* has chosen to make its home. It is also paradoxical that though the wind and the waters may carry this infectious spore for many miles, its ability to colonize and establish in its immediate neighborhood seems to be highly restricted for reasons yet unelucidated from our ecological work. As we seek *Coccidioides* from the creosote bush, the rodent burrow, the Indian mound, the fossil marine bed, no one can be sure by looking where *Coccidioides* will reside. Only through hard work in the laboratory can we detect the organisms at this time in nature. Let us hope that the generalities we have provided ourselves will guide future research and not handicap it by placing restrictions upon free thought for other avenues of investigation or sites or conditions for microenvironments in which this organism may also truly reside.

REFERENCES

1. Andrade, M.: Investigacion de la coccidioidomicosis en la capital de Guatemala por medio de la intradermo-reaccion a la coccidioidina. Tesis Facultad de Medicina, Universidad de San Carlos de Guatemala (1945).
2. Aronson, J. D., Gallagher, J. R.: Sensitivity to coccidioidin among boys in an eastern preparatory school. *Am J Pub Hlth, 32*:636, 1942.
3. Beck, M. D.: Epidemiology. Special Bull. No. 57, Calif. State Dept. Pub. Hlth., pp. 19-25, 1931.
4. Caldwell, G. T.: Coccidioidal granuloma: A report of three cases recognized in Texas. *Tex J Med, 28*:327, 1932.
5. Campins, H.: Coccidioidomycosis in Venezuela. Ajello, L.: Coccdioidomycosis, Proceedings of the 2nd Coccidioidomycosis Symp., Tucson (Arizona): Univ. Arizona Press, 1967.
6. Campins, H., Scharyj, M., Gluck, V.: Coccidioidomycosis (Enfermedad de Posadas). Su comprobacion en Venezuela. *Arch Venezol Pathol Trop Parasit Med, 1*:215, 1949.
7. Castro, A., Trejos, A.: Constatacion del primer caso centro Americano de coccidioidomycosis. *Rev Med Costa Rica, 18*:89, 1951.
8. Cicero, R. E.: El granuloma coccidioidal; presentacion de un caso clinico y consideraciones sobre esta enfermedad. *Gac Med Mex, 63*:132, 1932.

9. Converse, J. L., Reed, R. E., Kuller, H. W., Trautman, R. J., Snyder, E. M., Ray, J. G., Jr.: Experimental epidemiology of coccidioidomycosis I. Epizootiology of naturally exposed monkeys and dogs. Ajello, L. (Ed.): *Coccidioidomycosis*, 1967.
10. Cowper, H. H.: A coccidioidomycosis outbreak in Canoga Park, San Fernando Valley. *U S Naval Med Newsletter, 46*:18, 1965.
11. Davis, B. L., Jr., Smith, R. T., Smith, C. E.: An epidemic of coccidioidal infection (coccidioidomycosis). *JAMA, 118*:1182, 1942.
12. Dickson, E. C.: "Valley Fever" of the San Joaquin Valley and fungus *Coccidioides* (discussed by K. F. Myer). *Calif West Med, 47*:151, 1937.
13. Dickson, E. C., Gifford, M. A.: *Coccidioides infection* (coccidioidomycosis). II. The primary type of infection. *Arch Int Med, 62*:853, 1938.
14. Eckmann, B. H., Schafer, G. L., Huppert, M.: Bedside interhuman transmission of coccidioidomycosis via growth on fomites. An epidemic involving six persons. *Am Rev Respir Dis, 89*:175, 1964.
15. Edwards, P. Q., Palmer, C. E.: Prevalence of sensitivity to coccidioidin, with special reference to specific and nonspecific reactions to coccidioidin and histoplasmin. *Dis Chest, 31*:35, 1957.
16. Egeberg, R. O., Elconin, A. E., Egeberg, M. C.: Effects of salinity and temperature of *Coccidioides immitis* and three antagonistic soil saprophytes. *J Bact, 88*:473, 1964.
17. Elconin, A. F., Egeberg, R. O., Egeberg, M. P.: Significance of soil salinity on the ecology of *Coccidioides immitis. J Bact, 87*:500, 1964.
18. Emmons, C. W.: Isolation of *Coccidioides* from soil and rodents. *Pub Hlth Rep, 57*:109, 1942.
19. Emmons, C. W., Ashburn, L. I.: The isolation of *Haplosporangium parvum* n. sp. and *Coccidioides immitis* from wild rodents. Their relationship to coccidioidomycosis. *Pub Hlth Rep, 57*:1715, 1942.
20. Fennel, E. A.: Coccidioidal granuloma in Hawaii. Proc. Staff Meet. Clin., Honolulu, 6: No. 9, 1, 1935.
21. Gifford, M. A.: San Joaquin Fever. *Kern County Dept Pub Hlth Ann Rep*, 1935-1936.
22. Geller, R. D.: Coccidioidin sensitivity among southwestern American Indians. *Am J Respir Dis, 107*:301, 1973.
23. Gomez, R. F.: Endemism of coccidioidomycosis in the Paraguayan Chaco. *Calif Med, 73*:35, 1950.
24. Gonzalez-Ochoa, A.: Coccidioidomycosis in Mexico. Ajello, L. (Ed.): *Coccidioidomycosis*, 1967.
25. Guzman, B.: Informe de las actividades desarrolladas por el programa de control de la tuberculosis durante el ano de 1968. Tegucigalpa, Div. Tuberc., Ministerio de Salud Publica y Asistencia Social, Honduras, 1968.

26. Hirsch, E. F.: Introduction of coccidioidal granuloma in Chicago. *JAMA, 81*:375, 1923.
27. Hoekenga, M. T., Tucker, H. A.: Histoplasmina y coccidioidinea; sensibilidad a la histoplasmina y a la coccidioidinea en Honduras; informe sobre 300 enfermos. *Bol Ofic san panamer, 29*:1135, 1950.
28. Huppert, M., Sun, S. H., Bailey, J. W.: Natural variability in *Coccidioides immitis*. Ajello, L. (Ed.): *Coccidioidomycosis*, 1967.
29. Jacobson, H. P.: Coccidioidal granuloma; specific allergic cutaneous reaction; experimental and clinical investigations. *Arch Derm Syph, 18*:562, 1928.
30. Joffe, B.: An epidemic of coccidioidomycosis probably related to soil. *N Engl J Med, 262*:720, 1960.
31. Kritzer, M. D., Biddle, M., Kessel, J. F.: An outbreak of primary pulmonary coccidioidomycosis in Los Angeles, California. *Ann Int Med, 33*:960, 1950.
32. Lacy, G.: Soil ecology of *Coccidioides immitis* at archeological sites, Master's Thesis, California State College, Long Beach, Calif., 1971.
33. Lee, R. V.: Coccidioidomycosis: in the Western Flying Training Command. *Calif West Med, 61*:133, 1944.
34. Lipsitz, S. H.: Systemic blastomycosis and coccidioidal granuloma with a description of the first case of coccidioidal granuloma reported in Missouri. *J Mo M A*, 534, 1916.
35. Loofbourow, J. C., Pappagianis, D., Cooper, T. Y.: Endemic coccidioidomycosis in Northern California: An outbreak in the Capay Valley of Yolo County. *Calif Med, 111*:5, 1969.
36. MacNeal, W. J., Hjelm, C. E.: Note on a mould coccidioides immitis found in a case of generalized infection in man. *JAMA, 61*:2044, 1913.
37. Maddy, K. T.: Coccidioidomycosis of cattle in the Southwestern United States. *J Am Vet Med Assoc, 124*:456, 1954.
38. Maddy, K. T.: A study of one hundred cases of disseminated coccidioidomycosis in the dog. *Proc Symp Cocci U S Pub Hlth Serv Pub, 575*:107, 1957.
39. Maddy, K. T.: Ecological factors possibly relating to the geographic distribution of *Coccidioides immitis*. *Proc Symp Cocci U S Pub Hlth Bull, 575*:144, 1957.
40. Maddy, K. T.: Observations on *Coccidioides immitis* found growing naturally in soil. *Ariz Med, 22*:281, 1965.
41. Maddy, K. T., Crecelius, H. G.: Establishment of *Coccidioides immitis* in negative soil following burial of infected animals and animal tissue. Ajello, L. (Ed): *Coccidioidomycosis*, 1967.
42. Madrid, G. S.: Coccidioidomycosis en el Estado de Sonora. *Prensa med (Hermosillo) 10*:No. 3, 2, 1950.

43. Mayorga, P. R.: Coccidioidomycosis in Central America. Ajello, L. (Ed.): *Coccidioidomycosis,* 1967.
44. Moore, M.: Coccidioidal granuloma: a classification of the causative agent, *Coccidioides immitis. Ann Mo Bot Garden, 19*:397, 1932.
45. Nordstoga, K., Lindqvist, K., Strande, A.: Coccidioidomycosis. Report of a case in a dog. *Nordisk Verinaermedicin, 11*:461, 1959.
46. Perez-Guisasola, E., Rosal, J. E.: Coccidioidomicosis humana en Guatemala. Diagnostico micologico, histopathologico y comprobacion biologica del primer caso. *Rev Col Med (Guatemala), 11*:290, 1960.
47. Plunkett, O. A., Swatek, F. E.: Ecological studies of *Coccidioides immitis. Proc Armed Forces-VA Symp Cocci,* 1957.
48. Posadas, A.: Un nuevo caso de micosis fungoidea con psorospermias. *Ann Circ Med Argent, 15*:585, 1892.
49. Ragle, H. E.: Coccidioidal granuloma. *Tr Hawaii MA, 44*:47, 1934.
50. Ramras, D. G., Walch, H. A. A., Murray, J. P., Davidson, B. H.: An epidemic of coccidioidomycosis in the Pacific Beach area of San Diego. *Am Rev Respir Dis, 101*:975, 1970.
51. Rao, S., Biddle, M., Balchum, O. J., Robinson, J. L.: Focal endemic coccidioidomycosis in Los Angeles County. *Am Rev Respir Dis, 105*:410, 1972.
52. Riesman, D., Ahlfeldt, F. E.: Coccidioidal granuloma; review of the clinical data with report of Pennsylvania case. *Am J Med Sci, 174*: 151, 1927.
53. Riker, A. E.: For coccidioidomycosis—a possible source of infectious spores and of therapeutic agents. *Mycopath Mycol Appl, 34*:155, 1968.
54. Rixford, E.: Case for diagnosis presented before the San Francisco Medico-Chirurgical Society, March 5, 1894. *Occidental Med Times, 8*:326, 1894.
55. Roberts, P. L., Lisciandro, R. C.: A community epidemic of coccidioidomycosis. *Am Rev Respir Dis, 96*:766, 1967.
56. Robledo, V. M. A., Restrepo, M. M., Restrepo I. S., Ospina O. F., Gutierrez A.: Encuesta epidemiologica sobre coccidioidomicosis en algunas zonas aridas de Colombia. *Antioquia Med, 18*:505, 1968.
57. Shelton, R. M.: A survey of coccidioidomycosis at Camp Roberts, California. *JAMA, 118*:1186, 1942.
58. Sievers, M. L.: Coccidioidomycosis among southwestern American Indians. *Am Rev Respir Dis, 90*:920, 1964.
59. Smith, C. E.: Diagnosis of pulmonary coccidioidal infections. *Calif Med, 75*:385, 1951.
60. Smith, C. E., Beard, R. R., Rosenberger, H. G., Whiting, E. G.: Effect of season and dust control in coccidioidomycosis. *Am J Med Sci, 212*:652, 1946.

61. Sorensen, R. H.: Survival characteristics of diphasic *Coccidioides immitis* exposed to the rigors of a simulated natural environment. Ajello, L. (Ed.): *Coccidioidomycosis*, 1967.
62. Stewart, R. A., Meyer, K. F.: Isolation of *Coccidioides immitis* (stiles) from the soil. *Proc Soc Exp Biol Med, 29*:937, 1932.
63. Swatek, F. E., Omieczynski, D. T., Plunkett, O. A.: *Coccidioides immitis* in California. Ajello, L. (Ed.): *Coccidioidomycosis*, 1967.
64. Swatek, F. E., Plunkett, O. A.: Ecological studies on *Coccidioides immitis*; experimental infections of wild rodents and anmials other than mammals. *Proc Symp Cocci, U S Pub Hlth Bull, 575*:151, 1957.
65. Teel, K. W., Yow, M. D., Williams, T. W., Jr.: A localized outbreak of coccidioidomycosis in southern Texas. *J Pediatr, 77*:65, 1970.
66. Walch, H. A., Pribnow, J. F., Wyborney, V. J., Walch, R. K.: Coccidioidomycosis in San Diego County and the involvement of transported topsoil in certain cases. *Am Rev Respir Dis, 84*:359, 1961.
67. Werner, S. B., Pappagianis, D., Heindl, I., Mickel, A.: An epidemic of coccidioidomycosis among archeology students in northern California. *N Engl J Med, 286*:507, 1972.
68. Williams, J. J., Ellingson, H. V.: Studies on coccidioidomycosis at Air Force bases in the Southwestern United States, USAF School of Aviation Medicine, Unnumbered report, Dec., 1954.
69. Winn, W. A., Levine, H. B., Broderick, J. E., Crane, R. W.: A localized epidemic of coccidioidal infection. Primary coccidioidomycosis occurring in a group of ten children. *N Engl J Med, 268*:867, 1963.
70. Woolley, M. T.: Mycological findings in sputum. *J Lab Clin Med, 23*:553, 1938.

General References

Al-Doory, Y., Pairon, R.: A bibliography of Coccidioidomycosis. *Mycopath Mycol Appl, 46*:113, 1972.
Cheu, S.: Coccidioidomycosis bibliography. U. S. Veterans Hospital, Fresno, Calif., 1972.

Chapter 6

THE EPIDEMIOLOGY OF BLASTOMYCOSIS

Ernest W. Chick

Blastomycosis remains an enigma among the mycoses. We have knowledge of severe disease, but other than teasing tidbits we know little of mild disease and less of the possibility of asymptomatic cases. By analogy we may compare the present situation with that of histoplasmosis in the mid-1940's. It was not until after this period that appropriate skin-test and serologic antigens were developed, leading to an understanding of the full spectrum of infection and disease that histoplasmosis may take. Thirty years later we still do not have comparable antigens for *Blastomyces dermatitidis*. Comparably the natural habitats for *Histoplasma capsulatum* have long been identified, but the search continues for those of *B. dermatitidis*. Blastomycosis has been, and continues to be, a truly fascinating entity.

Clinical Aspects

To appreciate the epidemiological aspects of blastomycosis, one first should consider that blastomycosis (i.e. infection with *B. dermatitidis*) is a disease with protean manifestations. Clinically some cases may have signs and symptoms that can readily lead to the proper identification. In many instances, however, the signs and symptoms may be vague, variable, and misleading, indicative of the fact that blastomycosis can be a mimic of a wide variety of other diseases.

Consensus is that infection with *B. dermatitidis* is by inhalation leading to a primary pulmonary localization. The infection may remain in the lungs or may spread to virtually any organ of the body. The wide variety of symptoms found in the 198 collected cases by the Blastomycosis VA Cooperative Study (5) is indicative of the pattern, or lack of pattern, found throughout the literature (Table 6-I) and reflect the multiple organ involvement that may occur (Table 6-II).

The diagnosis of blastomycosis is by culture or by histologic demonstration of the fungus from tissue or clinical specimens (3). Unfortunately the skin-test reaction and serologic results are often inconsistent and transient, while cross-reactions with other fungi, primarily *H. capsulatum*, are common (6, 32). Thus

TABLE 6-I

SYMPTOMS LEADING TO EXAMINATION OR HOSPITALIZATION*

	Patients with Each Symptom	
Symptom	*Number*	*Percent*
Cough	71	35.8
Weight loss	55	27.8
Chest pain	52	26.2
Skin lesion	51	25.8
Fever	45	22.7
Hemoptysis	41	20.7
Localized swelling	27	13.6
Draining sinus	10	5.1
Night sweats	10	5.1
Genitourinary complaints	8	4.4
Mucous membrane lesion	7	3.5
Fatigue	6	3.3
Hoarseness	6	3.3
Painful joint	6	3.3
Gastrointestinal complaints	6	3.3
Malaise	5	2.0
Neurologic disturbance	5	2.0
Nodules	5	2.0
Chills	3	1.5
Dyspnea	2	1.0
Back pain	2	1.0
Pain in ear	1	0.5
Dysphagia	1	0.5

*Busey, et al. (1964).

the skin test and serologic tests do not have either the presumptive diagnostic significance or the epidemiologic usefulness in blastomycosis (10). A positive test should raise the index of suspicion for the possibility of blastomycosis. A negative test is meaningless and may represent either a true or false negative reaction.

Geographical Distribution

North America: The majority of cases of blastomycosis have occurred in the United States. Most have occurred in the states bordering and east of the Mississippi River (Fig. 6-1). This pattern of cases has been consistent over the years in case compilations derived by varying methods (5, 9, 35). Probably between one hundred and two hundred cases have been reported in Canada (20, 21, 28, 37, 41).

TABLE 6-II

SYSTEMS OR ORGANS INVOLVED IN 25 DEATHS FROM BLASTOMYCOSIS*

Organ or System	*Number*
Lungs	24
Skin	13
Liver	9
Kidneys	9
Prostate	9
Central nervous system	8
Spleen	8
Bone	7
Lymph nodes	6
Thyroid	4
Heart	3
Adrenals	3
Omentum	3
Gastroinestinal tract	2
Skeletal muscles	1
Pericardium	1
Testicle	1
Urinary bladder	1
Pancreas	1

*Busey, et al. (1964).

In a more recent study Furcolow et al. compiled data on 1,476 human and 384 canine cases of blastomycosis (18) (Table 6-III).

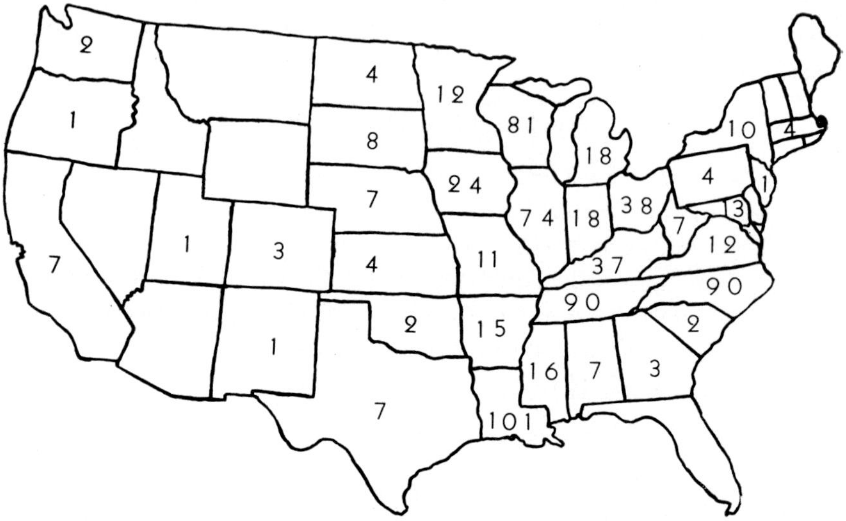

Figure 6-1. Distribution of 735 reported cases of Blastomycosis.

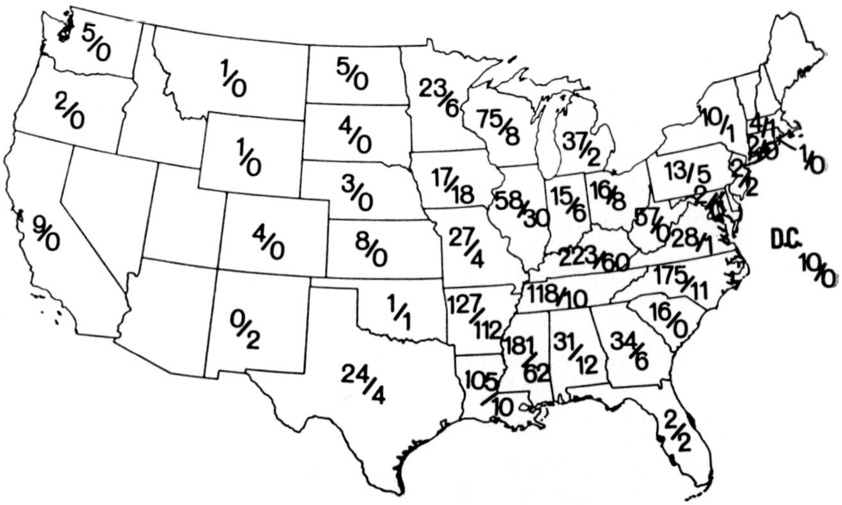

Figure 6-2. Blastomycosis in the United States, by states. Numbers represent the ratio of cases in humans to cases in dogs.

Again the same general pattern was apparent (Fig. 6-2) but more precise localization by county or residence revealed concentrations of cases not previously apparent within states (Fig. 6-3). Even in the five states with the highest prevalence rates, i.e. Mississippi, Kentucky, Arkansas, North Carolina, and Tennessee, definite clustering and patterning of cases is obvious (19).

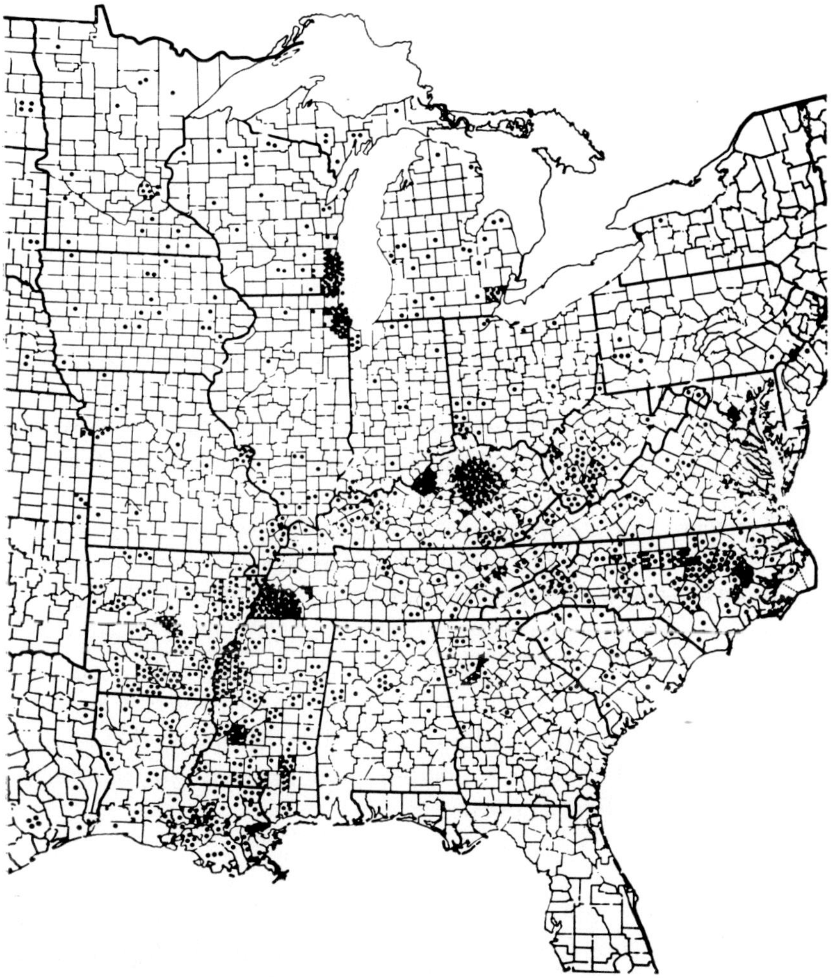

Figure 6-3. Location by county of 1,444 cases of human Blastomycosis. (Includes all but 20 U. S. cases.)

TABLE 6-III

HUMAN AND CANINE BLASTOMYCOSIS CASE RATE PER 100,000 POPULATION FOR LEADING STATES WITH HUMAN CASES*

	Case Rate	
State	*Human*	*Canine*
Mississippi	8.3	19.9
Kentucky	7.4	13.8
Arkansas	7.1	43.8
North Carolina	3.8	1.5
Tennessee	3.3	2.0

*Furculow, et al. (1970).

CASES OUTSIDE NORTH AMERICA: Vandepitte and Gatti (40) have reviewed seventeen cases of blastomycosis which occurred in Africa (Tunisia, Morocco, Zaire, Uganda, Tanzania, Mozambique, Rhodesia, Afrique de Sud). All seventeen were diagnosed by biopsy and twelve by culture. These cases were individually reported between 1952 and 1971 and are believed to be autochthonous.

At least one generally accepted case diagnosed by biopsy and culture has been reported in Venezuela (29). A scattering of other cases have been reported from Latin America (1, 2, 12). Da Fonscia (11) considers many cases reported in South America to be in error as regards the etiologic agent. Cases have been reported in England (15) and in Zurich, Switzerland (42), but have histories indicative of possible fomite transmission from the U. S. Many of the other reports of blastomycosis from Europe are felt to be due to other fungi, particularly *Cryptococcus neoformans*, to be inadequate in description of the etiologic agent, or to be based on a positive skin test without demonstration of the specific organism (9).

Age

Blastomycosis may occur in any age group. Cases have been reported from age five months (36) to the ninth decade of life (33). However, there is a definite clustering of cases between thirty and sixty. This pattern was also noted in the reports of many authors (23, 24, 35, 38).

Blastomycosis thus appears to be a clinical disease that occurs more often during the middle age span of life. It is of interest to contrast this with histoplasmosis in which the comparable chronic pulmonary form occurs during somewhat later ages of life and is generally felt to reflect a picture of reinfection.

Sex

A ratio of eight or nine males to each female with blastomycosis has been reported (7, 8, 24, 35). The extremes of this ratio have been reported by Schwarz and Baum (33), with a 15 to 1 ratio and by Smith et al. (36) with a very unusual 1 to 1 ratio. In looking at sex differences and type of disease Kunkel et al. (23) reported a 5 to 1 ratio in systemic cases and a 10 to 1 ratio in cutaneous cases.

Furcolow et al. (26) found 89 percent of 1,114 human cases were males. This contrasts with the concomitant 247 canine cases in which 67 percent males were found.

Race

In most series of reported cases the racial distribution has been thought to reflect the general population distribution. Thus series from northern U. S. have been predominantly white (86-93%) (7, 23, 35). In contrast, series from the southern U. S. report an increasing proportion of non-white (9, 22, 24), with 69 percent black patients in Memphis hospitals reported by Chick et al. (8).

In the overall series of 1,114 cases reported by Furcolow et al. (18), 810 were white and 304 non-white. At first note this appears in keeping with the above series. However, when these data were converted to ratios based on the 1960 census, the case rate for whites was 0.5/100,000 and for blacks was 1.6/100,000, a threefold difference. Unfortunately data were not available for appraisal of severity of disease in these two groups, so an appropriate comparison cannot be made with coccidioidomycosis in which disease is more severe in non-whites.

Occupation

It has become a tradition in discussing blastomycosis to attempt to correlate its occurrence with occupational status and/or living conditions. Many of the early cases reported by Stober, 1914 lived in damp conditions associated with dirty floors and rotting wood walls. Frequent correlations with manual labor, agricultural pursuits, construction, dust-exposure, etc. have been made by various workers (5, 8, 22, 35, 38).

Kunkel et al. (23), and Cherniss and Weisbren (7) found less correlation with outdoor occupation. Yet one cannot ignore the possibility (fact?) that housewives, lawyers, etc. do have outdoor pursuits, be it gardening, hiking, hunting, or whatever. Certainly there is little question that persons with indoor occupations have been infected with *H. capsulatum* or *Coccidioides immitis* as a result of a chance or casual exposure, as subsequently demonstrated by epidemiological investigation and soil studies. Certainly by analogy similar occurrences could happen in blastomycosis.

Transmission

To date no verified instances have been reported of human to human, animal to animal, or animal to human transmission of *B. dermatitidis*. Procknow (30) reported an instance of presumed human to human transmission.

All epidemiologic and clinical considerations indicate a probable soil to host transmission via the airborne route wth inhalation of infectious particles. A few cases have been documented for direct percutaneous inoculation of the fungus, but the consensus is that blastomycosis is a primary respiratory infection.

Clinically the lungs are most often involved, and in dissemination lesions in other organs often postdate the pulmonary lesions. Spread within the body may occur by hematogenous or lymphatic dissemination or by direct extension of the lesion.

There are continuing schools of thought as to the possibility of direct skin inoculation. Until the middle of the 1950's blastomycosis was thought to occur in three forms, the primary pulmonary, the primary cutaneous, and the systemic or disseminated. Schwarz and Baum (33, 34) in their studies of clinical and autopsy cases found the so-called cutaneous cases were identical with those in systemic cases and postulated that the cutaneous cases were secondary to a pulmonary focus as in the systemic cases. Wilson et al. (44), reported four cases of primary cutaneous involvement. Three of the cases resulted from trauma with cutaneous inoculation in autopsy performance and the fourth was a laboratory accident. All had a chancriform lesion with regional lymphangitis and lymphadenopathy. All had a strong tendency toward spontaneous recovery. This is quite different from the acanthotic, hyperkeratetic, and ulcerative lesions without lymph involvement usually found in blastomycosis. The observations of Schwarz and Baum and those of Wilson and his co-workers have become the basis for the present consensus of the rarity of the diagnosis of primary cutaneous lesions.

Thus it is believed that the host, be it human or lower animal, is infected by inhaling infectious particles of *B. dermatitidis*. As in every unfinished saga there is a point for questioning; where does *B. dermatitidis* exist and how does it get airborne? Epidemiologists have had, and for some time will continue to have "field days" with this question.

As highlighted in the sections dealing with age, sex, race, and occupation, patients with blastomycosis are usually active people who have opportunity to be in close contact with nature, i.e. soil. This has quite obvious similarity to coccidioidomycosis and histoplasmosis in which there is no question of infection occurring via inhalation from contaminated (infected) soil sources. The ecologic cycles for *C. immitis* and *H. capsulatum* are well documented in other chapters of this book.

The corresponding ecologic cycle for *B. dermatitidis* remains incomplete. The development of usable antigens for coccidioidomycosis and histoplasmosis was invaluable in developing an appreciation of the magnitude of asymptomatic cases, their relationship to clinical cases, and to localize clusters of infection for appropriate soil isolation studies. Without comparable antigens similar epidemiologic approaches have been impossible in blastomycosis.

Denton et al. reported in 1961 (13) the first isolation of *B. dermatitidis* from soil taken from a barn near Lexington, Kentucky. It is interesting that a dog had died of blastomycosis in this barn. In a subsequent study of 365 soil specimens taken near Augusta, Georgia, Denton and DiSalvo (14) cultured *B. derma-*

titidis from ten samples taken at five sites. All sites were within a 1.8 mile radius and included an unused cattle ramp, old chicken houses and rabbit pen, a mule stall, and an abandoned kitchen. Repeated culturing of the original samples and of the sites covered in both reports were negative.

B. dermatitidis can be grown on sterilized soil or tree bark under laboratory conditions (17, 25). Ajello (1) has reviewed the chemical and biological factors of soil which might relate to the frustrating inability to isolate this fungus repeatedly from soil.

Historically the report of Stober (39) is a teasingly "so near, yet so far." He examined the home conditions of a number of his patients and found a fungus growing on wet and decaying wooden walls. This fungus culturally resembled *B. dermatitidis.* He conservatively did not specifically so designate this fungus, but called attention to its similarity. It is regrettable that he did not do animal inoculations, since this may have shown conclusively the nature of this fungus.

Along with improved methods for soil sampling, it is hoped that appropriate antigens may soon be forthcoming which will have usefulness in epidemiologic studies. In their absence epidemiologic observations have been based, of necessity, on recognized clinical patients. By analogy this places the state of epidemiologic knowledge of blastomycosis and its transmission on a par with that of histoplasmosis in the early 1940's. This lack may be offset in some degree by more detailed studies of blastomycosis in animals.

Animal Infections

Ramsay and Carter (31) pointed out that blastomycosis in dogs is more frequent in areas where human cases are known to occur. Menges (26) reported 113 U. S. and three Canadian cases of canine blastomycosis. The greatest number of cases were found in Kentucky, twenty-one; Illinois, twenty-one; Iowa, thirteen; and Alabama, ten. Subsequently he reported seventy-nine canine cases in Arkansas (27).

Furcolow et al. (18, 19) reported 384 canine cases of blastomycosis. The greater number of cases were in Arkansas, 112;

Mississippi, sixty-two; and Kentucky, sixty. A general correlation is seen between the number of human and of canine cases in the various states (Fig. 6-2, Table 6-III). However, definite discrepancies are apparent. These relate to the intensity of and interest in case finding by (a) physicians, (b) veterinarians, or (c) both in any given state. Arkansas, for example, had a very intensive canine case finding program for some years which resulted in the surprising rate of 45.8/100,000 dogs. West Virginia, on the other extreme, has had little in the way of canine case finding and thus has a zero rate.

From these data it is apparent that the epidemiological and geographical distribution studies of blastomycosis could be intensified and expanded by a concerted medical-veterinary approach. Such a combined approach would suggest deficiencies in case finding if the rates were higher for human than dog, or vice versa. With adequate levels of case finding for human and dog, precise localizations of cases could be maintained and used for soil isolation and pathogenetic studies.

Other than dogs, Ajello (1) quotes cases of blastomycosis as occurring in a horse in Iowa (4), a captive Stellar's sea lion in Illinois (43), and a doubtful case in a Siamese cat (16).

Conclusions and Needs

Epidemiologic knowledge of blastomycosis is restricted to those cases which are severe enough to make them seek medical attention. Lack of appropriate antigens for skin testing and serologic studies has hampered documentation as to the true spectrum of disease, e.g. asymptomatic and/or spontaneously remitting cases. Thus knowledge based on what may well be an inadequately understood spectrum of disease may reflect such case bias.

At this point in the study of blastomycosis it is imperative to

a. develop better diagnostic antigens,
b. localize more precisely the geographic distribution,
c. determine the frequency of spontaneous remission of disease, and
d. determine the frequency of asymptomatic and mild infections.

Only then will we know if blastomycosis is a common infection with relative infrequency of severe disease, as histoplasmosis and coccidioidomycosis, or is truly an uncommon infection and usually a severe disease when it occurs.

REFERENCES

1. Ajello, L.: Comparative ecology of respiratory mycotic disease agents. *Bact Rev, 31*:6, 1967.
2. Arias Luzardo, J. J.: Micosis profundas mas frequentes en Mexico. Thesis. Univer. Nacion. Autonoma Mexico, Escuela Nacion. Med., 1962.
3. Baker, R. D.: The diagnosis of fungus diseases by biopsy. *J Chron Dis,* 5:552, 1957.
4. Benbrook, E. A., Bryant, J. T., Saunders, L. Z.: A case of blastomycosis in the horse. *J Am Vet Med Assoc, 112*:475, 1948.
5. Busey, J. F., Baker, R. D., Birch, L., Buechner, H., Chick, E. W., Justice, F. K., Matthews, J. H., McDearman, S., Pickar, D. N., Sutliff, W. D., Walkup, H. E., Zimmerman, S.: Blastomycosis. 1. A review of 198 collected cases in Veterans Administration hospitals. *Am Rev Respir Dis, 89*:659, 1964.
6. Campbell, C. C.: Serology in the respiratory mycoses, a review. *Sabouraudia, 5*:240, 1967.
7. Cherniss, E. I., Waisbren, B. A.: North American blastomycosis: A clinical study of forty cases. *Ann Intern Med, 44*:105, 1956.
8. Chick, E. W., Sutliff, W. D., Rakich, J. H., Furcolow, M. L.: Epidemiological aspects of cases of blastomycosis admitted to Memphis, Tennessee, hospitals during the period of 1922-1954. A review of eighty-six cases. *Am J Med Sci, 231*:253, 1956.
9. Chick, E. W., Peters, H. J., Denton, J. F., Boring, W. D.: Die Nordamerikanische Blastomykose. *Ergeb Algem Path Pathol Anat, 40*: 34, 1960.
10. Chick, E. W., Baum, G. L., Furcolow, M. L., Huppert, M., Kaufman, L., Pappagianis, D.: The use of skin tests and serologic tests in histoplasmosis, coccidioidomycosis, and blastomycosis. Scientific assembly statement. *Am Rev Respir Dis, 108*:156, 1973.
11. DaFonseca, O.: Deep skin and pulmonary mycoses in Brazil. In Sternberg, T. N., and Newcomer, V. D. (eds.), *Therapy of Fungus Diseases.* Boston, Little Brown, 1955.
12. DeMontemayor, L.: *Blastomyces dermatitidis*—Gilchrist & Stokes 1898 en Venezuela, Nota Previa. *Gac Med Caracas, 62*:675, 1954.
13. Denton, J. F., McDonough, E. S., Ajello, L., Ausherman, R. J.: Isolation of *Blastomyces dermatitidis* from soil. *Science, 133*:1126, 1961.
14. Denton, J. F., DiSalvo, A. F.: Isolation of *Blastomyces dermatitidis*

from natural sites in Augusta, Georgia. *Am J Trop Med Hyg, 13*: 716, 1964.

15. Dowling, G. B., Elsworthy, R. R.: Case of blastomycetic dermatitidis (Gilchrist). *Proc Roy Soc Med, 19*:4, 1926.
16. Easton, K. L.: Cutaneous North American blastomycosis in a Siamese cat. *Can Vet J, 2*:350, 1961.
17. Emmons, C. W.: Isolation of *Histoplasma capsulatum* from soil. *Pub Hlth Rep, 64*:892, 1949.
18. Furcolow, M. L., Chick, E. W., Busey, J. F., Menges, R. W.: Prevalence and incidence studies of human and canine blastomycosis. I. Cases in the United States, 1885-1968. *Am Rev Respir Dis, 102*:60, 1970.
19. Furcolow, M. L., Busey, J. F., Menges, R. W., Chick, E. W.: Prevalence and incidence studies of human and canine blastomycosis. II. Yearly incidence studies in three selected states, 1960-1967. *Am J Epid, 92*:121, 1970.
20. Gilles, M.: A case of blastomycosis. *Can Med Assoc J, 29*:183, 1933.
21. Grandbois, J.: La blastomycose Nord-Americaine au Canada. *Loval Med, 34*:714, 1963.
22. Howles, J. K., Black, C. I.: Cutaneous blastomycosis. A report of 58 unpublished cases. *J La Med Soc, 105*:72, 1953.
23. Kunkel, W. M., Jr., Weed, L. A., McDonald, J. R., Clagett, O. T.: Collective review: North American blastomycosis—Gilchrist's disease; clinicopathologic study of ninety cases. *Int Abstr Surg, 99*:1, 1954.
24. Martin, D. S., Smith, D. T.: Blastomycosis (American blastomycosis, Gilchrist's disease). II. A report of thirteen new cases. *Am Rev Tuberc, 39*:275, 1939.
25. Menges, R. W., Furcolow, M. L., Larsh, H. W.: Laboratory studies on histoplasmosis. I. The effect of humidity and temperature on the growth of *Histoplasma capsulatum*. *J Infect Dis, 90*:67, 1952.
26. Menges, R. W.: Blastomycosis in animals. *Vet Med, 55*:45, 1960.
27. Menges, R. W., Furcolow, M. L., Selby, L. A., Ellis, H. R., Haberman, R. T.: Clinical and epidemiologic studies on seventy-nine canine blastomycosis cases in Arkansas. *Am J Epid, 81*:164, 1965.
28. Poirier, P.: Blastomycose Nord-Americaine (Maladie de Gilchrist) *Un Med Can, 84*:287, 1955.
29. Polo, J. F., Brass, K., DeMontemayor, L.: Enfermeded de Gilchrist en Venezuela; primer case, estudio clinico; comprobacion histologica; aislamiento y determinacion de la primera cepa Suramericana de *Blastomyces dermatitides*. *Rev San (Caracas), 19*:217, 1954.
30. Procknow, J. J.: Disseminated blastomycosis treated successfully with the polypeptide antifungal agent x-5079C. Evidence for human to human transmission. *Am Rev Respir Dis, 94*:761, 1966.

31. Ramsay, F. K., Carter, G. R.: Canine blastomycosis in the U. S. *J Am Vet Assoc, 120*:93, 1952.
32. Salvin, S. B.: Immunologic aspects of the mycoses. *Prog Allergy, 7*:213, 1963.
33. Schwarz, J., Baum, G. L.: Blastomycosis. *Am J Clin Pathol, 21*:999, 1951.
34. Schwarz, J., Baum, G. L.: North American blastomycosis: (geographic distribution, pathology and pathogenesis). *Docum Med Geogr Trop, 5*:29, 1953.
35. Schwarz, J., Goldman, L.: Epidemiologic study of North American blastomycosis. *Arch Dermatol Syph (Chicago), 71*:84, 1955.
36. Smith, J. G., Jr., Harris, J. S., Conant, N. F., Smith, D. T.: An epidemic of North American blastomycosis. *JAMA, 158*:641, 1955.
37. Solway, L. J., Kohan, M., Pritzker, H. G.: A case of disseminated blastomycosis. *Can Med Assoc J, 41*:331, 1939.
38. Starrs, R. A., Klotz, M. L.: North American blastomycosis (Gilchrist's disease). I. A study of diseases from a review of the literature. *Arch Int Med, 82*:1, 1948.
39. Stober, A. M.: Systemic blastomycosis. *Arch Int Med, 13*:509, 1914.
40. Vandepitte, J., Gatti, F.: La Blastomycose Nord-Americaine en Afrique Son Existence en Republique de Zaire. Proc. Sec. Intern. Colloq. Med. Mycol. Prince Leopold Inst. Trop. Med. Antwerp, 1972.
41. Watson, S. H., Moore, S., Blank, F.: Generalized North American blastomycosis. *Can Med Assoc J, 78*:35, 1958.
42. Wegman, T.: Blastomykose und andere Pilzerkrankungen der lunge. *Dtsch Arch Klin Med, 199*:192, 1952.
43. Williamson, W. M., Lombard, L. S., Getty, R. E.: North American blastomycosis in a northern sea lion. *J Am Vet Med Assoc, 135*:513, 1959.
44. Wilson, J. W., Cawley, E. P., Weidman, F. D., Gilmer, W. S.: Primary cutaneous North American blastomycosis. *AMA Arch Dermatol, 71*:39, 1955.

Chapter 7

THE EPIDEMIOLOGY OF PARACOCCIDIOIDOMYCOSIS

DONALD L. GREER AND ANGELA RESTREPO

THE RECORDED HISTORY of paracoccidioidomycosis began in Brazil in 1908 with the report by Adolpho Lutz of two patients with a chronic mucocutaneous disease of unknown etiology. From these patients a slow-growing white mold was isolated. Lutz recognized that the malady was different from the mycoses that had been reported in the United States (blastomycosis) and Argentina (coccidioidomycosis), and he therefore considered the disease to be a "new pseudococcidioidic mycoses" (47). At about the same time Alfonso Splendore, working in Brazil as well, also undertook research on the agent of this disease. The two investigators clearly demonstrated that it was a dimorphic fungus, recognizing its yeast form *in vivo* and successfully growing its mold phase *in vitro*.

Despite this fruitful beginning, the history of paracoccidioidomycosis subsequently entered into a period of confusion. The importance of Lutz's and Splendore's work was not recognized at the time by other physicians, and the disease and its fungal agent remained equated with coccidioidomycosis and *Coccidioides immitis*. It was not until 1930 that the Brazilian scientist Floriano de Almeida definitively clarified the true nature of the disease and the taxonomy of its agent (3). As reported in his numerous publications, he studied the pathogenesis of the disease, succeeded in infecting animals, and determined that the fungus was a new agent, calling it *Paracoccidioides brasiliensis* (Splendore). His work stimulated others, and within a short time the distribution of the disease throughout Latin America was recognized and its diagnosis could be routinely confirmed in the laboratory.

Paracoccidioidomycosis is a progressive disease, mostly chronic, with an often fatal course if left untreated. Available data indicate that the primary lesion most frequently occurs in the lungs, with subsequent dissemination to other visceral organs. Lesions at the level of the mucosa, skin, and lymph nodes prompt patients to seek medical care, while the better-tolerated pulmonary manifestations may go unnoticed. It is difficult to determine precisely when the infection is acquired, as cases of long latency have been described. Besides the common full-blown disease, a benign self-limited infection has been documented in a few cases. Also, skin-test sensitivity indicates that a certain number of healthy individuals have had previous contact with the etiologic agent.

P. brasiliensis is a slow-growing mold which at room temperature produces a white colony with short aerial mycelia and a few microconidia. Under some conditions arthrospores and aleuriospores are also seen. In tissue or at 37 degrees C the fungus grows in the form of a spherical double-walled yeast cell and reproduces by multiple budding, exhibiting a large mother cell surrounded by small daughter cells, the classical "pilot wheel" (41).

GEOGRAPHICAL DISTRIBUTION

Paracoccidioidomycosis appears to be the only respiratory mycosis restricted to virtually a single continent. The disease is limited to Middle and South America, from Mèxico (23°N) to Argentina (34°S). However, it has not been reported in every one of the countries lying within these latitudes. The "negative" countries include Chile, Guyana, and Surinam, in South America, and El Salvador, Nicaragua, and Panama, in the Central American isthmus (52). The Caribbean islands have also been spared. Cases have been reported from countries outside the endemic area, but, as it will be discussed below, invariably the patients had at one time lived in Latin America.

Autochthonous cases have been recorded in fourteen countries

(Table 7-I) with Brazil ranking first, recording almost 4,000 cases (41, 45, 49) followed at a good distance by Venezuela (69, 76) and Colombia (32, 73). The remaining countries show smaller figures (28, 43, 64).

In all, there is a total of 5,445 published cases for the endemic area (52). A number of assumptions would indicate that it is low. In the first place, it is highly likely that not all the diagnosed cases have been reported in the literature. Moreover, some reports have undoubtedly appeared in journals of limited circulation and knowledge of them is not readily available. Finally, as the authors' own experience will testify, many cases of paracoccidioidomycosis are misdiagnosed as tuberculosis. On the other hand, some cases have been reported more than once, and this fact further prejudices the accuracy of the figures.

Paracoccidioidomycosis has been documented in countries outside the endemic area in patients who had previously resided in Latin America. While it is true that from Africa there have been reports of a presumed autochthonous patient, that is, a patient known to have never visited the recognized endemic regions, the

TABLE 7-I

DOCUMENTED AUTOCHTHONOUS CASES

Country	*No. Cases Reported*	*Year Reported*
Mexico	13	1957-1969
Guatemala	20	1968-1972
Honduras	5	1965
Costa Rica	3	1953
Colombia	561	1968-1972
Venezuela	686	1967-1969
French Guiana	1	1951
Brazil	3,771	1967-1972
Uruguay	40	1972
Paraguay	85	1965
Argentina	98	1965-1972
Peru	65	1961-1969
Ecuador	96	1971-1972
Bolivia	1	1966
Total	5,445	

data offered does not fully substantiate a diagnosis of paracoccidioidomycosis (48, 77). Of the twelve patients reported in the United States (38, 61), all but one gave histories of prolonged residence in endemic areas (Table 7-II). The exception was a Tennessee resident (27), who had lived for several years in Panama (where no cases have been recorded) and made only a short visit to Venezuela (where the disease is prevalent). The eleven patients (Table 7-III) reported from Europe, Asia, and Africa, all had lived previously in South America (7, 8, 22, 34, 37, 58, 59). Actually, in four instances the disease became manifest, although it was not always diagnosed, while the patient was still living in the endemic area.

TABLE 7-II

U. S. DOCUMENTED NON-AUTOCHTHONOUS CASES

Residence	*No. of Cases*	*Endemic Areas Visited*	*Years Between Visit to Endemic Areas and Lesions*	*Year Reported*
New York	1	Colombia Venezuela Brazil	Not Stated	1947
New York	1	Venezuela	Not Stated	1953
Oregon	1	Venezuela	3	1954
New York	1	Brazil	10	1962
Florida	1	Brazil	60	1966
California	1	Mexico	17	1968
Tennessee	1	Venezuela (Panama)	20	1969
Louisiana	1	Venezuela Costa Rica (Panama)	18	1971
New Jersey	1	Bolivia Argentina Peru	3	1972
New Jersey	1	Peru	5	1971*
Washington, D. C.	1	Ecuador	3	1973*
New York	1	Ecuador	20	1974

*Personal communication by Burgoon and Blank; Bennett (Skin and Cancer Hospital, Philadelphia; N.I.A.I.D., Bethesda, respectively).

A search of the literature has failed to disclose any recorded cases from Chile, Cuba, the Dominican Republic, El Salvador, Guyana, Haiti, Jamaica, Nicaragua, Trinidad and Tobago, or from the island of Puerto Rico (52). However, as Mackinnon has said, there is no assurance that countries which have not reported the disease to date will continue to retain their negative status in the future (52). Indeed, this assertion could probably be applied to other regions not considered endemic at the present as well.

The disease does not have an even geographical distribution within the endemic area, most cases being reported from regions within restricted climatic zones.

Among the different methods used effectively in delimiting the areas of endemicity for other mycoses, only the study of human morbidity reports have been fully investigated in paracoccidioidomycosis. The skin-test surveys conducted so far have been too modest in scope to offer any real answers. Although *P. brasiliensis* has been isolated from soil and the intestinal contents of bats (1, 15, 35, 62), these isolations have been sporadic and have not provided the real clue. As far as it is known to the authors,

TABLE 7-III

DOCUMENTED, NONAUTOCHTHONOUS CASES FROM EUROPE, ASIA, AND AFRICA

Country (City) Where Dx. Was Made	*No. of Cases*	*Endemic Areas Visited*	*Years Between Visit to Endemic Areas and Lesions*
Spain (Madrid)	1	Venezuela	10
Austria (Vienna)	1	Brazil	Not stated
Germany (Munich)	1	Peru	22
Italy (Genoa)	1	Brazil	Not stated
Italy (Naples)	1	Venezuela	3
Portugal (Coimbra)	1	Brazil	23
Portugal (unknown)	1	Brazil	37
Portugal (Coimbra)	1	Brazil	15
Republic of Bulgaria (Sofia)	1	Brazil	30
Japan (Tokyo)	1	Brazil	4
Africa (Casablanca)	1	Brazil	30
Total	11		

natural infections in animals have not been observed, although limited skin-test studies in horses (19) and cows (36) indicate that some of these animals have had previous contact with *P. brasiliensis*. Finally, there are no records of localized outbreaks.

All these factors have hindered progress in understanding the epidemiology of paracoccidioidomycosis, and the areas of endemicity have yet to be adequately pinpointed. The data available also show that paracoccidioidomycosis has a rather distinctive distribution with respect to the age, sex, and occupation of its victims.

AGE DISTRIBUTION

The disease is common in adults but rare in children. The age distribution pattern observed in different countries (Table 7-IV) shows that the proportion of cases is very small in the first ten years of life, continues to be low in the second decade, and then peaks in the following three decades. The greatest frequency is in patients between forty and fifty years of age; afterwards the curve tapers off.

The literature on paracoccidioidomycosis reveals only fifty-four cases in children under ten years of age (5, 41, 54, 80). Most were fatal disseminated cases.

TABLE 7-IV

DISTRIBUTION BY AGE IN SELECTED ENDEMIC COUNTRIES

Country	*Year Reported*	*No. of Cases*	*Ages* 0-10	11-20	21-30	31-40	41-50	51-60	61+
Brazil	1967	2,547*	45	249	458	565	690	381	159
Argentina	1965	75	0	3	6	22	22	18	4
Uruguay	1968	30	0	0	0	4	8	12	6
Venezuela	1961	62	0	2	3	12	21	15	9
Colombia	1970	101	0	4	10	28	30	20	9
	1972	39	0	0	0	9	12	13	5
Brazil	1971	130	0	4	17	39	46	18	6
	Total	2,984	45	262	494	679	829	477	198
	Percent	100	1.5	8.8	16.5	22.7	27.8	16.0	6.6

*Total number was 2,902, but in 355 cases age was not specified.

The explanation that has been offered is that youngsters have less contact with *P. brasiliensis* than older persons do. This idea probably has some validity, since the distribution of skin-test sensitivity in normal populations also tends to rise with age (71). The recognized chronic nature of the disease as well as its prolonged latency could also explain the age distribution pattern. It is still not clear, however, why adults in their third and fourth decades should be especially prone to develop this mycosis, particularly if one considers that most patients have lived in a uniform environment throughout their lives (67).

SEX DISTRIBUTION

Data from a number of authors all show that the disease affects males with a far greater frequency than females, in an average ratio of 13 to 1 (Table 7-V).

The explanation commonly offered is that men, because of their soil-related occupations, experience greater exposure to the microorganisms and are in a position to acquire the infection more often than females (40). This does not appear to be a valid explanation, however, since at the rural level, where most cases occur, women work in the fields as much as men do. Moreover, skin-test surveys (32, 71) have not revealed any significant sex

TABLE 7-V

DISTRIBUTION BY SEX IN SELECTED ENDEMIC COUNTRIES

Country	*Year Reported*	*No. of Cases*	*Sex*		*Ratio F:M*
			Female	*Male*	
Brazil	1967	2,837*	229	2,608	1:12
Argentina	1965	75	1	74	1:74
Uruguay	1968	30	0	30	—
Venezuela	1961	62	6	56	1:9
Colombia	1970	101	3	98	1:33
	1972	39	1	38	1:38
Brazil	1971	130	5	125	1:25
	Total	3,274	245	3,029	1:13
	Percent	100	7.5	92.5	

*Total number was 2,902, but in 55 patients sex was not specified.

difference in the incidence of positive reactions to paracoccidioidin. It will have to be concluded that other factors come into play.

It has been suggested that hormonal factors and phagocytic responses (65) could intervene to make the female a more resistant individual. *In vitro* estradiol and progesterone have been shown to have a certain inhibitory effect on the growth of *P. brasiliensis* (60). Also, experiments in mice have revealed a longer survival period for females. The studies along these lines, although promising, are still in the early stages and no real conclusions have yet been reached.

OCCUPATIONAL DISTRIBUTION

It was originally thought that paracoccidioidomycosis was a disease restricted to agricultural workers. Although patients with soil-related occupations still predominate, accounting for over 60 percent of the cases, reports of its occurrence in city dwellers such as clerks, industrial employees, and the like have recently been published (46, 73).

Lack of knowledge concerning the natural habitat of the fungus precludes a definitive statement. If *P. brasiliensis* could be repeatedly demonstrated as a soil microorganism, one could understand why the largest number of cases occur in agricultural workers, as well as the fact that city dwellers are also occasionally found to have the disease, since presumably they could have come in contact with the microorganism just by accident.

The authors' experience would indicate that the disease predominates in persons of low income. In a series of 140 cases, 114 patients were classified as being in the lowest of three income ranges, twenty-three corresponded to the middle bracket, and only three were in the upper category (32, 33). One wonders if malnutrition could facilitate the transition from infection to disease.

RACIAL DISTRIBUTION

Since it is difficult to precisely determine racial characteristics, especially in the case of Latin Americans, the race of the patients is not often recorded. Lacaz, in the largest series of cases that has been reported, classified 1,867 of the patients as Caucasians, 322 as yellow-skinned individuals, and 294 as Negroes or mulattoes (41). Other authors have stated that there is no real racial preference (6). It has been observed, however, that Asian and European immigrants tend to have a more serious form of the disease than persons native to the locale. A possible explanation for the phenomenon might be that lack of previous exposure to the fungus makes these individuals easy prey.

All the foregoing epidemiological characteristics could also be explained on different grounds. It has been demonstrated that although patients have normal immunoglobulin levels and proper humoral mechanisms (20) their cellular immunity appears to be impaired. It has been observed for years that a sizable percentage of patients fails to react to the paracoccidioidin skin test at the time of diagnosis. Later on, however, when the beneficial effects of treatment are apparent, most patients become positive (17). The lack of skin reactivity has recently been correlated with impairment of cellular immunity. A certain number of the patients tested not only failed to develop delayed hypersensitivity to paracoccidioidin, tuberculin, and other antigens but also lacked the capacity to become sensitized to DNCB. Furthermore, some patients exhibited a depressed response to phytohemagglutinin and at the same time were able to tolerate allografts better than normal individuals (56, 57).

If these results could be obtained in a larger number of patients, it would be possible to postulate that among infected individuals only those with impaired cellular immunity develop the classic manifestations of disease. In turn, this would subtly indicate that *P. brasiliensis* is also an opportunistic microorganism (14).

PREVALENCE AND INCIDENCE

Any tabulation to estimate the true prevalence or incidence of paracoccidioidomycosis is speculative. For lack of other sources of information, the data presented have been calculated from published reports of cases, which, for known reasons, are only a part of the total number of persons infected with the disease. Hence, it would appear, paradoxically, from the information available that the figures are lowest in those regions where the prevalence is known to be highest, since the disease is "common" in such places and only the unusual cases are published. In contrast, in areas that have only a few cases or in places outside the endemic zone, investigators tend to report every single patient. So it can be seen that the data compiled from the literature are at best only a relative gauge of the problem.

As it has been seen, Brazil alone accounts for 69 percent of the total number of cases reported. Venezuela and Colombia follow in second and third place, respectively. However, the order changes when the situation is considered from the standpoint of morbidity per 100,000 population (Table 7-VI).

Similar data among Brazil, Venezuela, and Paraguay was observed by Chirife (16) eight years earlier, even though there was an overall increase in prevalence during the intervening decade. The greatest advance over the period was reported in Colombia (32, 74). Obviously these changes must be viewed in relation to the increase in population, to the larger number of trained individuals interested in the study of the disease, and to the improvements in laboratory and clinical diagnosis.

An even bolder calculation to attempt is that of annual incidence. Fortunately, a number of investigators have reported

TABLE 7-VI

MORBIDITY PREVALENCE RATES BASED ON TOTAL REPORTED CASES OF PARACOCCIDIOIDOMYCOSIS IN SELECTED ENDEMIC COUNTRIES

Country	*Estimated Population 1972**	*Reported Cases*	*Case Rate Per 100,000*	
			1973	*1965†*
Brazil	97,800,000	3,771	3.9	2.5
Venezuela	10,800,000	686	6.4	4.9
Colombia	21,800,000	561	2.6	0.2
Argentina	24,400,000	98	0.4	0.5
Ecuador	6,300,000	96	1.5	0.7
Paraguay	2,500,000	85	3.4	4.5
Uruguay	2,900,000	40	1.4	0.7

*U.S.A.I.D., Office of Statistics and Reports. Latin American Growth Trends. 1972.

†Chirife and Del Rio (1965).

long-term studies from which a relative estimate of the number of cases occurring each year can be determined (9, 16, 39, 45, 63).

Table 7-VII summarizes the data recently reviewed by Mackinnon (52). From the information given, it is obvious that the Brazilian state of Sao Paulo is the area of highest incidence in Latin America, with an estimate of an annual rate of 0.92 per 100,000 population.

To demonstrate how the pattern of morbidity can vary within a given country, the tabulation of a series of 301 Colombian cases according to the patient's residence at the time of onset of illness is shown (Table 7-VIII). One sees, with a cursory glance, a range of from 0.1 to 4.8 cases per 100,000 inhabitants, with twelve of

TABLE 7-VII

ESTIMATED ANNUAL INCIDENCE REPORTED IN SELECTED ENDEMIC COUNTRIES

Country (State)	*Year Reported*	*Average Cases/Year*	*Incidence/ 100,000 Year*
Brazil (Sao Paulo)	1967	155	0.96
Brazil (Rio de Janiero)	1960	31	0.71
Brazil (Rio G. do Sul)	1968	—	0.10 0.40
Brazil (Rio G. do Sul)	1967	12	0.25
Argentina (Misiones)	1968 1972	2	0.45
Argentina (El Chaco)	1968 1972	5	0.80
Paraguay	1944 1972	12	0.80
Uruguay	1972	2	0.06
Colombia (Valle and Antioquia)	1973 1973	7 11	0.31 0.35

the eighteen states registering less than 1.0. It would appear that morbidity is impressively high in Antioquia and Valle; however, it should be realized that they are not only the largest states within the Colombian endemic area (71) but also the seats of the two centers where studies in medical mycology are being done on a regular basis.

As it has been said, paracoccidioidomycosis is not found in all the Latin American countries. Those countries that do report it are located within well-defined endemic zones. Still, within these zones its frequency varies remarkably. The observations that have been made on the basis of the limited material published so far are yet to be validated. An accurate account of the prevalence and incidence of this mycosis will be obtained only through the careful diagnosing and reporting of all cases that occur, both of infection and of disease. In the future precise data of this kind will be needed from all the Latin American countries if the im-

TABLE 7-VIII

MORBIDITY RATES OF PARACOCCIDIOIDOMYCOSIS IN COLOMBIA, REPORTED BY STATE

State	*Estimated Population 1971*	*No. of Cases*	*Case Rate Per 100,000*
Antioquia	3,117,600	149	4.8
Atlantico	929,900	1	0.1
Bolivar	872,800	1	0.1
Boyaca	1,225,500	2	0.2
Caldas	832,600	12	1.4
Cauca	714,800	4	0.6
Cesar	475,700	1	0.2
Choco	215,400	3	1.4
Cordoba	786,900	1	0.1
Cundinamarca	1,262,200	12	1.0
Huila	497,900	1	0.2
Guajira	255,900	1	0.4
Norte de Santander	631,600	5	0.8
Quindio	354,900	2	0.6
Risaralda	523,400	7	1.3
Santander	1,166,900	7	0.1
Tolima	928,700	2	0.2
Valle	2,172,800	90	4.1

portance of this respiratory mycosis is to be imposed upon public health officials.

INFECTION VERSUS DISEASE

In paracoccidioidomycosis the importance of subclinical infections yet remain to be determined (26). Skin-test studies conducted in selected endemic zones (17, 21, 26) have established the presence of the hypersensitive state. Table 7-IX summarizes the findings from various skin-test surveys. With the exception of the results obtained for Albornoz (2), showing that 52 percent of the population tested was positive in Venezuela, the sensitivity in general has been low. However, as Campbell has admonished, "it

TABLE 7-IX

RESULTS OF SKIN TEST SURVEYS WITH PARACOCCIDIOIDIN IN NORMAL POPULATION OF ENDEMIC AREAS

Country	*Year Reported*	*No. Tested*	*Percent Positive*	*Antigen Used*
Brazil	1951	330	7.8	MF
Argentina	1952	64	4.6	MF
Uruguay	1953	537	2.0	YF
Brazil	1953	475	4.2	MF
Brazil	1955	230	3.9	MF
Chile	1957	137	0.0	YF
Uruguay	1957	30	0.0	YF
Uruguay	1957	12	25.0	YF
Uruguay	1957	12	41.6	YF
Brazil	1958	300	8.0	MF
Brazil	1959	529	4.7	YF
Brazil	1961	372	26.0	EYC
Brazil	1961	66	20.0	EYC
Colombia	1968	3,938	9.6	EPF (Y&M)
Colombia	1968	1,659	8.3	EPF (Y&M)
Brazil	1969	136	33.0	EYC
Brazil	1969	122	20.6	EYC
Brazil	1969	81	3.7	EYC
Brazil	1970	43	11.2	YF
Venezuela	1971	686	52.0	EYC
Venezuela	1971	418	6.1	EYC
Colombia	1972	162	12.0	EPF (M)

MF = Mycelial filtrate.
YF = Yeast filtrate.
EYC = Extract of yeast cells.
EPF = Etanol-precipitated fraction.
(Y) = Yeast phase.
(M) = Mycelial phase.

is extremely important to remember that negative skin tests—regardless of how good or specific the antigen—do not always tell us that a given area is free of the fungus. They may signify that a microfocus has not yet been disturbed in that particular area" (14).

Mackinnon's group (53) was the first to suggest the existence of mild infections in paracoccidioidomycosis. Using properly standardized antigens, he demonstrated 2 percent positive reactivity in a normal population. Shortly thereafter Lacaz and his team (42) observed twenty-five positive reactions in a group of 529 healthy persons tested with paracoccidioidin. Of these, two had detectable circulating antibodies to *P. brasiliensis* and nine revealed abnormal lung X-ray pictures. On the basis of these findings the authors postulated the existence of two entities, *blastomycosis infection* and *blastomycosis disease,* the first characterizing the situation of those persons who have had contact with *P. brasiliensis* but have not developed any clinical illness and the second the clinical manifestation of the disease.

In surveys carried out by Restrepo et al. (71) in a group of 3,938 apparently normal persons, 455 reacted to paracoccidioidin, 126 of them to this antigen alone and 329 to both paracoccidioidin and histoplasmin. Even if it is accepted that there are cross-reactions between the two antigens, there is no question that the 126 persons who were reactive to paracoccidioidin alone must have had a previous infection with *P. brasiliensis.*

Recently Angulo-Ortega (4) reported two postmortem findings of residual calcified nodules containing the fungus in patients who had not exhibited any of the characteristic manifestations of paracoccidioidomycosis. Similarly, other studies (26) found fibrotic nodules in the lungs of three untreated patients who had died of other causes. Such cases, although they are rare, clearly indicate the existence of self-limited infections.

Also, the fact that patients have been diagnosed in places far from the endemic area, many years after leaving it, prove that *P. brasiliensis* must have had access to the tissues (the lungs?) but managed to remain dormant. These cases amount, in effect, to a natural experiment that demonstrates the existence of subclinical infections. Another unexplained peculiar feature is that no laboratory acquired infections have been reported in persons working with *P. brasiliensis.* Although in many ways this disease resembles the better-studied systemic mycoses, especially in its clinical aspects, it does not completely fit into the preformed picture. Why is this? Campbell (14) has commented that "it is easy to be diverted by our biases and our analogies with what we know about the habitats of other fungi. . . ." Much remains to be learned, and at present one can only accept that subclinical infections, though they are rare and difficult to demonstrate, do occur in paracoccidioidomycosis.

SOURCE OF INFECTION

The source of infection is still a matter of debate. *P. brasiliensis* is presumed to have an external habitat, one that has not yet been extensively or repeatedly demonstrated. As a result, many questions still puzzle us, for instance, the route of infection, the site of the primary lesion, and the relationship between the patient's occupation and susceptibility to the disease.

Chaves Batista and co-workers (15) reported on the isolation of *P. brasiliensis* from two soil samples from Brazil; however, the isolates were reclassified later as *Aspergillus peniciliodes* (11).

Grose and Tamsitt (35) described the isolation of the fungus from the intestinal contents of three fructivorous bats (*Artibeus lituratus*) and Negroni (62) has reported success in isolating *P. brasiliensis* from soil from the endemic area of El Chaco, Argentina.

More recently Albornoz inoculated mice with eighty-seven soil samples collected in an endemic area of Venezuela (1). Animals injected with three of these samples developed lesions in various internal organs. Tissue sections and cultures revealed the presence of *P. brasiliensis.*

At the same time, various workers have reported their failure to isolate *P. brasiliensis* from soil, plant debris, and bat guano (31, 55, 75).

It is quite possible that in searching for the natural habitat of *P. brasiliensis* one has been governed by preconceived ideas that do not apply in this case. Padilha-Goncalves (67) has suggested that the fungus in its saprophytic phase might assume a third, as yet unknown form (sexual?), which would require a totally different approach for its study.

Do animals play any role in the ecology and epidemiology of paracoccidioidomycosis? So little is known that it is unsafe to answer the question. Borelli (10, 12) has set forth an interesting hypothesis based in part on the restricted geographical distribution of the disease. He suggests that perhaps a heterothermic animal, confined to and native of the endemic area, serves as the reservoir for the fungus. Since *P. brasiliensis* does not sporulate freely in its mycelial phase, it would be unable to compete with other more prolific soil microorganisms and would therefore need a "protector" to keep it alive in the yeast phase. He believes that the protector does not fly, sail, or swim in salt water, at least not for long distances, or else otherwise it would have established itself in the Caribbean islands, which are now free of the disease. Ectoparasites feeding on this neotropical reservoir would acquire the fungus and, acting as vectors, transmit the infection to humans (12).

PORTAL OF ENTRY

How *P. brasiliensis* gains entrance into the human host is another question still unanswered. Recent reviews (29, 81) list more than eight different hypotheses accounting for the fungus' penetration into the body of man. This is an unusually large number for any single disease. It would appear that the diversity of ideas about the portal of entry stems largely from the observation of a limited number of cases, or, at times, even a single case. The theories stating that penetration occurs probably as a result of trauma in the area of the nasal mucosa, the gastrointestinal tract, the conjunctiva, the tonsils, the larynx, or the pharynx, the anoractal mucosa and perianal zone, or the teeth and gums are not supported by sufficient evidence to make a rule out of these exceptional cases.

Lutz' first publication (47), which described two patients with mucocutaneous lesions, indicated that the oral mucosa was the most likely portal of entry. This hypothesis has been perpetuated until today by various investigators (25, 41).

There is no doubt that the patient seeking medical attention most frequently is the one who has painful mucocutaneous lesions. However, it is the *pathogenesis* of a lesion and *not its frequency* that classifies it as primary or secondary. The mucosal portal of entry began to be questioned in the 1950's by investigators who noticed that in some patients the oral lesion appeared years after the pulmonary infection was first observed (30). It was also noted that the simultaneous multiple oral lesions appeared without giving rise to the expected symptoms of the primary complex (64). Primary infection through the oral or rectal mucosa can indeed occur and can be induced experimentally (44, 50); however, as a natural portal of entry this route does not fully explain the pathogenesis of the classical progressive disseminated disease.

The most natural and probable means of penetration would be by inhalation of spores, resulting in a primary lung infection which may or may not disseminate. Gonzalez-Ochoa was the first to formulate the hypothesis of inhalation as the most probable portal of entry (30). During the 1960 to 1970 decade the evidence in support of this hypothesis was strengthened, and reports of cases of primary pulmonary infections continue to increase (46, 49, 68, 73). Today such a theory is accepted by most of the workers in the field.

Disseminated cases with no mucosal lesions have also been recorded (70). Studies on the prevalence of pulmonary and oral mucosal lesions have shown that the lungs are infected with the same or greater frequency than the oral mucosa (46, 49, 63, 73). Furthermore, in several series of autopsies the lungs have been involved in virtually all the cases (6, 13, 76). In this connection, Teixeira et al. (79) observed that rats inoculated intradermally with *P. brasiliensis* developed lung lesions. However, neither parasites nor lesions were demonstrated at the site of the original inoculation.

TRANSMISSION OF INFECTION

Greer (32) in his studies of two groups of families made up of patients and controls found that the rate of infection was equal in males and females in both groups and that the prevalence of positive skin-test reactions was statistically higher in patients' families than in the controls (Table 7-X). It was also shown that the wives were three to five times more likely to acquire the infection than other adult women living in the same household. Positive reactivity among the wives was 53 percent, compared with 12 percent in the population at large in the same endemic zone of Colombia. These findings supported earlier studies by Fava-Netto and Raphael (23), who found that the patients and their wives reacted to paracoccidioidin at a similar rate. The conclusion is that the transmission of infection might have occurred from person to person. It should be mentioned that Greer was not able to demonstrate disease in any of the family members of patients.

The reports of disease within the same household are scarce (24, 66). Fourteen cases of familiar paracoccidioidomycosis were reviewed by Fava-Netto (24), ten in brothers and four in fathers and sons. The author proposed that disease might be accounted for by genetic susceptibility, a common source of infection, or interhuman transmission of infection. Genetic susceptibility could explain the discrepancy between dermal sensitivity rates and the few cases reported. Family members without the genetic trait

TABLE 7-X

PARACOCCIDIOIDIN SENSITIVITY IN RELATIVES OF PATIENTS AND CONTROL FAMILIES

	Positive Reactions			
	*Mycelial Antigen**		*Yeast Phase Antigen†*	
	Total	*Percent*	*Total*	*Percent*
Patients				
Husband	21	81	79	87
Wives	17	53	20	85
Relatives	166	19	24	50
Controls				
Husband	20	35	Not done	
Wives	27	19	Not done	
Relatives	115	6	Not done	

*Greer et al. (1974).

†C. Fava-Netto and A. Raphael (1961).

would develop only the infection, whereas those susceptible would become ill. This hypothesis would favor multiple cases in families and a high rate of disease among given ethnic groups, which have not been shown to be the case in paracoccidioidomycosis.

The most common explanation is that the infection was acquired from a common source in the environment. Since the exact habitat of *P. brasiliensis* remains obscure, one could argue that the common source is a microhabitat within the home, unrelated to the patient himself. The *common source* hypothesis would expect everyone in the household to have a positive skin-test reaction. However, Greer (32) showed that the control families living in the same environment had lower skin-test reactivity than did the relatives of patients. Moreover, only the wives of patients showed an exceptionally high sensitivity rate. These findings indicate that interhuman transmission of the infection is possible but that it is not an easy process, and that probably close and prolonged contact with an active case is required.

ECOLOGICAL CHARACTERISTICS

The information available on the exogenous habitat of *P. brasiliensis* is inadequate to permit a clear understanding of the relationship existing between the fungus and the environment.

If only the patients' residential histories are taken into consideration, it is found that most cases have been reported in the wet, forested regions of the endemic countries. However, these records must be judiciously interpreted, for often an infection has been acquired in areas far from the place of diagnosis. Thus, ". . . the memory of infection is lost and so is the spatial relationship. . . ." (12). Table 7-XI summarizes some of the climatic characteristics that predominate in a number of the endemic zones in South America.

What are the most important observed climatic conditions? Without doubt, temperature and humidity. The former ranges between extremes of 12 degrees and 28 degrees C, with a mean of 20 to 23 degrees C, and the latter between 800 and 2,000 mm a year. A third factor, altitude, does not appear to be as significant,

TABLE 7-XI

SOME CLIMATIC CONDITIONS PREVAILING IN VARIOUS OF THE ENDEMIC AREAS IN SOUTH AMERICA

Country	*Year Reported*	*Average Temperature (°C)*	*Mean Annual Rainfall (mm)*	*Altitude (m)*
Venezuela	1964	18-23	800-2,000	500-1,500
Brazil	1967	20-28	1,350-2,000	500-1,200
Brazil	1972	14-25	1,350-1,800	150- 400
Paraguay	1965	14-24	500-2,000	—*
Colombia	1968	17-24	1,000-4,000	900-2,100
Uruguay	1968	16-19	1,000-1,400	—
Argentina	1968	15-30	500-1,000	—
Venezuela	1971	23	1,400	648

*Altitude not given.

but it could also exert some influence; it ranges from 300 to 1,000 meters above sea level. Experimentally, temperature and humidity have been shown to affect the viability of *P. brasiliensis* (18, 51, 72, 78).

Although not all the complex factors that intervene to create an ecologic area must necessarily be present, it is very likely that at least some are required in order to make a satisfactory habitat for *P. brasiliensis*. It is also possible that these conditions only attain their optimum range in certain restricted localities (point-source, reservarea, microniche) strategically distributed in the endemic areas (10, 26).

All this speculation clearly shows that the relationship between the fungus and its environment is sufficiently subtle to have so far escaped detailed scientific analysis. (Or perhaps the answer to the riddle is so simple that it has been overlooked!) Until these answers are known, the chain that accidentally joins the only known host, man, to the dimorphic fungus *P. brasiliensis* will have a missing link, and the prevention of the human illness paracoccidioidomycosis, which should be a major concern to public health authorities, will remain a difficult task.

ACKNOWLEDGMENT

Sincere appreciation is expressed to Mrs. M. Vasconcellos for her kind and expert cooperation in the preparation of the manuscript.

REFERENCES

1. Albornoz, M.: Isolation of *P. brasiliensis* from rural soil in Venezuela. *Sabouraudio,* 9:248, 1971.
2. Albornoz, M. Albornoz, R.: Estudio de la sensibilidad especifica en residentes de un area endemica a la paracoccidioidomicosis en Venezuela. *Mycopath Mycol Appl, 45*:65, 1972.
3. Almeida, F. P.: Estudos comparativos do granuloma coccidioidico nos Estados Unidos e no Brasil; novo genero para o parasito brasileiro. *Ann Fac Med Sao Paulo, 5*:125, 1930.
4. Angulo-Ortega, A.: Calcifications in paracoccidioidomycosis: Are they the morphological manifestation of subclinical infections? Proc Symp Paracoccidioidomycosis. PAHO No. 254, 1972, p. 129.
5. Angulo-Ortega, A., Pollak, L.: Paracoccidioidomicosis en ninos. Communication to the VII Congreso Latinoamericano de Patologia, P. Rico, 1967.
6. Angulo-Ortega, A., Pollak, L.: Paracoccidioidomycosis. In Baker (Ed.), *Human Infections with Fungi, Actinomycetes and Algae.* Berlin, Springer-Verlag, 1970, p. 507.
7. Balabanov, K., Balabanoff, V. A., Angelov, N.: Blastomycose sud-americaine chez un laboureur bulgare revenu depuis 30 ans du Bresil. *Mycopath Mycol Appl, 24*:265, 1964.
8. Baptista, A. P., Goncalo, S.: A blastomicose sul-americana. *Trab Soc Port Dermatol, 29*:117, 1971.
9. Bopp, C., Bernardi, C. D.: Geopatologia da blastomicose sulamericana no Rio Grande do Sul. *Hospital (Rio), 71*:1613, 1967.
10. Borelli, D.: Hipotesis sobre ecologia de Paracoccidioides. *Dermatol Venez, 3*:130, 1963.
11. Borelli, D.: Lobomicosis; nomenclatura de su agente. *Med Cut, 2*:151, 1968.
12. Borelli, D.: Algunos aspectos ecologicos de la paracoccidioidomicosis. *Dermatol Venez, 13*:1190, 1971.
13. Brass, K.: Observacion sobre la anatomia patologica, patogenesis y evolucion de la paracoccidioidomicosis. *Mycopath Mycol Appl, 37*:119, 1969.
14. Campbell, C. C.: The "pilot wheel"; a change in course. Proc. Symp. Paracoccidioidomycosis, PAHO No. 254, 1972, p. 306.
15. Chaves-Batista, A., Shome, S. K., Santos, F. M.: Pathogenicity of *P. brasiliensis* isolated from soil. *Pub Inst Micol Recife, 373*:3, 1962.
16. Chirife, A. V., Del Rio, C. A.: Geopatologia de la blastomicosis sud-americana. *Prensa Med Argent, 52*:54, 1965.
17. Conti-Diaz, I. A.: Skin tests with paracoccidioidin and their importance. Proc. Symp. Paracoccidioidomycosis, PAHO No. 254, 1972, p. 197.
18. Conti-Diaz, I. A., Mackinnon, J. E., Furcolow, M. L.: Effect of drying on *P. brasiliensis. Sabouraudia,* 9:69, 1971.

19. Conti-Diaz, I. A., Alvarez, B. J., Gezuele, E., Gonzalez-Marini, H., Duarte, J., Falcon, J.: Encuesta mediante intradermorreacciones con paracoccidioidina e histoplasmina en caballos. *Rev Inst Med Trop Sao Paulo, 14*:372, 1972.
20. Correa, A., Giraldo, R.: Study of immune mechanisms in paracoccidioidomycosis. I. Changes in immunoglobulins (IgG, IgM, and IgA). Proc. Symp. Paracoccidioidomycosis, PAHO No. 254, 1972, p. 245.
21. Farinas, L. N., Hospedales, A., Torres, E., Villarroel, J.: Estudio de la sensibilidad cutanea a la paracoccidioidina en poblacion estudiantil de Caripe y sus alrededores. *Dermatol Venez, 11*:329, 1972.
22. Farris, C.: Contributo personal alla conoscenza della paracoccidioidosis (cosi-detta "blastomicosis brasiliana"). *Gior Ital Dermatol, 96*:321, 1955.
23. Fava-Netto, C., Raphael, A.: A reacao intradermica com polissacaride do *P. brasiliensis* na blastomicose sulamericana. *Rev Inst Med Trop Sao Paulo, 3*:161, 1961.
24. Fava-Netto, C., Martins-Castro, R., Padilha-Goncalves, A., Dillon, N. L.: Ocorrencia familiar da blastomicose sulamericana; a proposito de 14 casos. *Rev Inst Med Trop Sao Paulo, 7*:332, 1965.
25. Furtado, T.: Mechanism of infection in South American blastomycosis. *Dermatol Trop, 2*:27, 1963.
26. Furtado, T.: Infection vs. disease in paracoccidioidomycosis. In Proc. Symp. Paracoccidioidomycosis, PAHO No. 254, 1972, p. 271.
27. Fountain, F. F., Sutliff, W. D.: Paracoccidioidomycosis in the United States, *Am Rev Respir Dis. 99*:89, 1969.
28. Gonzalez-Ochoa, A.: Las micosis pulmonares en Mexico y Centroamerica; aspectos epidemiologicos. *Rev Invest Salud Publica, 29*: 179, 1969.
29. Gonzalez-Ochoa, A.: Theories regarding the portal of entry of *P. brasiliensis*. In Proc. Symp. Paracoccidioidomycosis, PAHO No. 254, 1972, p. 278.
30. Gonzalez-Ochoa, A., Dominguez-Soto, L.: Blastomicosis sudamericana; casos Mexicanos. *Rev Inst Salubr Enfer Trop* (Mexico), *17*:97, 1957.
31. Greer, D. L.: Unpublished data.
32. Greer, D. L., Estrada, D., Trejos, L.: Dermal sensitivity to paracoccidioidin and histoplasmin in family members of patients with paracoccidioidomycosis. *Am J Trop Med Hyg, 23*:87, 1974.
33. Greer, D. L., Restrepo, A.: Unpublished data.
34. Gotz, H.: Klinische und experimentelle Studies uber das Granuloma Paracoccidioides (Morbus Lutz-Splendore de Almeida) *Arch Dermatal Syph, 198*:508, 1954.
35. Grose, E., Tamsitt, J. R.: *P. brasiliensis* recovered from the intestinal tract of three bats *(A. lituratus)* in Colombia, S. A. *Sabouraudia, 4*:124, 1965.

36. Gutierrez, A., Ceballos, G., Ferrer, H. I., Rangel, O.: Encuesta sobre tuberculosis, histoplasmosis y paracoccidioidocicosis en ganado lechero del Valle de Aburra. *Antioquia Med, 24*:339, 1974.
37. Koya, G.: An autopsy case of mixed infection of *L. donovani* and *Blastomyces brasiliensis,* with emphasis on the histopathogenesis of reticuloendotheliosis. *Acta Pathol Jap, 14*:223, 1964.
38. Kroll, J. J., Walzer, R. A.: Paracoccidioidomycosis in the United States. *Arch Dermatol, 106*:543, 1972.
39. Lacaz, C. S.: South American blastomycosis. *Ann Fac Med Sao Paulo, 29*:9, 1956.
40. Lacaz, C. S.: Aspectos clinicos e epidemiologicos das micoses profundas na America do Sul. *Rev Inst Med Trop Sao Paulo, 1*:150, 1959.
41. Lacaz, C. S.: Compendio de Micologia Medica. Sao Paulo, Edit. Univ. Sao Paulo, 1967.
42. Lacaz, C. S.: Passos-Filho, M. C. R., Fava-Netto, C., Macaroon, B.: Contribuicao para o estudo de "blastomicose-infeccao"; inquerito com a paracoccidioidina; estudo serologico e clinico-radiologico dos paracoccidioidina-positivos. *Rev Inst Med Trop Sao Paulo, 1*:245, 1959.
43. Leon, L. A.: La paracoccidioidomicosis tegumentaria en el Ecuador. *Dermatol Venez, 13*:1225, 1971.
44. Linares, L., Friedman, L.: Experimental paracoccidioidomycosis in mice. *Infect Immunol, 5*:681, 1972.
45. Londero, A. T.: Aspectos de la blastomicose sudamericana en Rio Grande do Sul, Brasil. *Torax, 17*:56, 1968.
46. Londero, A. T.: Paracoccidioidomycosis; a clinical and mycological study of 41 cases observed in Santa Maria, R. S. Brazil. *Am J Med, 52*:771, 1972.
47. Lutz, A.: Uma mycose pseudo-coccidioidica localizada na boca e observada no Brasil; contribuicao ao conhecimento das hyphoblastocoses americanas. *Brasil Med, 22*:121, 1908.
48. Lythcott, C. I., Edgcomb, J. H.: The occurrence of South American blastomycosis in Accra, Ghana. *Lancet, 1*:916, 1964.
49. Machado-Filho, J., Miranda, J. L.: Consideracoes relativas a blastomicose sulamericana; evolucao, resultados terapeuticos e molestias associadas em 394 casos. *Hospital (Rio), 60*:375, 1961.
50. Mackinnon, J. E.: Blastomicose sudamericana experimental evolutiva por via pulmonar. *Ann Fac Med Montevideo, 44*:355, 1959.
51. Mackinnon, J. E.: The effect of temperature on the deep mycoses. In Wolstenholme, G. E. W. and Porter, R. (Eds.): *Systemic Mycoses.* London, J. & A. Churchill, 1968, p. 164.
52. Mackinnon, J. E.: Geographical distribution and prevalence of paracoccidioidomycosis. Proc. Symp. Paracoccidioidomycosis, PAHO No. 254, 1972, p. 45.

53. Mackinnon, J. E., Artagaveytia-Allende, R. C., Arroyo, L.: Sobre la especificidad de la intradermorreaccion con paracoccidioidina. *An Fac Med Montevideo, 38*:363, 1953.
54. Marcano, H., Hernandez, R. S., Cabrera, C.: Paracoccidiosis brasiliensis infantil de evolucion poco comun. *Rev Tisiol Neumol (Caracas), 5*:87, 1963.
55. Mendelovici, M., Salfelder, K., Mendelovici, E., Roman, A. R. de: Intento de aislamiento del *P. brasiliensis* del suelo. *Mycopath Mycol Appl, 52*:65, 1974.
56. Mendez, E., Raphael, A.: Impaired delayed hypersensitivity in patients with South American blastomycosis. *J Allergy Clin Immunol, 47*: 17, 1971.
57. Mendes, N. F., Musatti, C. C., Leao, C., Mendes, E., Naspitz, C. K.: Lymphocyte cultures and skin allograft survival in patients with South American blastomycosis. *J Allergy Clin Immunol, 48*:40, 1970.
58. Merchan, S. A., Escudero, R., Lavin, R.: Un caso de blastomicosis sudamericana observada en Espana. *Med Cut, 5*:631, 1970.
59. Molese, A., Pane, A., Vingiani, A., Pagano, A.: Su di un caso di granulomatosi paracoccidiodea (malatti di Lutz-Splendore-de Almeida). *Rifor Med, 70*:1009, 1956.
60. Muchmore, H. G., McKown, B. A., Mohr, J. A.: Effect of steroid hormones on the growth of *P. brasiliensis.* Proc. Symp. Paracoccidiodomycosis, PAHO No. 254, 1972, p. 300.
61. Murray, H. W., Littman, M. L., Roberts, R. B.: Disseminated paracoccidioidomycosis (South American Blastomycosis) in the United States. *Am J Med, 56*:209, 1974.
62. Negroni, P.: Estudios sobre la ecologia del *P. brasiliensis* en la Argentina. *Torax, 17*:60, 1968.
63. Negroni, R.: Las micosis broncopulmonares en la Republica Argentina. *Torax, 19*:67, 1970.
64. Negroni, P., Negroni, R.: Aspectos clinicos e inmunologicos de la blastomicosis sudamericana en la Argentina. *Torax, 17*:63, 1968.
65. Nicol, T., Vernon-Roberts, B., Quantock, D. C.: The influence of various hormones on the reticuloendothelial system; endocrine control of body defense. *J Endocrinol, 33*:365, 1965.
66. Padilha-Goncalves, A.: *Adenopatia da Micose de Lutz.* Dissertation for full professorship, Univ. Rio de Janeiro, Rio Copicentro, 1971.
67. Padilha-Goncalves, A.: Epidemiological factors in paracoccidioidomycosis. Proc. Symp. Paracoccidioidomycosis, PAHO No. 254, 1972, p. 53.
68. Passos-Filho, M. C. R.: Blastomicose sul-americana; comentarios em torno de 83 casos de localizacao pulmonar; classificacao radiologica. *Hospital (Rio), 70*:109, 1966.

69. Pollak, L., Angulo-Ortega, A.: Las micosis broncopulmonares en Venezuela. *Torax, 16*:135, 1967.
70. Porto, J. A., Rodrigues, J. S.: Micose de Lutz. *J Brasil Med, 6*:192, 1962.
71. Restrepo, A., Robledo, M., Ospina, S., Restrepo, M., Correa, A.: Distribution of paracoccidioidin sensitivity in Colombia. *A. J Trop Med Hyg, 17*:25, 1968.
72. Restrepo, A., Moncada, L. H., Quintero, M.: Effect of hydrogenion concentration and of temperature on the growth of *P. brasiliensis* in soil extracts. *Sabouraudia, 7*:207, 1969.
73. Restrepo, A., Robledo, M., Gutierrez, F., Sanclemente, M., Castaneda, E., Calle, G.: Paracoccidioidomycosis (South American blastomycosis); a study of thirty-nine cases observed in Medellin, Colombia. *Am J Trop Med Hyg, 19*:68, 1970.
74. Restrepo, A., Greer, D. L., Moncada, L. H.: Relationship between the environment and paracoccidioidomycosis. Proc. Symp. Paracoccidioidomycosis, PAHO No. 254, 1972, p. 84.
75. Rogers, A. L., Beneke, E. S.: Human pathogenic fungi recovered from Brazilian soil. *Mycopath Mycol Appl, 22*:15, 1964.
76. Salfelder, K., Doehnert, G., Doehnert, H. R.: Paracoccidioidomycosis; anatomic study with complete autopsies. *Virchows Arch Pathol Anat, 348*:51, 1969.
77. Salles, C. A., *Blastomyces (Paracoccidioides) brasiliensis* in Africa. *Nature, 204*:1211, 1964.
78. Tesh, R. B., Schneidau, J. D., Erwin, C. A.: Effect of freezing and storage at 24°C on the survival of pathogenic fungi in excised tissue. *Am J Clin Pathol, 48*:100, 1967.
79. Teixeira, G. A., Machado-Filho, J., Lisboa-Miranda, J.: Blastomicose sul-americana experimental; estudo em ratos, com consideracoes relativas a patogenia das lesoes. *Hospital (Rio), 68*:1081, 1965.
80. Urdaneta, E., Belfort, E.: Micosis sistemicas en el nino. II. Paracoccidioidomicosis. *Arch Venez Puericult Pediatr, 29*:390, 1966.
81. Yarzabal, L. A.: Pathogenesis of paracoccidioidomycosis in man. Proc. Symp. Paracoccidioidomycosis, PAHO No. 254, 1972, p. 261.

Chapter 8

THE EPIDEMIOLOGY OF CRYPTOCOCCOSIS

MORRIS A. GORDON

CRYPTOCOCCOSIS IS THE TERM applied to any human or animal disease attributable to the yeast-like fungus *Cryptococcus neoformans* (Sanfelice) Vuillemin, 1901. Cryptococcosis is synonymous with torulosis, European blastomycosis, and Busse-Buschke's disease. Synonyms for *C. neoformans* include *C. hominis* Vuillemin, 1901, and *Torula histolytica* Stoddard and Cutler, 1916. Cryptococcal infection comes to medical attention most frequently as a meningitis or cerebral abscess, accompanied by the appearance in cerebrospinal fluid of spherical to subspherical, usually single-budding, yeast-like cells with a thick, gelatinous capsule. However, the fungus enters the body almost exclusively through the respiratory tract, and primary pulmonary cryptococcosis is not uncommon, although lesions are often inapparent or found with difficulty. Frank pulmonary cryptococcosis may take the form of a cryptococcoma, in which the cryptococci are walled off and generally not expelled in sputum, or a more diffuse involvement of one or both lungs. There have been a number of reports of solitary cutaneous or subcutaneous cryptococcal nodules without evidence of involvement of any other part of the body, and also of disseminated cryptococcosis in which bones or internal organs have been involved.

The human population at risk of cryptococcosis is a specialized one in that the majority of cases occur in compromised hosts, most prominently those suffering from lymphomas, particularly

Hodgkin's disease, or less frequently leukemias. Dissemination of cryptococcosis within the body is also promoted by steroid therapy and other immunosuppressive measures, and this raises the question of whether some cases may be of endogenous origin. However, many cases of cryptococcal meningitis occur in apparently normal, healthy young adults with no known immunodeficiency. Possibly these individuals have been exposed to overwhelming dosages of cryptococcal cells.

Although there are well-established reservoirs of *C. neoformans* in nature, particularly pigeon droppings and soil contaminated with these or other organic materials, few case histories reveal the proximate source of the cryptococcal cells presumed to have been inhaled by the patient.

Contagion

Cryptococcosis in any of its manifestations must be considered a nontransmissible disease. There has been no authenticated report of its transfer from person to person, from animal to person, or between animals, although viable cryptococci may be excreted in sputum, urine, exudates of lesions, and in cow's milk.

Opportunism: The Special Risk

The epidemiology of cryptococcosis must be understood in terms of the ubiquitousness of the incitant microorganism (with consequent frequent exposure of a large proportion of the population), the comparatively small number of clinical cases, and the fact that the majority of these cases occur in compromised hosts. These facts, together with the occurrence of healed pulmonary cryptococcal lesions discovered inadvertently, indicate that most people have a strong innate resistance to cryptococcal infection. The available evidence indicates that the defenses are predominantly cellular (21, 25, 32, 34). Several investigators (3, 53) have demonstrated anticryptococcal factors in normal human serum, but these seem to play little if any role in protective immunity. Most frequently cited predisposing factors to human cryptococcosis are diseases in which the cellular immune defenses are compromised, especially Hodgkin's disease, other lymphomas, and leukemia (29, 33). Sera from patients with such diseases are reported to have a lower than normal inhibitory effect on *C. neoformans* (20). Further evidence of the primacy of cellular immunity is given in reports of nonspecific resistance to cryptococcosis conferred by activated macrophages in bacterial and protozoal infections (21) and of predisposal to cryptococcosis in patients on long-term steroid therapy (7).

Cryptococcosis has been found in patients of all ages, but approximately two-thirds of the victims are males between thirty and fifty years old (32).

Occurrence and Distribution

Cryptococcosis is the most widespread and geographically indiscriminate of the systemic mycoses. Although it is by far the most common deep-seated fungal disease of man in Europe, the term European blastomycosis once applied to it is a misnomer, since numerous cases have been reported from every continent (43). It occurs most frequently in the United States of America and secondly in Australia, but there has been no particular concentration of cases except in microenvironments, and no highly endemic areas are known. *C. neoformans* is practically ubiquitous in man's environment. There are particularly numerous reports of its isolation from soils, especially those contaminated with bird manure, but it is abundant only in pigeon droppings and in soils containing this material (19, 47, 49). Curiously, it was first identified as an isolate from peach juice (44), and it has been found in such substrates as plant exudate (16) and cow's milk (10). In our experience, searches for *Histoplasma capsulatum* in sites associated with outbreaks of histoplasmosis have turned up more isolates of *C. neoformans* than of *H. capsulatum* (24). Emmons, who was the first to discover *C. neoformans* in pigeon nests and droppings (13), has recovered the organism also from window ledges on which pigeons have roosted (14).

C. neoformans probably does not occur normally on the skin or in the intestinal tract of man, although closely related avirulent species have been recovered from such habitats (4, 18, 41). There is, however, a suggestion that *C. neoformans* may be a transient colonizer of the pulmonary tract (22). Support for this is the occurrence, in asymptomatic cases, of subpleural pulmonary granulomas and other healing pulmonary foci which ordinarily are overlooked (28, 56). Skin tests have not been helpful in determining carrier states, since reliable reagents for this purpose are not yet available (2, 6, 37, 46). In one survey (38) reactions to cryptococcin occurred in a high percentage of pigeon breeders, but no correlation has been reported between skin sensitivity and pulmonary lesions. A leukocyte migration-inhibition test (35) may prove useful in detecting delayed hypersensitivity as a possible indicator of exposure to *C. neoformans.*

Highly reliable serologic tests are available for diagnosis and prognosis of active cryptococcosis (23), and there is suggestive evidence that serology may be useful in detection of past infection (58, 59).

Occurrence in Lower Animals

Overt cryptococcosis has been reported in a number of mammalian species, both feral and domestic (62). Naturally occurring cryptococcosis of pigeons or other birds is unknown, although infection has been established in pigeons, with difficulty, via unusual modes of inoculation (31, 48). Epizootics of bovine mastitis have provided the greatest number of cases (40, 45, 50), with infection occurring via the teat canals from contaminated milking machines or by injection of contaminated antibiotics. Cryptococcal mastitis has also occurred in sheep (1). There was no contagion to persons who handled the infected cattle or their products nor to consumers of milk from these animals. This is partially attributable to the fact that *C. neoformans* is killed by standard milk pasteurization methods (40, 50).

With cryptococcosis in the cat, of which numerous cases have been reported (also in the dog and horse), lesions have occurred mainly in the facial region, especially about the nose and palate. In other instances there has been pulmonary involvement without external lesions. Bats have been found to harbor *C. neoformans* (26), but no animal is known to be a reservoir of infection.

Source of Infection

There are remarkably few reported cases of cryptococcosis for which a source of infection has been indicated. However, the widespread occurrence of *C. neoformans* in soil and dusty areas frequented by pigeons or sometimes other birds, its abundance in pigeon droppings, and the compelling evidence that the respiratory tract is the almost exclusive portal of entry of this microorganism in man strongly suggest that avian habitats, especially those of pigeons, are the prime source of human infection, as argued by Littman and Borok (30). If this is the case, pigeons cannot be considered as vectors or even disseminators of the disease, but simply as preparers of the environment for proliferation of the microorganism. *C. neoformans* remains viable in desiccated pigeon droppings for long periods of time, and there are now a number of reports offering highly suggestive evidence that the disease was initiated through inhalation of dried pigeon excreta (32, 36). Yamamoto (63) demonstrated this association in a case of pulmonary cryptococcosis in a cat which had frequented pigeon habitats, and *C. neoformans* has been isolated from the air in a pigeon loft (51).

Utilizing a serologic technique combining immunofluorescence and complement fixation, Walter and Atchison (59) demonstrated cryptococcal antibodies in 22 percent of 134 pigeon breeders, as compared with 3 percent of thirty-six non-pigeon breeders. Emmons (15) has suggested that certain epidemics of pneumonitis associated with pigeon manure, although presumed to have been due to histoplasmosis, may have been caused by *C. neoformans*. There is evidence (17) that the cryptococcal capsule exists in an attenuated form in soil and that this form is more infectious for the human host than is the fully encapsulated cell.

It has been thought that in some cases cryptococcal infection might be endogenous (33, 43), but although encapsulated cryptococci have been recovered in large numbers and on several occasions from the normal human skin and intestinal tract, these have generally been shown to be avirulent or relatively so (4, 5, 18, 41, 64). So-called *C. neoformans* var. *innocuous* (33) should be considered separate species, since they are not only avirulent but differ from *C. neoformans* in biochemistry and in temperature relationships; we have identified some of these strains as *C. albidus* and *C. diffluens*. *C. neoformans* is often cultured from urine (but not from feces) in disseminated cases, but there is no evidence that urine is a source of contagion. Likewise, no conclusive evidence for neonatal cryptococcosis has been presented.

There have been no epidemics of human cryptococcosis, and the only epizootics known were common source infections resulting in bovine mastitis, as noted above.

Portal of Entry

The portal of entry of almost all cases of cryptococcosis is generally agreed to be the respiratory tract. Much of the evidence is given above. Focal cryptococcal lesions found in the lungs and pleura of patients with cryptococcal meningitis (28, 56) support this concept, as do the incidental finding in noncryptococcal patients of solitary pulmonary nodules (28, 52), and the demonstration that *C. neoformans* may exist in the pulmonary tract as a temporary colonizer (57, 60). Primary pulmonary cryptococcosis is not uncommon, and in some cases the infection has evolved into meningitis (9, 27, 55).

Most cases of cutaneous cryptococcosis undoubtedly proceed by hematogenous spread from pulmonary lesions. In a study of 110 patients with cryptococcal meningitis (11), thirteen had lesions of the skin. Apparent primary cutaneous cryptococcosis has also been reported (8, 42), but in many of these cases there may have been a "silent" primary focus elsewhere. An analogous situation exists in the phenomenon of apparently solitary bone lesions (39).

There is suggestive evidence that the nasopharynx may act as a portal of entry for cryptococcosis (12). Cryptococcal meningitis and pulmonary disease have been produced experimentally in Marmoset monkeys through oral ingestion of live cryptococci (54), but other feeding experiments have failed to produce infection (40, 47).

Laboratory Infections

In a recent review (61), there were no reported laboratory-acquired human infections with *C. neoformans.* This is in sharp contrast to the 108 cases of coccidioidomycosis, eighty-one cases of histoplasmosis, and eight cases of blastomycosis so reported.

REFERENCES

1. Abdallah, I. S.: Study of sheep mastitis as caused by *Cryptococcus neoformans* in Egypt. *Vet Med J Giza, 16*:203, 1969.
2. Atkinson, A. J., Jr., Bennett, J. E.: Experience with a new skin test antigen prepared from *Cryptococcus neoformans. Am Rev Resp Dis, 97*:637, 1968.
3. Baum, G. L., Artis, D.: Characterization of the growth inhibition factor for *Cryptococcus neoformans* in human serum. *Am J Med Sci, 246*: 53, 1963.
4. Benham, R. W.: Cryptococci—their identification by morphology and by serology. *J Infect Dis, 57*:255, 1935.
5. Benham, R. W., Hopkins, A. M.: Yeastlike fungi found on the skin and in the intestines of normal subjects; a survey of one hundred persons. *Arch Dermatol Syph (Chicago), 28*:532, 1933.
6. Bennett, J. E., Hasenclever, H. F., Baum, G. L.: Evaluation of a skin test for cryptococcosis. *Am Rev Resp Dis, 91*:616, 1965.
7. Bennington, J. L., Haber, S. L., Morgenstern, N. L.: Increased susceptibility to cryptococcosis following steroid therapy. *Dis Chest, 45*:262, 1964.
8. Brier, R. L., Coleman, M., Stone, J.: Cutaneous cryptococcosis. Presentation of a case and a review of previously reported cases. *Arch Dermatol, 75*:262, 1957.
9. Campbell, G. D.: Primary pulmonary cryptococcosis. *Am Rev Resp Dis, 94*:236, 1966.
10. Carter, H. S., Young, J. L.: Note on the isolation of *Cryptococcus neoformans* from a sample of milk. *J Pathol Bact, 62*:271, 1950.
11. Cawley, E. P., Grekin, R. H., Curtis, A. C.: Torulosis. A review of the cutaneous and adjoining mucous membrane manifestations. *J Invest Derm, 14*:327, 1950.
12. Cox, L. B., Tolhurst, J. C.: *Human Torulosis*. A clinical, pathological and microbiological study with a report of thirteen cases. Melbourne: Melbourne Univ. Press, 1946.
13. Emmons, C. W.: Saprophytic sources of *Cryptococcus neoformans* associated with the pigeon (*Columba livia*). *Am J Hyg, 62*:227, 1955.
14. Emmons, C. W.: Prevalence of *Cryptococcus neoformans* in pigeon habitats. *Publ Hlth Rep (Washington), 75*:362, 1960.
15. Emmons, C. W., Binford, C. H., Utz, J. P.: *Medical Mycology*, 2nd ed. Philadelphia, Lea & Febiger, 1970.
16. Evenson, A. E., Lamb, J. W.: Slime flux of mesquite as a new saprophytic source of *Cryptococcus neoformans. J. Bact, 88*:542, 1964.
17. Farhi, F., Bulmer, G. S., Tacker, J. R.: *Cryptococcus neoformans* IV. The not-so-encapsulated yeast. *Infect Immun, 1*:526, 1970.

18. Felsenfeld, O.: Yeast-like fungi in the intestinal tract of chronically institutionalized patients. *Am J Med Sci, 207*:60, 1944.
19. Frey, D., Durie, E. B.: The isolation of *Cryptococcus neoformans (Torula histolytica)* from soil in New Guinea and pigeon droppings in Sydney, New South Wales. *Med J Aust, 25*:947, 1964.
20. Gadebusch, H. H.: Anticryptococcal serum factors in malignant reticuloendothelioses in man. 1965. *Antimicrob Ag Chemother*—1964, p. 640.
21. Gentry, L. O., Remington, J. S.: Resistance against Cryptococcus conferred by intracellular bacteria and protozoa. *J Infect Dis, 123*:22, 1971.
22. Gordon, M. A., Buckley, H. R.: When is the *Cryptococcus* dangerous? *Lancet, 2*:1162, 1969.
23. Gordon, M. A., Vedder, D. K.: Serologic tests in diagnosis and prognosis of cryptococcosis. *JAMA, 197*:961, 1966.
24. Gordon, M. A., Ziment, I.: Epidemic of acute histoplasmosis in western New York State. *N Y State J Med, 67*:235, 1967.
25. Goren, M. B.: Experimental murine cryptococcosis: Effect of hyperimmunization to capsular polysaccharide. *J Immunol, 98*:914, 1967.
26. Grose, E., Marinkelle, C. J., Striegel, C.: The use of tissue cultures in the identification of *Cryptococcus neoformans* isolated from Colombian bats. *Sabouraudia, 6*:127, 1968.
27. Hatcher, C. R., Jr., Sehdeva, J., Waters, W. C., III, Schulze, V., Logan, W. D., Jr., Symbas, P., Abbott, O. A.: Primary pulmonary cryptococcosis. *J Thorac Cardiovasc Surg, 61*:39, 1971.
28. Haugen, R. K., Baker, R. D.: The pulmonary lesions in cryptococcosis with special reference to subpleural nodes. *Am J Clin Pathol, 24*:1381, 1954.
29. Hutter, R. V. P., Collins, H. S.: The occurrence of opportunistic fungus infections in a cancer hospital. *Lab Invest, 11*:1035, 1962.
30. Littman, M. L., Borok, R.: Relation of the pigeon to cryptococcosis: Natural carrier state, heat resistance and survival of *Cryptococcus neoformans. Mycopath Mycol Appl, 35*:329, 1968.
31. Littman, M. L., Borok, R., Dalton, T. J.: Experimental avian cryptococcosis. *Am J Epidem, 82*:197, 1965.
32. Littman, M. L., Walter, J. E.: Cryptococcosis: Current status. *Am J Med, 45*:922, 1968.
33. Littman, M. L., Zimmermann, L. E.: *Cryptococcosis, Torulosis or European Blastomycosis*. N. Y. and London: Grune & Stratton. 1956.
34. Louria, D. B., Kaminski, T., Finkel, G.: Further studies on immunity in experimental cryptococcosis. *J Exp Med, 117*:509, 1963.
35. Mohr, J. A., Muchmore, H. G., Felton, F. G., Rhoades, E. R., McKown, B. A.: The effect of cryptococcin on leukocytic migration. *Infect Dis, 122*:454, 1970.

36. Muchmore, H. G., Rhoades, E. R., Nix, G. E., Felton, F. G., Carpenter, R. E.: Occurrence of *Cryptococcus neoformans* in the environment of three geographically associated cases of cryptococcal meningitis. *N Engl J Med, 268*:1112, 1963.
37. Muchmore, H. G., Felton, F. G., Salvin, S. B., Rhoades, E. R.: Delayed hypersensitivity to cryptococcin in man. *Sabouraudia, 6*:285, 1968.
38. Newberry, W. M., Jr., Walter, J. E., Chandler, J. W., Jr., Tosh, F. E.: Epidemiologic study of *Cryptococcus neoformans. Ann Int Med, 67*:724, 1967.
39. Ong, T. H., Parthap, K.: Localized osseous involvement in cryptococcosis: Case report and review of the literature. *Aust N Z J Surg, 40*:186, 1970.
40. Pounden, W. D., Amberson, J. M., Jaeger, R. F.: A severe mastitis problem associated with *Cryptococcus neoformans* in a large dairy herd. *Am J Vet Res, 13*:121, 1952.
41. Ravits, H. G.: Cutaneous cryptococcosis. A survey of cryptococcus on normal and pathologic skin. *J Invest Derm, 12*:271, 1949.
42. Ruiter, M., Ensink, G. J.: Acute primary cutaneous cryptococcosis. *Dermatologica (Basel), 128*:185, 1964.
43. Salfelder, K., Schwarz, J., Romero, A., de Liscano, T. R., Zambrano, P., Z., Diaz, P., I.: Habitat de *Nocardia asteroides, Phialophora pedrosoi* y *Cryptococcus neoformans* en Venezuela. *Mycopathol (Den Haag), 34*:144, 1968.
44. Sanfelice, F.: Contributo alla morfologia e biologia dei blastomichetiche si sviluppano nei succhi di alcuna frutti. *Ann d'Ig, 4*:463, 1894.
45. Scholer, H. J., Schneider, P. A., Bertschinger, H. U.: Nachweis von *Cryptococcus neformans* und anderen Hefen aus Milch von Kuhen mit Mastitis. *Pathol Microbiol (Basel), 24*:803, 1961.
46. Seeliger, H. P. R:. Use of serological methods for the diagnosis of cryptococcosis. A review. *Ann Soc Belge Med Trop, 44*:657, 1964.
47. Sethi, K. K.: Pigeons and mycoses. *N Engl J Med, 276*:62, 1967.
48. Sethi, K. K., Schwarz, J.: Experimental ocular cryptococcosis in pigeons. *Am J Ophthal, 62*:95, 1966.
49. Silva, M. E., Paula, L. A.: Isolation of *Cryptococcus neoformans* from excrement and nests of pigeons (*Columbia livia*) in Salvador, Bahia (Brasil). *Rev Inst Med Trop S Paulo, 5*:9, 1963.
50. Simon, J., Nicholas, R. E., Morse, E. V.: An outbreak of bovine cryptococcosis. *J Am Vet Med Assoc, 122*:31, 1953.
51. Staib, F., Bethauser, G.: Zum Nachweis von *Cryptococcus neoformans* im Staub von einem Taubenschlag. *Mykosen. 11*:619, 1968.
52. Steele, J. D.: The solitary pulmonary nodule. Report of a cooperative study of resected asymptomatic solitary pulmonary nodules in males. *J Thorac Cardiovasc Surg, 46*:21, 1963.

53. Szilagyi, G., Reiss, F., Smith, J. C.: The anti-cryptococcal factor of blood serum. A preliminary report. *J Invest Derm, 46*:306, 1966.
54. Takos, M. J., Experimental cryptococcosis produced by the ingestion of virulent organisms. *N Engl J Med, 254*:598, 1956.
55. Taylor, E. R.: Pulmonary cryptococcosis. Analysis of fifteen cases from the Columbia area. *Ann Thorac Surg, 10*:309, 1970.
56. Terplan, K.: Pathogenesis of cryptococcic (Torula) meningitis. *Am J Pathol, 24*:711, 1948.
57. Tynes, B., Mason, K. N., Jennings, A. E., Bennett, J. E.: Variant forms of pulmonary cryptococcosis. *Ann Intern Med, 69*:1117, 1968.
58. Vogel, R. A.: The indirect fluorescent antibody test for the detection of antibody in human cryptococcal disease. *J Infect Dis, 116*:573, 1966.
59. Walter, J. E., Atchison, R. W.: Epidemiological and immunological studies of *Cryptococcus neoformans*. *J Bact,* 92:82, 1966.
60. Warr, W., Bates, J. H., Stone, A.: The spectrum of pulmonary cryptococcosis. *Ann Intern Med, 69*:1109, 1968.
61. Wedum, A. G., Kruse, R. H.: Assessment of risk of human infection in the microbiological laboratory (2nd ed.). Miscellaneous publication No. 30 Department of the Army, 1969.
62. Weitzman, I., Bonaparte, P., Guevin, V., Crist, M.: Cryptococcosis in a field mouse. *Sabouraudia, 11*:77, 1973.
63. Yamamoto, S., Ishida, K., Sato, A.: Isolation of *Cryptococcus neoformans* from pulmonary granuloma of a cat and from pigeon droppings. *Jap J Vet Sci, 19*:179, 1957.
64. Zimmermann, L. E., Rappaport, H.: Occurrence of cryptococcosis in patients with malignant disease of reticuloendothelial system. *Am J Clin Pathol, 24*:1050, 1954.

Chapter 9

THE EPIDEMIOLOGY OF CANDIDOSIS

H. I. Winner

The epidemiology of *Candida* infections has been little studied until recent years. The main factors responsible for its prominence today can be summarized: 1) The relative diminution of importance of bacterial infections since the introduction of antibacterial antibiotics. Opportunistic infections, of which Candidosis is among the most prominent, have simultaneously grown in importance. 2) The increased availability of, and reliance on, laboratory investigations in the diagnosis of disease. This has brought about the more frequent detection of Candidas in clinical specimens. 3) The recognition of the importance of *Candida* infections in immunologically depressed persons, and 4) The recognition of *Candida* species as important causes of sexually transmitted infections.

This chapter deals with infections by all the pathogenic species of *Candida.* About 90 percent of infections are caused by *Candida albicans,* while the remainder shared by *C. guilliermondii, C. parapsilosis, C. krusei, C. tropicalis, C. stellatoidea, C. pseudotropicalis, C. viswanathii.*

SOURCES AND HABITAT

The commonest natural habitat of *Candida* ("*Candida*" here refers to all the pathogenic species) appears to be the surfaces of the human body exposed to the environment. *Candida* has also been found occurring naturally or as a cause of spontaneous disease in several other animal species, but it does not appear to be as prevalent in any other species as it is in man. Subhuman primates (monkeys and baboons) may also be infected. Apart from primates, turkey, chick, fowl, pigeon, parrot, partridge, cattle, sheep, pig, dog, cat, hedgehog, guinea pig, and mouse are among the most important animal species liable to natural infection. *Candida* is also found in the soil and in vegetable sources. In human beings *Candida* is found most often in:

1. The vagina: Various surveys show it to be carried by up to 35 percent of symptomless normal women in various parts of the world (30). Different surveys naturally vary in the results. Its incidence may be increased by pregnancy, menstrual changes, diabetes and other systemic diseases, the use of oral contraceptives, and other factors (3, 9, 13, 17, 18, 25).
2. The mouth: Surveys of oral thrush in the newborn show an incidence ranging from 0.5 to 18.8 percent (30). It varies with the degree of maternal infection, the maturity of the infant at birth, the method of feeding, and the prevailing social conditions.
3. The sputum: Surveys range from 0.6 to 77 percent (30).
4. The gut: The incidence of *C. albicans* in the feces has ranged in various surveys from 10 to 85 percent (30).
5. The skin: Less commonly than in the above-mentioned sites (11, 30).

TRANSMISSION

1. Person to person: *Candida* can be transferred by direct physical contact, or by indirect contact from clothing and fomites (15). During the act of parturition various surveys have shown in different communities that a widely varying proportion of newborn infants is infected at birth (7, 24, 28). Such infections may be inapparent, or they may lead to disease of greater or lesser severity in the infant. There is an inverse relation with the material standard of living of communities. As this tends to show a progressive improvement with the passage of time, the incidence of neonatal

Candida shows a corresponding fall (19). Also, *Candida* can be transmitted during nursing, from the skin of the mother's breast and hands. Further, epidemics due to imperfect sterilization of babies' feeding bottles may occur in maternity hospitals (30).

Candida can also be transmitted from person to person by sexual contact, and it is an important cause of conjugal and venereal infection (19, 31). For many years the husband with *Candida* balanitis was regarded as the "forgotten man" (29). Within the same person, the gut is perhaps the most important reservoir of *Candida* in the human being. From it the organism can be transferred to other sites by faecal contamination. This would account for the frequent persistence or recurrence of vaginal thrush in women (18). It would also account for the occurrence of *Candida* napkin eruption in infants (2, 5, 6, 20). Also, *Candida* may be transferred by sucking from the mouth of people with latent or clinical oral thrush to the hands.

2. Environment: *Candida* has been recovered from the air of hospital wards (4, 12, 16). It is found more often than elsewhere in the air of wards in which there are patients whose immunity is less than that of the general population, either for natural reasons, newborn infants, and people with immunological disorders, or because of therapy for malignant disease or as a prelude to organ transplantation (10). Much sophisticated *hospital apparatus*, such as cardiac and renal dialysis apparatus, is difficult to sterilize and has access to the bloodstream of patients with possible immunological depression. Such apparatus can be a good source of transmission. Because *Candida* can grow almost anywhere where there is a readily available source of carbohydrate, it is an important infecting organism in parenteral fluids. Further, Candidosis of the skin occurs frequently in circumstances in which the skin is liable to be macerated, that is, damaged by moisture. Thus, it occurs as a napkin eruption in infants and as an occupational infection in adults (30).

3. Food, drink and drugs: Apart from the milk and feeding bottles of bottle-fed infants, no appreciable incidence in food and drink has been reported. *Candida* infection has occurred in "main-line" drug addicts who give themselves injections with infected syringes or needles (26).
4. Animals: The author knows of no reported cases of transmission from animals to man. Transmission from man to animals, such as domestic pets, is probably more important.

FACTORS FAVORING INFECTION

Many factors may have an effect on the likelihood of a given infectivity of individuals with *Candida.* Little is known regarding the effect of variations in virulence of the organism.

However, certain types of exposure may increase the numbers of *Candida,* such as in broad-spectrum of antibiotic therapy and in heavy case-to-case infection (newborn infant by the mother) (8, 21, 23, 27, 30).

Other factors which may increase the susceptibility of the individual is immunological depression duets: pregnancy, infancy, endocrine or steroid therapy, oral contraceptive, irradiation, maceration of skin, malnutrition and malabsorption syndrome, blood dyscrasias, malignancy, allergy of skin, diabetic, and a few others.

REFERENCES

1. Ainsworth, G. C., Austwick, P. K. C.: Fungal Diseases of Animals. Commonw. Agricul. Bureau, Slough, England, 1973.
2. Blaschke-Hellmessen, Renate, Hubner, Ursula, Seebacher, C.: Vergleichende Untersuchungen zum Vorkommen von Sprosspilzen auf gesunder und krankhaft veranderter Haut. 2. Zur Epidemiologie der Ausbreitung von Sprosspilzen auf gesunder und kranker Haut. *Mykosen, 15*:83, 1972.
3. Catterall, R. D.: Influence of gestogenic contraceptive pills on vaginal candidosis. *Br J Vener Dis, 47*:45, 1971.
4. Clayton, Y. M., Noble, W. C.: Observations on the epidemiology of *Candida albicans. J Clin Pathol, 19*:76, 1966.
5. Dixon, P. N., Waring, R. P., English, M. P.: Role of *Candida albicans* infection in napkin rashes. *Br Med J, 2*:23, 1969.
6. Fergusson, A. G., Fraser, N. G., Grant, P. W.: Napkin dermatitis with psoriasiform "ide." A review of fifty-two cases. *Br J Derm, 78*:289, 1966.

7. France, Diana R.: Survival of *Candida albicans* in hand creams. *N Z Med J, 67*:552, 1968.
8. Holt, R. J., Newman, R. L.: *Candida* in the faeces of children receiving oral tetracycline and phenoxymethyl penicillin. *J Clin Pathol, 20*:80, 1967.
9. Jensen, H. K., Hansen, P. A., Blom, J.: Incidence of *C. albicans* in women using oral contraceptives. *Act Obstet Gynecol Scand, 49*: 293, 1970.
10. Kaufmann, H. J.: *Candida* oesophagitis in children with malignant disorders. Sem. Hosp. Paris, *Ann Radiol, 13*:157, 1970.
11. Marcelou-Kinti, O., Marioli, S., Saxoni-Anastassopoulou, P.: Frequency of *Candida* in both in and outpatients of the dermatological clinic. *Acta Microb Hellen, 16*:325, 1971.
12. Midgley, G., Clayton, Y. M.: Distribution of dermatophytes and spores in the environment. *Br J Dermatol, 86*:69, 1972.
13. Pumpianski, R., Ganor, S.: Recurrent candidal vaginitis. *J Isr Med Assoc, 79*:311, 1970.
14. Phillips, A. W.: *Candida albicans* in the gnotobiotic animal. IX Int. Cong. Microb., Moscow, 349, 1966.
15. Rahim, G. F.: Candidiasis in the family. *J Med Liban, 17*:97, 1964.
16. Refai, M., El-Monsoury, H., Osman, M. A.: Incidence of yeasts in sputa and urine in chest and urinary diseases. *Mykosen, 14*:299, 1971.
17. Rieth, H.: *Candida*-Balanitis und *Candida*-Fluor nach langerem Einnehmen oraler Kontrazeptiva. *Mykosen, 10*:151, 1967.
18. Rohatiner, J. J., Grimble, A.: Genital candidiasis and oral contraceptives. *J Obstet Gynecol Br Commonw, 77*:1013, 1970.
19. Saggese, V., Di Marco, A.: Le micosi da *Candida ablicans* con particolare riguardo all'infanzia. *Minerva Paediat, 22*:611, 1970.
20. Seebacher, C., Hubner, Ursula, Blaschke-Hellmessen, Renate: Vergleichende Untersuchungen zum Vorkommen von Sprosspilzen auf gesunder und krankhaft veronderter Haut. II. Mitteilung: Das Vorkommen von Sprosspilzen auf gesunder und kranker Haut. *Mykosen, 14*:371, 1971.
21. Sellig, M. S.: Mechanisms by which antibiotics increase the incidence and severity of candidiasis and alter the immunological defenses. *Bact Rev, 30*:442, 1966.
22. Smith, J. M. B.: Candidiasis in animals in New Zealand. *Sabouraudia, 5*:220, 1967.
23. Smits, B. J., Prior, A. P., Arblaster, P. G.: Incidence of *Candida* in hospital in-patients and the effects of antibiotic therapy. *Br Med J, 1*:208, 1966.
24. Somerville, D. A.: *Candida albicans* in a maternity hospital. *N Z Med J, 63*:592, 1964.

25. Spellacy, W. N., Zaias, N., Buhi, W. C., Birk, S. A.: Vaginal yeast growth and contraceptive practices. *Obst Gyn N Y, 38*:343, 1971.
26. Symmers, W. St. C.: in Symposium on *Candida* Infections, ed. Winner and Hurley, Edinburgh, Livingstone, 1966.
27. Toala, P., Schroeder, S. A., Daly, A. Kathleen, Finland, M.: *Candida* at Boston City Hospital. Clinical and epidemiological characteristics and susceptibility to eight antimicrobial agents. *Arch Intern Med, 126*:982, 1970.
28. Wedum, A. G., Kruse, R. H.: *Assessment of Risk of Human Infection in the Microbiological Laboratory,* 2nd ed. Frederick, Md., Misc. Pub. 30, Dept. of the Army, Fort Detrick, 1969.
29. Weisman, M.: Genital moniliasis as a conjugal infection. *Arch Dermatol Syph (Chicago), 70*:718, 1954.
30. Winner, H. I., Hurley, R.: *Candida Albicans.* London, Churchill, 1964.
31. Wisdom, A.: *Colour Atlas of Venereology.* London, Wolfe Medical Books, 1973.

Chapter 10

CLINICAL ASPECTS OF CANDIDA INFECTIONS

MARCUS L. DILLON, JR.

THIRTY YEARS AGO clinical candida infection was recognized to exist primarily in the mouth and adjacent skin, the nails and surrounding areas, the moist creases formed by folds of skin, and the mucous surfaces of the vagina and the glans penis. *Candida albicans* was recognized as the only pathogenic species. Visceral candidosis was practically an unrecognized entity while oral candidosis (thrush) was and is still characterized by marked hyperemia and edema from the superficial infection and may have erosions of the mucous membrane, deep fissures in the corners of the mouth, and fuzzy white patches at areas of erosion (Fig. 10-1). Extension of the infection into the esophagus with the formation of lesions is not unusual (Fig. 10-2). The few reported visceral lesions were medical oddities and were characterized with acute inflammatory responses and abscess formation (Fig. 10-3). It was recognized also that *Candida* vulvovaginitis was common in the diabetic female while *Candida* balanitis occurred in the male as infection from sexual contact. However, the pathogenicity of *Candida* is so weak the organism is tolerated as a normal inhabitant of the gastrointestinal tract in the majority of people and in the vagina of many women without inflammatory response.

The incidence of *Candida* infections increased with the advent of the broad spectrum of antibiotics twenty years ago. Antibiotics

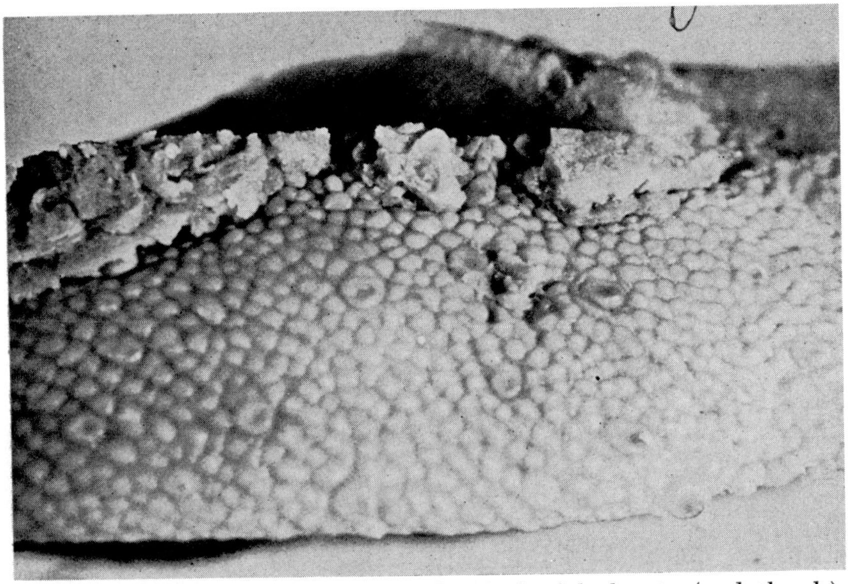

Figure 10-1. Tongue of a patient who died of leukemia (and thrush). Growth of *Candida* is clearly seen on the surface of the tongue.

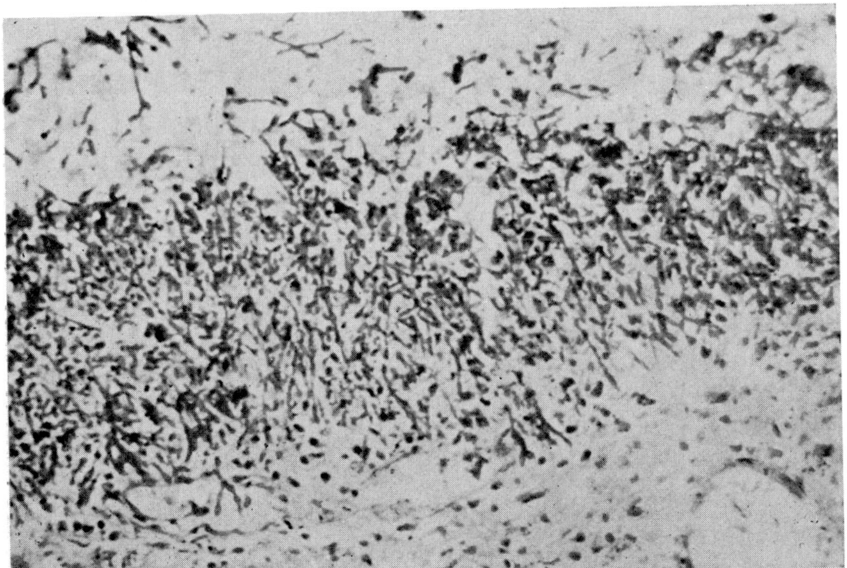

Figure 10-2. Candidosis of the esophagus. The growth of *Candida* appears in the superficial ulcer. There is relatively little cellular reaction to this invasion.

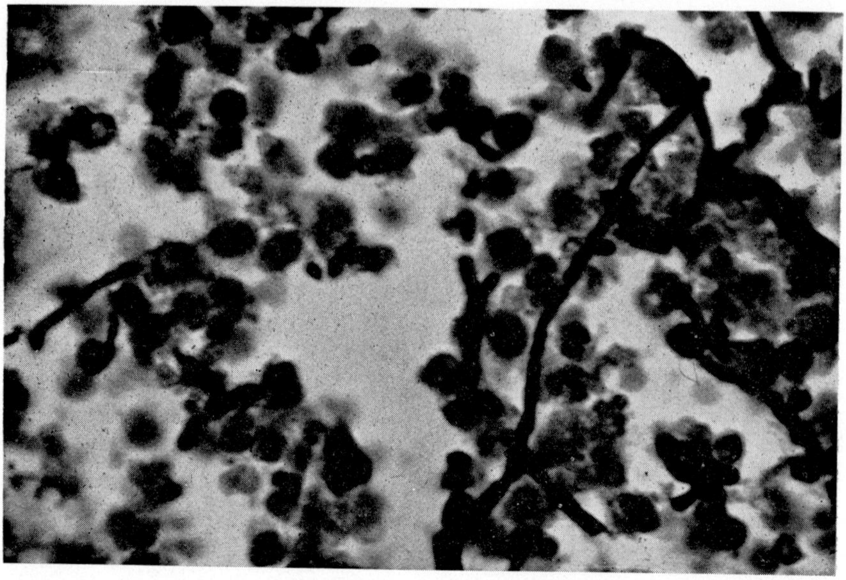

Figure 10-3. *Candida* pseudohyphae in an acute abscess in the brain of a patient who had *Candida* sepsis for fifteen months from an infected aortic valve prosthesis. Valve replacement and continuous amphotericin B therapy failed to control the infection.

may alter the intestinal flora so that *Candida* becomes the predominant organism. During a clinical trial of the efficacy of tetracycline as an antituberculous drug in 1954, it was observed that after three weeks on oral tetracycline, sputum cultures for *Mycobacterium tuberculosis* were overgrown with *Candida.* The patients developed thrush while women developed thrush and vulvovaginitis. *Candida* grew in cultures from the sputum, stool, gastric contents and the vagina of these patients.

The rapid rate of change in medical care during the past fifteen years has added factors at increasing frequency which contribute to the development of *Candida* infections. The use of contraceptive pills, cancer chemotherapeutic agents, and many potent forms of steroids have resulted in reduced host resistance to *Candida* and it is suspected that some antibiotics also have this capability.

Although emphasis has been placed on the risk of fungacemia from hyperalimentation, the development and general use of many types of catheters for the vascular system has provided routes of entry for *Candida* into the blood stream more frequently than those used for hyperalimentation.

The increasing number of people involved in taking hard drugs has made fungal tricuspid endocarditis a significant problem in some centers. Many of the first reported cases of fungal endocarditis were in drug addicts and they continue to comprise a significant percentage of those who develop fungal endocarditis.

Development in the past ten years of open heart surgery, organ transplantation with immunosuppression, and intravenous hyperalimentation has contributed to both the frequency and severity of *Candida* infections. A review of the clinical problems will reveal the severe consequences which can occur with *Candida* infections and identify some high risk groups.

HEART SURGERY

Inherent in the management of patients with operative heart disease are a sequence of events which predispose to the possibility of blood stream infection with resulting endocarditis. Valvular heart disease supplies a focus of least resistance within the blood stream for setting up and maintaining a subacute bacterial endocarditis. The treatment of bacterial endocarditis requiring six weeks of intravenous antibiotic therapy provides a route for inoculation with *Candida* that may well come from the patient's gastrointestinal tract as a result of overgrowth from use of broad spectrum antibiotics for long periods of time. Additional sources of entry to the vascular system are provided by the preoperative catheterization for hemodynamic evaluation of the valvular disease, the pump oxygenator system with the large volume of blood and fluids used to prime the system, and the frequent sampling of blood and injection of multiple medications via the intravenous route in the postoperative period. Fungal endocarditis following heart surgery was first reported in 1956 and was due to *C. albicans*. Only seventeen cases of endocarditis had previously been reported at that time due to *Candida* and seven of these were in drug addicts. Table 10-I outlines the reported postoperative heart surgery *Candida* infections since 1956 and tends to reflect the difficulties encountered clinically. The association with bacterial infection is not reflected in the table, but it was frequent. The delay in making the diagnosis is apparent and is frequently made at autopsy. Delay in diagnosis leads to an anatomically incurable condition because of involvement of aortic and/or heart wall or distant vital organs. The number of reports have increased over the years with a decrease in the past two years. The principles of treatment in order to obtain a cure are emphasized by early diagnosis, institution of antifungal therapy and removal of the cardiac focus of infection (30, 44). Since cultures tend to be negative or transiently positive until late in the course of the disease, other indications must be used to

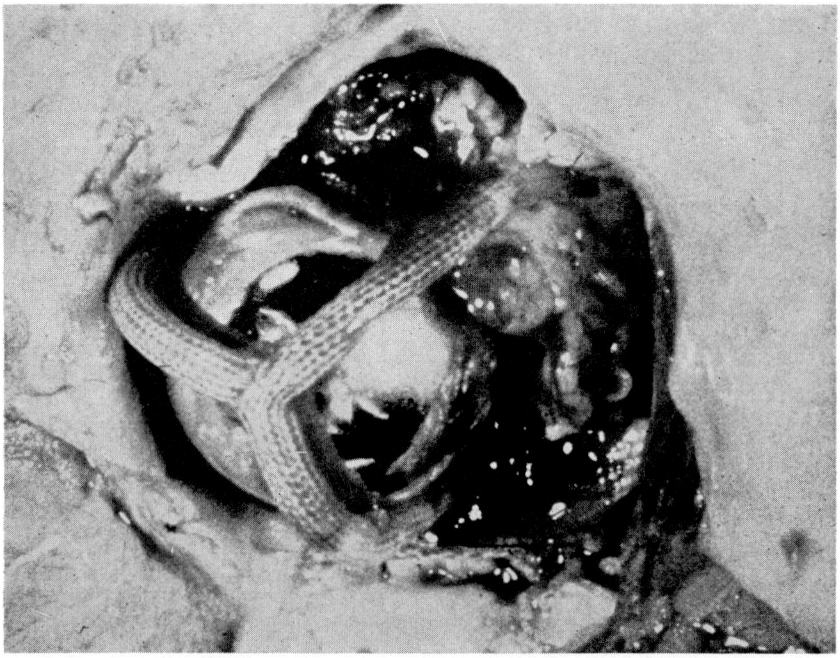

Figure 10-4. The aortic surface of the Starr-Edwards valve with ingrowth of vegetations that restrict the ball motion. Culture of the material grew *Candida* and *S. aureus*.

initiate treatment. These indications essentially consist of a high index of suspicion from the clinical course combined with serologic precipitin and agglutinin titers for *Candida* (21, 29, 44). Early initiation of amphotericin B treatment at lower doses may give further confirmation or rejection of the suspected diagnosis and be less risky for the patient than allowing invasion of vegetations into areas that are not curable.

One of our patients illustrates a typical course of *Candida* infection. A sixty-one-year-old male with aortic stenosis developed a *Staphylococcus aureus* septicemia following cardiac catherterization. He was treated for six weeks with intravenous antibiotics and in March 1968 his aortic valve was replaced with

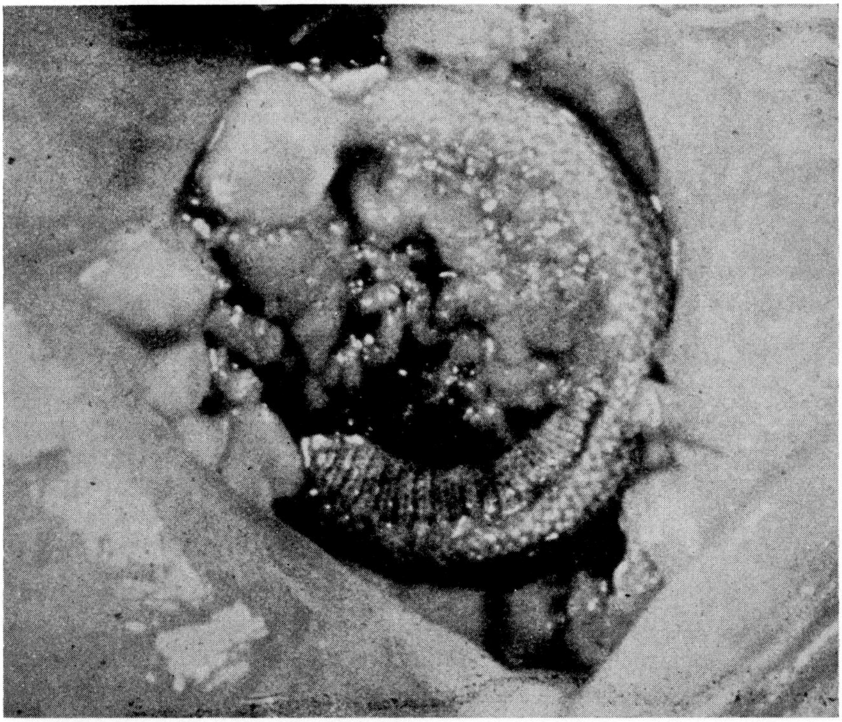

Figure 10-5. The ventricular side of the Starr-Edwards valve (shown in Fig. 10-4) with the fall and vegetations producing almost complete outflow obstruction. Two areas of paravalvular leak are seen at the top and bottom of the valve ring.

a Starr-Edwards prosthesis. No vegetations were found on the aortic valve at operation and no growth was obtained from culture. Treatment for subacute bacterial endocarditis was not continued in the postoperative period; however, his postoperative course was complicated by a right lower lobe lung abscess. Sputum cultures grew *S. aureus, Proteus* and *Escherishia coli.* The lung abscess resolved with treatment. Two months after discharge he returned to the emergency room in shock and failed to respond to resuscitative measures. Figures 10-4 and 10-5 show the gross vegetations on the Starr-Edwards valve which restricted the ball motion and obstructed the orifice. The largest channel for blood to pass was by way of paravalvular defects. The aortic valve vegetation grew *C. albicans* and *S. aureus.* Figure 10-6 shows a portion of the aortic wall invaded by *Candida* and experience has demonstrated that such areas must be excised to effect a cure.

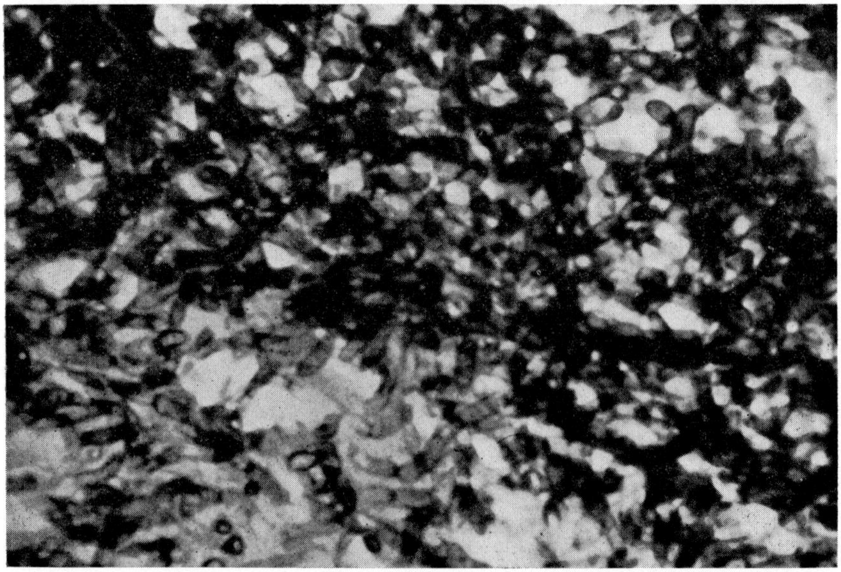

Figure 10-6. A photomicrograph of the aortic wall adjacent to the valve (shown in Figs. 10-4, 10-5) shows the aorta invaded by *Candida.*

TABLE 10-I

POSTOPERATIVE HEART SURGERY CANDIDA INFECTIONS

Reference	*Date of Report*	*Interval for Diagnosis*	*Operation*	*Organism*	*Result*
31	1956	3 months	Aortic valvulotomy	*C. albicans*	Died 3½ months
27	1960	3 months	Mitral valvulotomy	*C. albicans*	Died 3 months
		1 month	Aortic valvulotomy	*C. albicans*	Died 2 months
		1 month	Aortic valvulotomy	*C. albicans*	Died 3 months
		1 month	Aortic valvulotomy	*C. albicans*	Died 2½ months
33	1960	1 month	Mitral valvulotomy	*C. albicans*	Died 17 months
52	1961	8 days	Mitral valvulotomy	*C. parakrusei*	Died 3 weeks
11	1961	10 weeks	Mitral valvulotomy	*C. parakrusei*	Died 14 weeks
		3½ months	Mitral anuloplasty	*C. guilliermondi*	Died 4 months
		7 weeks	Aortic valvulotomy	*C. guilliermondi*	Died 5 months
37	1961	4 months	Aortic valvulotomy	*C. parakrusei*	Died 4 months
1	1962	6 months	Aortic valvulotomy	*C. guilliermondi*	Died 10 months
		1½ months	Mitral valvulotomy	*C. parakrusei*	Died 3½ months
		3½ months	Mitral valvulotomy	*C. parakrusei*	Died 3½ months
		1½ months	Mitral valvulotomy	*C. albicans*	Died 5 months
43	1962	1 month	Aortic valvulotomy	*C. albicans*	Died 1 month
		—	VSD (Teflon)	*C. albicans*	Well, 1 year
28	1963	2 months	Mitral valvulotomy	*C. stellaloidae*	Died 2 months
46	1963	4 months	Mitral valvulotomy	*C. albicans*	Died 5 months
9	1965	1 month	Aortic homograft	*Candida sp.*	Died 2 months
47	1966	—	Mitral prothesis	*C. albicans*	Died 2 months (est.)

TABLE 10-I—Continued

POSTOPERATIVE HEART SURGERY CANDIDA INFECTIONS

Reference	*Date of Report*	*Interval for Diagnosis*	*Operation*	*Organism*	*Result*
10	1966	4 months	Aortic prosthesis	*C. albicans*	Died 4 months
7	1967	10 days	Aortic prosthesis	*C. tropicalis*	Died 24 months
				C. parapsilosis	
35	1967	16 months	Aortic valvulotomy	*C. albicans*	Died 16 months
34	1967	2 months	Aortic homograft	*C. albicans*	Died 5 months
		1 month	Aortic homograft	*C. albicans*	Died 4 months
		1 month	Aortic homograft	*C. albicans*	Died 3 months
51	1968	2 months	Aortic prosthesis	*C. parapsilosis*	Died 5 months
39	1968	2 weeks	Aortic homograft	*C. albicans*	Died 2 weeks
30	1968	3 weeks	Aortic prosthesis	*C. albicans*	Died 31 months
50	1968	2 weeks	Mitral prosthesis	*Candida sp.*	Died 3 weeks (est.)
49	1968	—	Aortic homograft	*C. albicans*	Died . . .
		—	Aortic homograft	*C. albicans*	Died . . .
		—	Aortic homograft	*C. albicans*	Died . . .
		—	Aortic homograft	*C. albicans*	Died . . .
		—	Aortic homograft	*C. albicans*	Died . . .
		—	Aortic homograft	*C. albicans*	Living . . .
13	1969	10 months	Pacemaker (IV)	*Candida sp.*	Died 10 months
25	1969	2 months	Aortocarotid endart.	*C. albicans*	Died 2 months
		3 months	Aortic prosthesis	*C. albicans*	Died 4½ months
42	1969	1 month	Mitral homograft	*Candida sp.*	Sepsis at 8 months

TABLE 10-I—Continued

POSTOPERATIVE HEART SURGERY CANDIDA INFECTIONS

Reference	*Date of Report*	*Interval for Diagnosis*	*Operation*	*Organism*	*Result*
8	1970	2 months	Aortic homograft	*C. albicans*	Died 2 months
		2 months	Aortic & mitral prosthesis	*C. albicans*	Died 2 months
38	1970	2 months	Aortic prosthesis	*Candida sp.*	Died 2 months
24	1970	1 year, 5 mos.	Mitral prosthesis	*C. albicans*	Died 3 months after dx. of liver necrosis
		2 months	Aortic prosthesis	*C. albicans*	Died 4 months
22	1970	4 months	Aortic homograft	*C. albicans*	Living 2 months
18	1971	1 week	Aortic prosthesis	*Candida sp.*	Died 7 months
53	1971	6 weeks	Mitral prosthesis	*C. krusei*	Died 2 months
40	1971	3 months	Aortic prosthesis	*C. parapsilosis*	Died 6 months
36	1971	3 days	Aortic prosthesis	*C. albicans*	Died 9 months
		1 month	Aortic prosthesis	*C. albicans*	Died 1 month
		3 months	Aortic prosthesis	*C. albicans*	Died 4 months
23	1972	5 months	Aortic homograft	*C. parapsilosis*	Living 22 months
		—	Aortic homograft	*Candida sp.*	Living 6 months
		—	Aortic homograft	*Candida sp.*	Died . . .
26	1972	1 month	Aortic prosthesis	*C. krusei*	Died 1 month
		10 months	Aortic prosthesis	*C. krusei*	Living 11 months

ORGAN TRANSPLANTATION

These patients with altered immunity present a different clinical picture than the operative heart patients. The portal of entry is more commonly respiratory and gastrointestinal and the infection is truly more opportunistic from their disease than iatrogenic from catheter inoculation.

The susceptibility of these patients illustrated by the findings of Rifkind et al. (41) who analyzed the data on 107 recipients of renal transplantation. Systemic fungal infection was present in twenty-three of fifty-one patients who died between three and forty months following transplantation. *Candida* was found in twelve, *Aspergillus* in five, *Nocardia* in two, *Histoplasma* in one and a combination of these fungi in three. Pulmonary involvement was the most common location and was found in eighteen, the gastrointestinal tract in nine, central nervous system in eight, kidney in four and other organs ten. *Candida* showed a predilection for the gastrointestinal tract which may be a reflection of the reservoir of *Candida.* Concomitant bacterial, viral or parasitic infection was present in twenty of the twenty-three patients with fungus infection. Table 10-II shows pulmonary fungal infection which occurred in the first 112 renal transplant patients at Duke Medical Center (14). *Candida* was the most common in these eighteen patients (16%). The relatively high survival rate was obtained by giving smaller doses than usual of amphotericin B for longer periods of time and early surgical resection of unresponsive localized lesions.

TABLE 10-II

PULMONARY FUNGAL INFECTIONS IN 112 PATIENTS

Number	*Organism*	*Result*
3	*Cryptococcus*	Died
3	*Cryptococcus*	Living
2	*Candida*	Died
8	*Candida*	Living
1	*Aspergillus*	Living
1	*Nocardia*	Living

IMMUNODEFICIENCY

During the past fifteen years many immunodeficiency states have been recognized and some understanding has been gained of the defects present, i.e. agammaglobulinemia, phagocytic dysfunction syndromes, impaired cell-mediated immunity syndromes. Some of these defects are associated with resistant mucocutaneous candidosis. Arvanitakis and Knouss have reported two patients with chronic mucocutaneous candidosis who had hypopituitarism and impaired cell-mediated immunity (3).

The complexities of management of such patients is illustrated by a nine-year-old boy who had a life-long history of multiple infections and allergies. He developed mucocutaneous candidosis with involvement of his fingernails before the age of one year following a course of chloromycetin for Staphylococcal infection of the skin. At five years of age he developed chronic diarrhea at times as many as twenty bowel movements a day. Cultures from the mouth grew *C. albicans* but no *Candida* was grown from stool cultures. Precipitin test for *Candida* were positive but skin tests were negative. The child was diagnosed as having a malabsorption syndrome and improved on a glutin free diet although a jejunal biopsy was normal. At seven years of age a diagnosis of Addison's disease was made on the basis of no response to ACTH stimulation and thymic dysplasia was suspected. He was started on steroid therapy and within four days of discharge from the hospital returned with abdominal pain from fecal impaction. At nine years of age new *Candida* lesions appeared on his neck. He was given about half of a planned fourteen-day treatment with amphotericin B at 25 mgm per day and had his involved fingernails removed. Skin test to *Candida* was now positive. Four months later he was admitted with severe anemia with edema and ascitries. His hemoglobin was 2.2 gms and hematocrit 8.5 vol. %. This was found to have a megaloblastic anemia which responded well to B_{12} injections. When last seen two months later he still had thrush which did not respond to mycostatin and one nail bed was clear but the others were variably involved. He received transfer factor two months before with no obvious effect on the *Candida* infection. Figures 10-7 and 10-8 illustrate the mucocutaneous lesions of the mouth and hands. The practical clinical importance of such lesions is that it is an indication of more serious underlying disease.

Immunodeficiency may occur as a result of other diseases and be recognized only in terms of increased frequency of *Candida* infections as with the leukemias, Hodgkins, aplastic anemia, tuberculosis and diabetes mellitus (54, 15). *Candida* lesions of the mitral valve are shown in Figure 10-9 from a newborn infant who had a premature birth and early respiratory distress. She was kept on a respirator and on the twenty-fourth day of life *Candida* was cultured from the blood. She developed anemia, splenomegaly, hepatomegaly, congestive heart failure, and died on the forty-fifth day. Urine cultures taken three days before

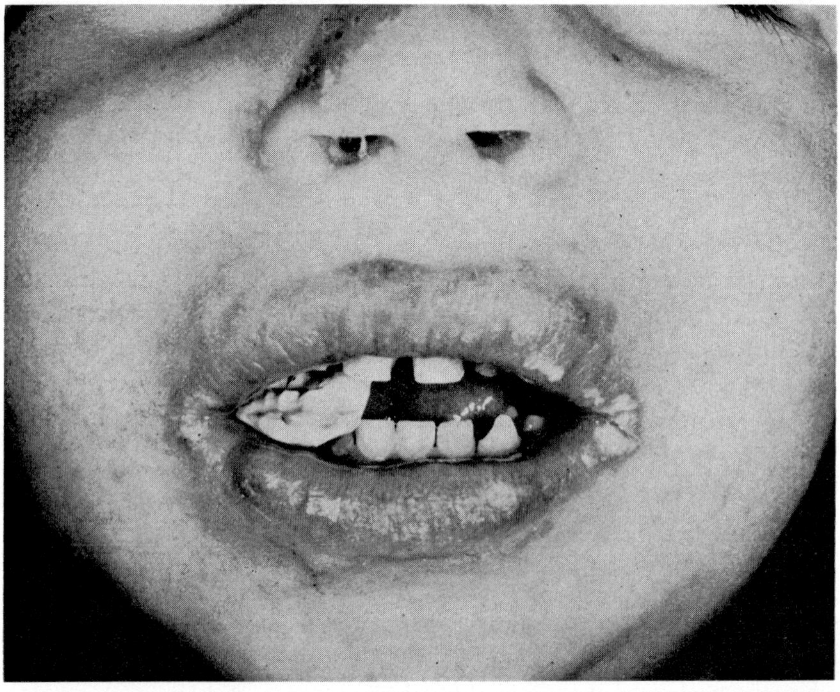

Figure 10-7. *Candida* lesions of the mouth and face with fissures in the mucous membranes of the mouth and white patches of the lips. (Courtesy of Ullen Leavell, M.D., Univ. Kentucky).

death grew cytomegalovirus. An autopsy showed *C. albicans* septicemia and endocarditis with cytomegalic inclusion disease. There may be some unrecognized immune defect other than prematurity which allowed both diseases to develop in this infant.

INTRAVENOUS HYPERALIMENTATION

In 1968 Dudrick et al. demonstrated that not only could a positive nitrogen balance be maintained by intravenous feeding but normal growth and development could be obtained in children (16). This intravenous hyperalimentation requires a central venous catheter for long periods of time. Vic-Dupont et al. from a review of thirty patients with *Candida* septicemia felt that the portal of entry in eighteen to be the intravenous catheter (50). With removal of the catheter the culture reverts to negative

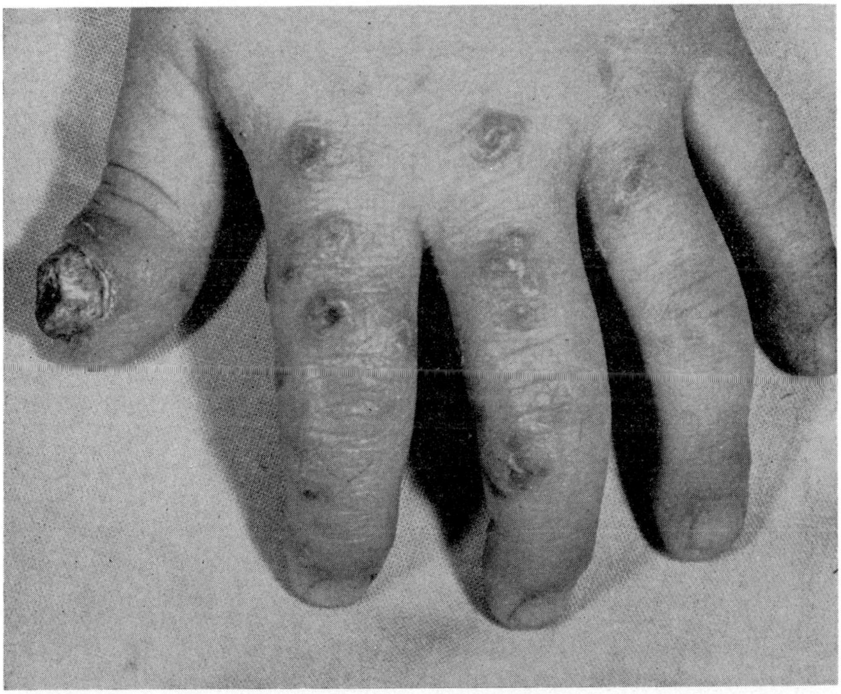

Figure 10-8. *Candida* involvement of the skin and nails of the hand. The thumb nail is markedly thickened and swelling of the cuticle is apparent. (Courtesy of Ullen Leavell, M.D., Univ. Kentucky).

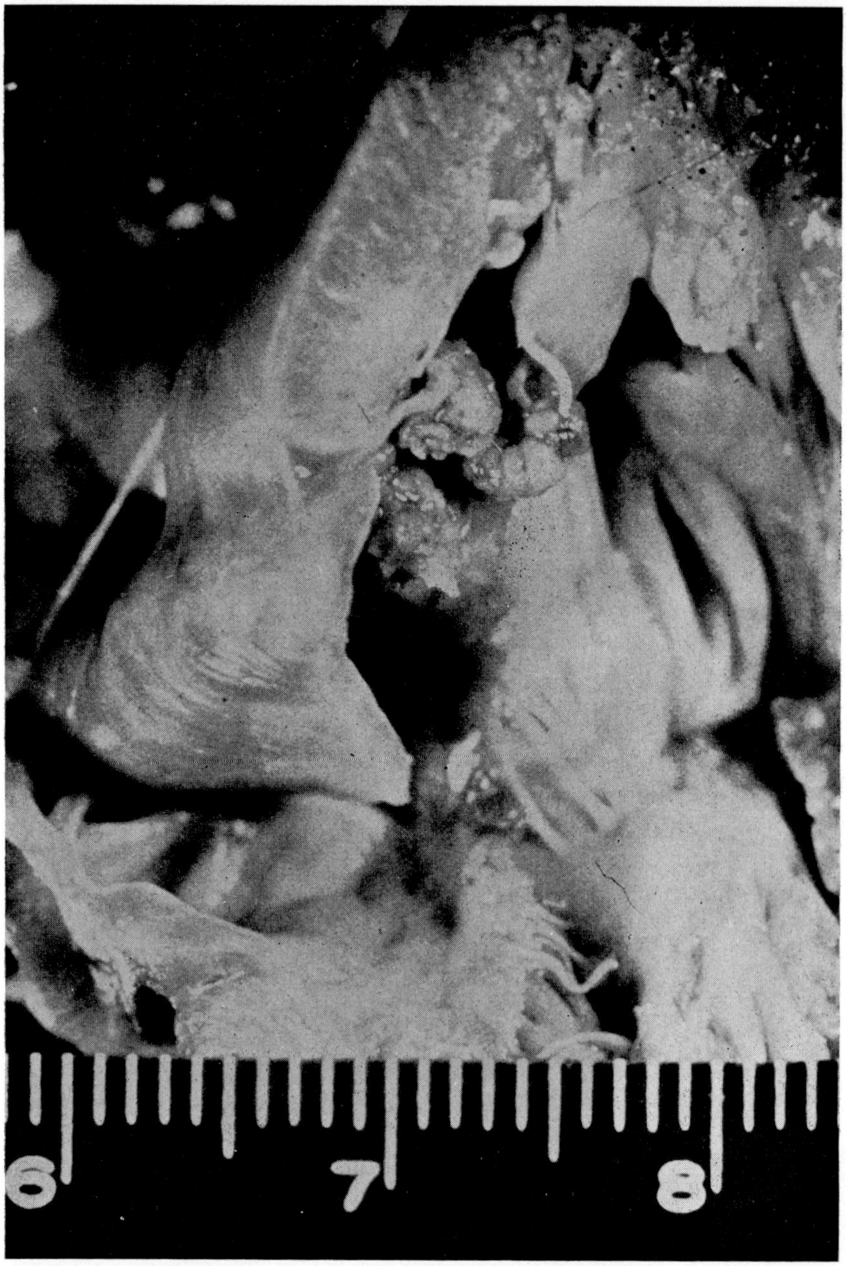

Figure 10-9. Heart from a five-day-old infant with cytomegalic inclusion disease and *C. albicans* vegetations on the mitral valve.

immediately but fever usually persists for several days. The ability of the human to clear the blood stream of *Candida* was discussed by Eras et al. by demonstrating the rapid onset of fungemia when *Candida* was administered orally to a normal subject (17). He noted that the fungemia and funguria were completely cleared by normal host defenses in three hours. *Candida* passes through the normal intestinal wall probably by "persorption," a process by which particles up to 120 μ in diameter pass through the intestinal wall. The incidence of funicemia from intravenous hyperalimentation has varied widely. Kropelin et al. reported ten patients on long-term subclavian vein intravenous therapy (32). Five had fibrile episodes and *Candida* cultured from the blood, catheter or both. One patient with no fever had *Candida* isolated from the catheter tip. Ashcraft and Leape found *Candida* sepsis in five of twenty-two patients, two died of the infection (2). Boechman and Krill found *Candida* sepsis in six of fifteen patients (5). There were twenty-six serious complications in twelve patients. *Candida* sepsis was the cause of death in three patients, but two of the three survivors of sepsis required only catheter removal. The three patients free of bacterial or fungal sepsis had intravenous catheterization of short duration (10, 12 and 21 days), had no open abdominal wounds, had received no steroids and only one received antibiotics. Curry and Quie found that of twenty-two patients with fungal septicemia from IV hyperalimentation, seventeen were due to *Candida* and that the incidence of septicemia relates both to the duration of hyperalimentation and to the time since the last catheter change (12). Strunin et al. reported a prospective study of one hundred patients with prolonged intravenous therapy from three to ninety-five days with no fungal septicemia and *Candida* cultured from the skin around the catheter in only one patient (48). Fischer et al. reported on 375 patients with a sepsis rate of less than three percent in lines used for hyperalimentation alone (19). They stress the importance of following details in protective devices, both in manufacture and administration. Since the use of hyperalimentation will undoubtedly increase, it is important to be aware of the work of Brennen et al. who by using 1 ml of 1 mgm of amphotericin B twice a week to flush the intravenous line have had no *Candida* sepsis (6). One of their patients who had had five previous episodes of candidemia was maintained for an additional 460 days with no further episodes using the flush technique.

SPECIAL STUDIES

There are advocates of using precipitin and agglutinen titers as an indication of deep fungus infection, especially to obtain an early diagnosis when treatment is most effective (44, 21, 29).

Balandran et al. have reported two patients with leukemia who developed a disseminated maculonodular rash as a manifestation of systemic candidosis (4). Biopsies showed subepithelial pseudohyphae and *Candida* was cultured from one.

Silverman et al. reported a patient who was first found to have *Candida* sepsis by examination of a smear of venous blood stained with Wright's stain (45). Culture of the central venous pressure catheter tip revealed *C. albicans.*

Freeman et al. point out that *Candida* endophthalmitis is serious and complicates with a high incidence of visual loss and mortality (20). The presence of pain or other visual disturbances combined with the characteristic fundoscopic appearance of "cotton wool" exudates are absolute indications for prompt administration of amphotericin B. They also advocate routine daily fundoscopic examination in any patient who is a suspect for fungal overgrowth.

REFERENCES

1. Andriole, V. T., Kravetz, H. M., Roberts, W. C., Utz, J. P.: *Candida* Endocarditis. *Am J Med, 32*:251, 1962.
2. Ashcraft, K. W., Leape, L.: *Candida* sepsis complicating parenteral feeding. *JAMA, 212*:454, 1970.
3. Arvanitakis, C., Knouss, R. F.: Selective hypopituitarism; impaired cell-mediated immunity and chronic mucocutaneous candidiasis. *JAMA, 225*:1492, 1973.
4. Balandran, L., Rothschild, H., Pugh, N., Seabury, J.: A cutaneous manifestation of systemic candidiasis. *Ann Int Med, 78*:400, 1973.
5. Boeckman, C. R., Krill, C. E.: Bacterial and fungal infection complicating parenteral alimentation in infants and children. *J Pediatr Surg, 5*:117, 1970.

6. Brennen, M. F., Goldman, M. T., O'Connell, R. C., Kundsin, R. B., Moore, F. D.: Prolonged parenteral alimentation: *Candida* growth and the prevention of candidemia by amphotericin instillation. *Ann Surg, 176*:265, 1972.
7. Carey, J. S., Hughes, R.: Cardiac valve replacement for the narcotic addict. *J Thor Card Surg, 53*:663, 1967.
8. Chaudhuri, M. R.: Fungal endocarditis after valve replacement. *J Thorac Card Surg, 60*:207, 1970.
9. Climie, A. R. W., Rachmanioff, N.: Fungal (*Candida*) endocarditis following open heart surgery. *J Thor Card Surg, 50*:437, 1965.
10. Cohn, L. H., Roberts, W. C., Rockoff, S. O., Morrow, A. G.: Bacterial endocarditis following aortic valve replacement. *Circulation, 33*: 209, 1966.
11. Cooper, T., Morrow, A. G., Roberts, W. C., Herman, L. G.: Postoperative endocarditis due to *Candida*: Clinical observations and the experimental production of the lesion. *Surgery, 50*:341, 1961.
12. Curry, E. R., Quie, P. G.: Fungal septicemia complicating intravenous hyperalimentation. *N Engl J Med, 285*:1221, 1971.
13. Davis, J. M., Moss, A. J., Schenk, E. A.: Tricuspid *Candida* endocarditis complicating a permanently implanted transvenous Pacemaker. *Am Heart J, 77*:818, 1969.
14. Dillon, M. L.: Discussion in: Surgical management of localized Thoracic infections in immunosuppressed patients. *Ann Thor Surg, 12*:471, 1971, by Williams, G. D., Flanigan, W. J., Campbell, G. S.
15. Dillon, M. L., Postlethwait, R. W.: Phychomycosis. *J Ind Med Prof, 11*:4950, 1964.
16. Dudrick, S. J., Wilmore, D. W., Vars, H. M., Rhoades, J. E.: Long term total parenteral nutrition with growth, development and positive nitrogen balance. *Surgery, 64*:134, 1968.
17. Eras, P., Goldstein, M. J., Sherlock, P.: *Candida* infection of the gastrointestinal tract. *Medicine, 51*:367, 1972.
18. Fass, F. J., Perkins, R. L.: 5-Fluorocytosine in the treatment of *Cryptococcal* and *Candida* mycoses. *Ann Int Med, 74*:535, 1971.
19. Fischer, J. E., Abbott, W. M., Abel, R. M.: Fungal septicemia complicating intravenous hyperalimentation. *Lancet, 1*:640, 1972.
20. Freeman, J. B., Davis, P. L., Maclean, L. D.: *Candida* endophthalmitis associated with intravenous hyperalimentation. *Arch Surg, 108*:237, 1974.
21. Gaines, J. D., Remington, J. S., Sanford, C. A.: Diagnosis of deep infection with *Candida*; a study of *Candida* precipitins. *Arch Int Med, 132*:699, 1973.
22. Gonzales-Lavin, L., Scappatura, E., Lise, M., Roso, D. N.: Mycotic aneurysms of the aortic root. *Ann Thor Surg, 9*:551, 1970.
23. Grehl, T. M., Cohn, L. H., Angell, W. W.: Management of *Candida* endocarditis. *J Thor Card Surg, 63*:118, 1972.

24. Hairston, P., Lee, W. H.: Management of infected prosthetic heart valves. *Ann Thor Surg, 9*:229, 1970.
25. Hairston, P., Lee, W. H.: Mycotic (fungal) endocarditis after cardiovascular surgery. *Am Surg, 35*:135, 1969.
26. Harris, P. D., Yeoh, C. B., Breault, J., Meltzer, J., Katz, S.: Fungal endocarditis secondary to drug addiction. Recent concepts in diagnosis and therapy. *J Thor Card Surg, 63*:980, 1972.
27. Hyun, B. H., Collier, F. C.: Mycotic endocarditis following intracardiac operations: Operation report of four cases. *N Engl J Med, 263*:1339, 1960.
28. Jamshidi, A., Pope, R. H., Friedman, N. H.: Fungal endocarditis complicating cardiac surgery. *Arch Int Med, 112*:370, 1963.
29. Jones, S. A., Brennan, M., Kundsin, R. B.: *Candida* serology: An aid in diagnosis of deep organ candidiasis. *J Surg Res, 14*:235, 1973.
30. Kay, J. H., Bernstein, S., Tsuji, H. K., Redington, J. V., Milgram, M., Brem, T.: Surgical treatment of *Candida* endocarditis. *JAMA, 203*:621, 1968.
31. Koelle, W. A., Pastor, B. H.: *Candida albicans* endocarditis after aortic valvulotomy. *N Engl J Med, 225*:997, 1956.
32. Kropelin, K., Mossner, G., Gibhardt, W.: The subclavian catheter as a focus of fungal infection. *German Med Monthly, 13*:486, 1968.
33. Louria, D. B., Dineen, P.: Amphotericin B in treatment of disseminated moniliasis. *JAMA, 174*:273, 1960.
34. McConnell, E. M., Roberts, C.: Pathological findings in three cases of fungal endocarditis complicating open heart surgery. *J Clin Pathol, 20*:555, 1967.
35. Newsom, S. W. B., Lee, W. R., Rees, J. R.: Fatal fungal infection following open heart surgery. *Br Heart J, 29*:457, 1967.
36. Ostermiller, W. E., Dye, W. S., Weinberg, M.: Fungal endocarditis following cardiovascular surgery. *J Thor Card Surg, 61*:670, 1971.
37. Persellin, R. H., Haring, O. H., Lewis, J. F:. Fungal endocarditis following cardiac surgery. *Ann Int Med, 54*:127, 1961.
38. Purandare, S. M., Deshpande, C. K.: Mycotic endocarditis following open heart surgery. *J Postgrad Med, 15*:206, 1970.
39. Ratcliffe, J. G., Pryce, D. M.: Disseminated candidiasis following aortic valve homograft replacement and tracheostomy. *J Med Microb, 1*:220, 1968.
40. Record, C. O., Skinner, J. M., Sleight, P., Speller, D. C. E.: *Candida* endocarditis treated with 5-fluorocystosine. *Br Med J, 1*:262, 1971.
41. Rifkind, D., Marchioro, T. L., Schneck, S. A., Hill, R. B.: Systemic fungal infections complicating renal transplantation and immunosuppressive therapy. *Am J Med, 43*:28, 1967.
42. Rothlin, M., Baymann, P. C., Ratti, R., Senning, A.: Infectious endocarditis following cardiac surgery. *German Med Monthly, 14*:539, 1969.

43. Sanger, P. W., Taylor, F. H., Robicsek, F., Germuth, F., Senterfit, L., McKinnon, G.: *Candida* infections as a complication of heart surgery, *JAMA, 181*:88, 1962.
44. Sellig, M. S., Speth, C. P., Kozinn, P. J., Toni, E. F., Taschdjian, C. L.: *Candida* endocarditis after cardiac surgery; clues to earlier detection. *J Thor Card Surg, 65*:583, 1973.
45. Silverman, E. M., Norman, L. E., Goldman, R. T., Simmons, J.: Diagnosis of systemic candiasis in smears of venous blood stained with Wright's stain. *Am J Clin Pathol, 60*:473, 1973.
46. Simmons, N. A., Turner, P.: *Candida* endocarditis after cardiac surgery. *Br Med J, 11*:1041, 1963.
47. Stein, P. D., Harken, D. E., Dexter, L.: The nature and prevention of prosthetic valve endocarditis. *Am Heart J, 71*:393, 1966.
48. Strunin, L., Colvin, M. P., Blogg, C. E., Savege, T. M.: Fungal septicemia complicating parenteral feeding. *Lancet, 1*:201, 1972.
49. Temple, L. J., Molloy, P.: Heart valve homografts succumb to *Candida. World Med,* May 23, 1968.
50. Vic-Dupont, V., Coulaud, J. P., Delrieu, F.: Les septicemies A. Candida; aspects etiologiques, cliniques et therapeutiques, D'apres thirty observations. *Presse Med, 76*:747, 1968.
51. Watanakunakorn, C., Carlton, J., Goldberg, L. M., Hamburger, M.: *Candida* endocarditis surrounding a Starr-Edwards prosthetic valve, recovery of *Candida* in hypertonic medium during treatment. *Arch Int Med, 121*:243, 1968.
52. Wilson, R. M.: *Candida* endocarditis. *JAMA, 177*:332, 1961.
53. Yeoh, Chin: Discussion in urgent open heart surgery for endocarditis of mitral valve. *N Y State J Med, 71*:2651, 1971 (by Khonsari, S., Bahabozorgui, S., Cook, W. A., Frater, R. W. M.)
54. Zimmerman, L. E:. Fatal fungus infections complicating other diseases. *Am J Clin Pathol, 25*:46, 1955.

Chapter 11

THE EPIDEMIOLOGY OF ENTOMOPHTHOROMYCOSES

Betty M. Clark

The entomophthoromycoses are a group of fungous infections caused by Phycomycetes or Zygomycetes, belonging to the order Entomophthorales, family Entomophthoraceae. The taxanomy of the Phycomycetes has been a subject of debate by many authorities for many years. This chapter is not the place for a discussion of this subject, except where it is relevant to the etiology and epidemiology of the entomophthoromycoses.

The entomophthoromycoses differ from mucormycosis, in that they usually occur in otherwise apparently healthy individuals. However, none of these patients has been fully investigated for possible immunological defects. Unlike the Mucoraceae, involvement of the vasculature by the Entomophthoraceae has seldom been reported (72, 91, 94). The entomophthoromycoses are seldom fatal.

The two most common clinical and mycological types of entomophthoromycosis, are subcutaneous phycomycosis caused by a species of *Basidiobolus*, currently considered to be *B. haptosporus*, and rhino-entomophthoromycosis caused by *Entomophthora coronata.* A case of mediastinal entomophthoromycosis caused by an unidentified species of *Entomophthora* has been reported (26, 38).

Due to the fact that the entomophthoromycoses cannot be differentiated histologically, the possibility of infection with other genera and species cannot be excluded, when mycological cultures have not been obtained. An example of this is that in the past, cases which were clinically typical of rhino-entomophthoromycosis were frequently diagnosed as subcutaneous phycomycosis of the face (15, 74). Furthermore the eosinophilic granuloma, which has often been considered to be histologically pathognomonic of the entomophthoromycoses, may occasionally be found in other mycotic and parasitic infections (84, 94).

SUBCUTANEOUS PHYCOMYCOSIS

Subcutaneous phycomycosis is a chronic, granulomatous lesion of the subcutaneous tissues, caused by *B. haptosporus.* This disease is also called Primary subcutaneous phycomycosis (94) and basidiobolomycosis (100). Deeper tissues may also be involved, therefore the name basidiobolomycosis is more accurate, providing the etiological fungus has been identified.

It is universally agreed that the etiological fungus of basidiobolomycosis, belongs to the genus *Basidiobolus,* but the identity of the pathogenic species is still controversial.

Natural Habitat

It is not possible to give an accurate account of the natural habitat and saprophytic life of the human pathogen. This is due to the lack of concurrence among mycologists, on the taxonomy of the genus *Basidiobolus.* For this reason, the species identification used by the original authors, are retained herein.

Basidiobolus species are saprophytes of soil, decaying vegetation, the gastrointestinal tract and excreta of reptiles, amphibia and fish. *Basidiobolus* species identified as *B. ranarum, B. haptosporus* or *B. meristosporus,* have been isolated from one or several of these sources, in many parts of the world.

Saprophytic isolates have been reported from Indonesia (55), India (87), Malagasy (10), Zaire (18), Nigeria (15), Czechoslovakia (99), Germany (28), Belgium (19), U.S.A. (24, 25, 41), Jamaica (15) and Colombia (40).

Basidiobolus is ingested by reptiles, amphibia and fish with their food. Spherical spores of *Basidiobolus* which have arisen from the sporangia (conidia), have been observed in the gastrointestinal contents of lizards (70) and frogs (68). Here the sporangiospores multiply by fission, and are returned to the soil in the excreta of these animals (68). Given suitable conditions, such as moisture and decaying vegetation, the sporangiospores germinate to produce the mycelial form, and the cycle is repeated.

There is evidence to suggest that insects are the vehicle whereby *Basidiobolus* enters the digestive tract of reptiles and amphibia (18, 68). It is not known whether the insects ingest the fungus, or act as vehicles as a result of contamination. Nor has it been established that insects are the only vehicle, whereby *Basidiobolus* gains access to the digestive tract. The possibility that insects might supply an essential source of nutriment for the fungus in this environment, has not been excluded.

B. meristosporus has been isolated from ants from Zaire (18). Other attempts to isolate *Basidiobolus* from insects, have been unsuccessful (15, 19, 41).

Geographical Distribution

Since the first report of subcutaneous phycomycosis from Indonesia in 1956 (56), over 170 cases have been diagnosed but mycological confirmation of basidiobolomycosis has not been obtained in all these cases (Table 11-I). All the proven cases of basidiobolomycosis have been from tropical regions; the Australian case was from Northern Territory (39). The largest number of cases of subcutaneous phycomycosis have been reported from Uganda, but the number in which mycological confirmation was obtained is not known.

B. ranarum was isolated from a granulating wound on the leg of a horse in Java (102). *B. haptosporus* was isolated from a granulomatous lesion of the eye of another horse in Queensland, Australia (17). Histological evidence of subcutaneous phycomycosis was found in a dog in Britain (94).

It has been suggested that the geographical distribution of basidiobolomycosis is related to that of lizards, of the family Agamidae (18). Other factors which have to be considered include the ability of the fungus, regardless of species, to grow

TABLE 11-I

CASES OF SUBCUTANEOUS PHYCOMYCOSIS

Country	*No.*	*Cases*	*References*
Uganda	50	(?)	11, 12, 49, 52, 53, 104, 106
Nigeria	26	(16)	15, 16, 27, 29, 34, 46, 51, 76
Kenya	20	(6)	13, 79
Sudan	2	(1)	30, 72
Ivory Coast	2	(1)	3, 103
Chad	2	(0)	23, 86
Senegal	2	(0)	5
Cameroun	1	(1)	36
Congo	1	(1)	90
Zaire	1	(1)	37, 101
Ghana	1	(0)	11
Rep. Central Africa	1	(0)	23
Malawi	1	(0)	50
Upper Volta	1	(0)	67
Malagasy	1	(0)	9
India	12	(7)	1, 42, 43, 60, 64, 65, 73, 77, 78, 98
Burma	4	(4)	88
Thailand	2	(1)	14, 95
Indonesia	18	(9)	47, 54, 55, 56, 57, 91, 92, 96, 97
Australia	2	(1)	39, 110
England	1	(0)	93
Germany	1	(0)	94

( ) = No. of mycologically proven cases of basidiobolomycosis.

well at 37 degrees C. It is unlikely that a saprophytic strain, which has become adapted to low temperatures, would be capable of establishing infection in man. The environmental conditions and habits of people living in tropical countries may also contribute to the incidence of the disease. It is, however, difficult to explain why basidiobolomycosis has not been reported from the western hemisphere.

Pathogenesis and Clinical Features

Basidiobolus probably gains access to the subcutaneous tissues by minor trauma, which is frequently forgotten, by the time the patient becomes aware of the lesion. A history of previous infection (47, 77), trauma (93), mosquito bite (97) and caterpillar "bite" (15), at the site of the lesion, has been obtained in a few cases.

In the majority of cases, including those associated with insect bites, the trauma is probably mechanical. The fungus may have been implanted in the tissues, as a result of the patient scratching the area of the insect bite. Mechanical trauma associated with direct contact with the soil, has been suggested as the commonest mode of infection, particularly in children (18).

The gastrointestinal tract has been suggested as a portal of entry (31). The only evidence to support this theory is a report of the isolation of *B. ranarum* from human feces. There was no indication that the fungus was acting as a pathogen in this case.

The incubation period is not known. In two cases the lesion was noticed two to three months after a history of trauma at the site of infection (15, 93).

Subcutaneous phycomycosis is characterized by a chronic, painless, firm, well-demarcated swelling of the subcutaneous tissues. Early lesions are firmly attached to the skin, but are freely movable over deeper tissues. The skin over the lesion is usually intact, but ulceration, abscess formation and secondary infection may occur. In more advanced lesions, infiltration of muscle and occasionally deeper tissues may occur. *Basidiobolus* was isolated from the subcutaneous tissues, as well as the muscles of the neck and the pharynx of a Nigerian child.

Lesions may occur on any part of the body including the face. They may be localized, or may involve an extensive area. The buttocks and thighs are most frequently involved. The legs are more frequently affected than the arms, and the proximal end is affected more often than the distal.

In a few cases multiple isolated lesions have been observed (46, 76, 97) (Fig. 11-1). Histological evidence of extension to the viscera was reported in one case (27), but there was no evidence of haematogenous dissemination. A case of disseminated infection by a Phycomycete in a woman from Iraq (84) was once considered to be subcutaneous phycomycosis (15). The absence of mycological proof and the atypical clinical picture suggests that this is more likely to have been a case of mucormycosis (75).

Age and Sex

Subcutaneous phycomycosis is predominantly a disease of childhood and adolescence, but it occurs in all age groups. The youngest case was six months old (98), and the eldest eighty

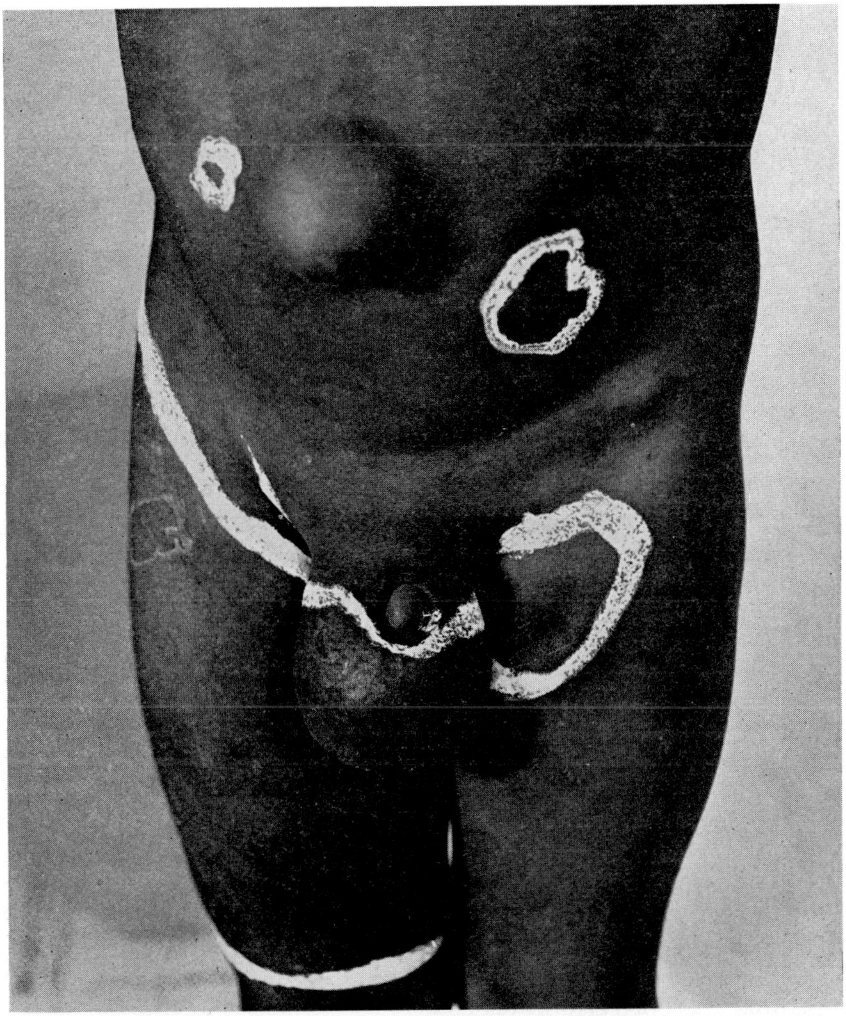

Figure 11-1. Basidiobolomycosis in a five-year-old boy. Extensive lesion involving the right thigh and scrotum. Smaller isolated lesions on the left thigh and abdomen.

years old (1). Of 116 cases of which the age was known, 50 percent were ten years or less, and 80 percent were not more than twenty years of age. Coremans-Pelseneer (18) found that the highest incidence was amongst children aged five to nine years, and that 75 percent of the patients were less than fifteen years of age.

It has been suggested that the high incidence of subcutaneous phycomycosis in children may be due to the fact that adults have acquired immunity as a result of subclinical infection (71). It has also been attributed to the tendency of children, particularly boys in the tropics, to go about naked or scantily clad (96).

The disease occurs more frequently in males than in females. Of 116 patients whose sexes are known, 69 percent were males. A higher male incidence of 80 percent has been reported (18).

RHINO-ENTOMOPHTHOROMYCOSIS

Rhino-entomophthoromycosis is a chronic granulomatous lesion of the upper respiratory tract and face. It is caused by *Entomophthora coronata.* This disease is also called Rhinophycomycosis Entomophthorae (76), Phycomycosis Entomophthorae (32), and Entomophorosis (101).

Natural Habitat

E. coronata occurs in soil and decaying vegetation. It has been isolated in the U.S.A. (20), Colombia (40), Nigeria (15), Australia (35), New Guinea and the Bismarck Archipelago (63). It has also been isolated from soil collected from flower pots in greenhouses in Sweden (44).

E. coronata is a pathogen of insects, which probably facilitate the dissemination of the fungus. It has been isolated from termites in Cuba (61) and the U.S.A. (108), from aphids in the U.S.A. (45) and Sweden (44), and from mosquitoes in the U.S.A. (69). The fungus has never been isolated from the gastrointestinal tract of vertebrates.

Experimental studies indicate that the growth of *E. coronata* is strongly influenced by environmental conditions. It has been found that the optimum temperature for germination of the conidia, varied with the substrate. Maximum germination was obtained at 16 degrees C on a nutrient substrate, whereas on glass it was obtained at 30 degrees C. Conidial germination did not occur below a humidity of 95 percent and was maximum at 100 percent (107). These findings are relevant to the geographical distribution of rhino-entomophthoromycosis.

Geographical Distribution

Rhino-entomophthoromycosis occurs in tropical regions, particularly in areas of high humidity. The first mycologically proven case in man was reported in 1965 (7). Since then over thirty cases have been diagnosed (Table 11-II). Mycological confirmation has not been obtained in all cases, and some of these were diagnosed retrospectively (15, 76, 105).

TABLE 11-II

CASES OF RHINO-ENTOMOPHTHOROMYCOSIS

Country	*No.*	*Cases*	*References*
Nigeria	19	(11)	15, 16, 46, 74, 75, 76
Zaire	3	(2)	81, 105
Cameroun	3	(1)	6, 15, 66, 75
Rep. Central Africa	1	(0)	15, 80
Senegal	1	(0)	5, 15
India	3	(0)	15, 64
Cayman Islands	1	(1)	7
Brazil	1	(1)	2
Colombia	1	(1)	82
Puerto Rico ?	1	(0)	15, 89, 109
?	2	(1)	4, 15, 94

( ) = No. of mycologically proven cases of rhino-entomophthoromycosis.

E. coronata was first reported as a cause of granulomatous lesions of the nostril and lip of horses in Texas (8, 33). Since then similar mycologically proven lesions have been reported in horses from Colombia (83) and Australia (48, 58), and in mules from Brazil (59) and Colombia (83). Rhino-entomophthoromycosis has also been reported in a chimpanzee from Tanzania (85).

Pathogenesis and Clinical Features

The primary site of infection is the submucosa of the nostril, usually the inferior turbinate (75). The incubation period is not known, and the means whereby the fungus gains access to the submucosa is uncertain. Inhalation of spores, given suitable conditions for their germination, and invasion of the mucosa has been postulated. Insect bites or accidentally self-inflicted wounds have also been suggested (76).

The lesion in the nose is a firm granuloma, which causes nasal obstruction, and symptoms common to many other nasal diseases. The fungus spreads internally and externally. Internally the nasopharynx, palate oropharynx and paranasal sinuses are involved. Lesions in the pharynx may be sufficiently extensive to cause compression of the larynx. Externally, the lesion usually first appears on the dorsum of the nose. From here, it spreads to the glabella, central region of the forehead, nasolabial fold, cheek and upper lip.

The lesions on the face are firm, with well defined edges, similar to those of subcutaneous phycomycosis. In contrast, early lesions of rhino-entomophthoromycosis are firmly fixed to deeper structures, but the skin is movable over them. As the lesions become larger, the skin is gradually immobilized. Ulceration usually does not occur.

The tissues of the face lateral to the zygoma and below the angle of the mouth, are not involved. Neither are the supra-orbital region nor the temporal fossa. Extension beyond these limits occurs only in cases of surgical interference at the edge of the lesion (74, 75, 76) (Fig. 11-2).

There is no mycological evidence of lymphatic or haematogenous dissemination. In a fatal case of proven rhino-entomophthoromycosis in which there was secondary bacterial infection, lesions histologically similar to those of the nose and sinuses were found in the lower lobes of the lungs (94).

Age and Sex

Rhino-entomophthoromycosis is predominantly a disease of adults, but occasionally adolescents and children are affected. Of thirty-three cases in which the ages are known, the youngest was an eight-year-old girl from Brazil (2), and the eldest a sixty-year-old Nigerian woman (15, 46). Only three patients were less than twenty years of age (2, 4, 7, 15). Of the remaining thirty cases, 60 percent were between twenty and twenty-nine years of age.

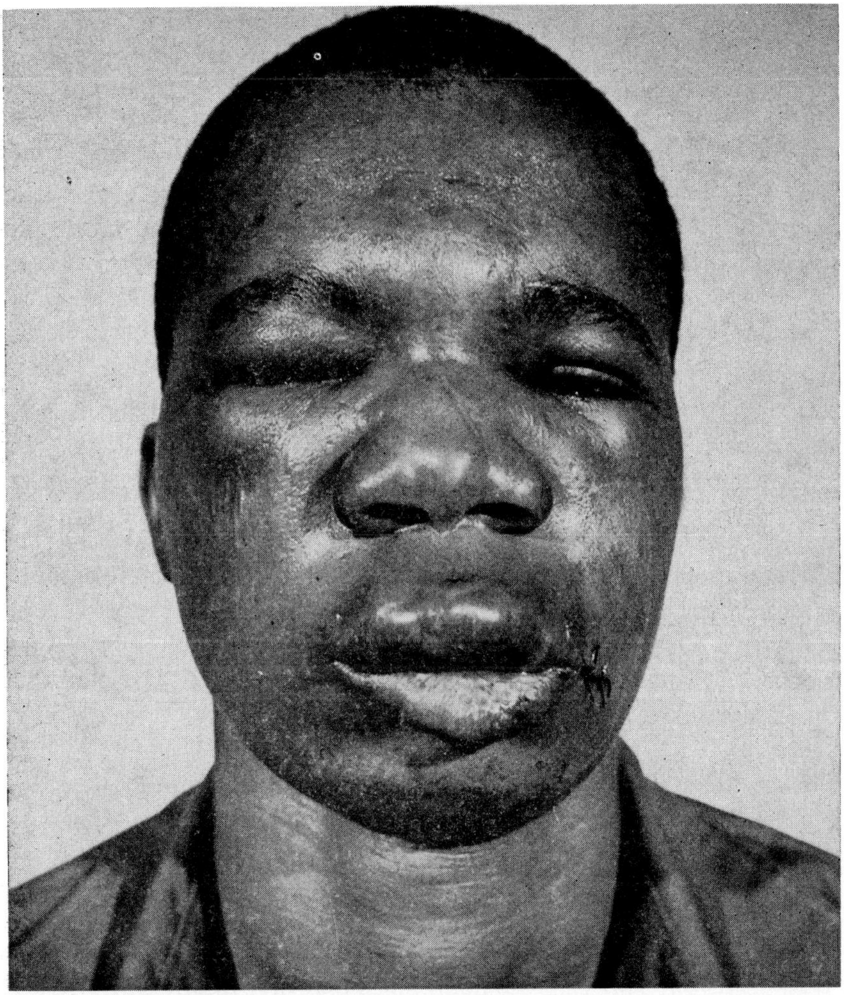

Figure 11-2. Rhino-entomophthoromycosis. Extension of the lesion to the lower lip, as a result of a biopsy taken at the angle of the mouth.

Rhino-entomophthoromycosis is seen more frequently in males than females. Of thirty-five patients of whom the sexes are known, 83 percent were males.

An association of the incidence of rhino-entomophthoromycosis with outdoor occupations has previously been inferred (15). This does not explain the higher incidence of this mycosis in adult males. Women frequently assist in agriculture, and children spend a lot of time outdoors. The high incidence in males also makes it difficult to attribute the prevalence of the mycosis in adults to the loss or lack of immunity acquired in childhood.

PROGNOSIS, THERAPY AND DIFFERENTIAL DIAGNOSIS

The duration of both rhino-entomophthoromycosis and the lesion of subcutaneous phycomycosis, varies from one month to years (55, 75). It is not always possible to follow-up the patients until the final outcome of the infection. Spontaneous recovery has not been reported in rhino-entomophthoromycosis possibly because many of the patients have been treated (75). But, however, such recovery has been reported in subcutaneous phycomycosis (55, 56), as well as recovery after complete or partial excision of the lesion (12, 55, 72). Also complete recovery following therapy with potassium iodide has been reported (12, 46, 55). However, the reports on the response to partial excision, and treatment with chemotherapeutic agents in rhino-entomophthoromycosis have been with variable results.

Two fatal cases have been reported in rhino-entomophthoromycosis. In one the cause of death was not stated (94), and in the other case it was attributed to pneumonia caused by a bacteria.

Subcutaneous phycomycosis is seldom fatal. In one case death occurred as a result of intestinal obstruction (27), and in a second case in a Nigerian child, death was probably due to pharngo-laryngeal obstruction. Death from tetanus occurred in a third Nigerian child, the infection was probably secondary to severe ulceration of the affected leg. Four other fatal cases have been recorded, but there was no evidence that death was attributable to the mycosis (5, 47, 57, 97).

The anatomical distribution of the lesions of rhino-entomophthoromycosis, differentiates it clinically from subcutaneous phycomycosis (74, 75, 76).

Two reports of probable rhino-entomophthoromycosis, have been included under subcutaneous phycomycosis. Both cases lacked mycological confirmation, and the distribution of the lesions was atypical. The case from Malagasy was originally reported as subcutaneous phycomycosis of the face (9). It was subsequently suggested that this might have been a case of rhino-entomophthoromycosis (21). The second case was that of an eleven-year-old boy from Chad (23).

OTHER ENTOMOPHTHOROMYCOSES

There is one mycologically proven case of entomophthoromycosis, caused by a fungus which was neither a *Basidiobolus* nor *Entomophora coronata.* This was a case of a mediastinal granuloma, which involved the root of both lungs and the pericaridium. The lesion occurred in a fifteen-month-old boy, who lived in the temperate zone in the U.S.A. The fungus isolated was identified as a species of *Entomophthora,* which was definitely not *E. coronata.* The patient was successfully treated with amphotericin B. The mode of infection was not known, but it was suggested that it might have resulted from the inhalation of an infected insect (16, 26, 38).

Four cases of entomophthoromycosis of the face, which have been reported in the literature, have not been included under subcutaneous phycomycosis or rhino-entomophthoromycosis in this chapter. The reasons for this are that none of these cases were confirmed mycologically, and the descriptions of the anatomical distribution of the lesions are inadequate. They include two males aged fifty and fifty-five years, from Cameroun (22), a thirty-two-year-old male from the Republic of Central Africa (23) and a twenty-five-year-old male from Zaire (105).

Two cases of entomophthoromycosis of the face in Kenyans have also not been included, because of lack of adequate information of the anatomical distribution of the lesions. In one of these cases, an unidentified species of *Entomophthora* was isolated from a lesion on the forehead of a forty-nine-year-old male. There was no mycological diagnosis in the second case.

A histological picture, similar to that of entomophthoromycosis, was seen in a fatal case of phycomycosis, in a three-year-old boy in the U.S.A. (62). The evolution of the disease and the autopsy findings suggest that this was probably a case of mucormycosis.

Our present knowledge of the epidemiology of the entomophthoromycosis is still grossly inadequate. This is partially due to lack of clinical awareness of these mycoses, and the lack of adequate laboratory facilities in some areas. The tendency of some patients to avoid seeking medical attention, except when the lesions are physically incapacitating, or are causing disfigurement, is also a contributing factor.

Population surveys of the incidence of hypersensitivity are not yet possible. Precipitin antibodies have been demonstrated in patients with proven basidiobolomycosis (16). This technique has not been sufficiently standardized or tested, to establish whether or not it could be used in diagnosing early cases of entomophthoromycosis.

A detailed assessment of the immunological status and a mycological diagnosis of patients with clinical lesions is also essential.

The lack of agreement among mycologists, on the validity of criteria used in identifying fungi belonging to the family Entomophthoraceae, is also a major contributing factor. This problem will not be solved until we know more about the factors which affect the variation, adaptability and possibly mutation of these fungi.

Until these problems have been overcome, it will not be possible to give an accurate account of the epidemiology of the entomophthoromycoses. Nor will it be possible to explain why, although *Basidiobolus* and *E. coronata* are such ubiquitous fungi, there is not a higher incidence of basidiobolomycosis and rhinoentomophthoromycosis, particularly in the tropics.

REFERENCES

1. Abrol, B. M., Mohapatra, L. N.: Personal communication.
2. Andrade, Z. A., Paula, L. A., Sherlock, I. A., Cheever, A. W.: Nasal

granuloma caused by *Entomophthora coronata*. *Am J Trop Med Hyg, 16*:31, 1967.

3. Angate, Y., Ouedraogo, H., Diarra, S., Camain, R.: Sur un cas de phycomycose en Cote-d'Ivoire. *Bull Soc Pathol Exot, 56*:112, 1963.
4. Ash, J. E., Raum, M.: An atlas of otolaryngic pathology. Washington, D. C.: *Armed Forces Instit Pathol*, 1956.
5. Bassett, A., Camain, R., Lariviere, M.: Trois cas senegalais de phycomycose. *Bull Pathol Exot, 56*:108, 1963.
6. Blache, R., Destombes, P., Nazimoff, O.: Nouvelles mycoses souscutanees au Sud-Cameroun. *Bull Soc Pathol Exot, 54*:56, 1961.
7. Bras, G., Gordon, C. C., Emmons, C. W., Prendegast, K. M., Sugar, M.: A case of phycomycosis observed in Jamaica: infection with *Entomophthora coronata. Am J Trop Med Hyg, 14*:141, 1965.
8. Bridges, C. H., Romane, W. M., Emmons, C. W.: Phycomycosis of horses caused by *Entomophthora coronata. J Am Vet Med Assoc, 140*:673, 1962.
9. Brygoo, E. R.: Service d'epidemiologie et de parasitologie. *Arch Inst Pasteur Madagascar, 33*:174, 1964.
10. Brygoo, E. R.: Inventaire des agents de mycoses des vertebres a Madagascar. *Arch Inst Pasteur Madagascar, 36*:29, 1967.
11. Burkitt, D. P., Wilson, A. M. M., Jelliffe, D. B.: Subcutaneous phycomycosis. *E Afr Med J, 40*:34, 1963.
12. Burkitt, D. P., Wilson, A. M. M., Jelliffe, D. B.: Subcutaneous phycomycosis: a review of thirty-one cases seen in Uganda. *Br Med J, 1*:1969, 1964.
13. Cameron, H. M., Gatti, D., Bremner, A. D.: Personal communication. Cameron, H. M., 1972.
14. Chantarakul, N., Talax, P., Vareenil, J.: Subcutaneous phycomycosis. *J Med Assoc, Thailand 48*:740, 1965.
15. Clark, B. M.: *In* Ciba Foundation symposium on systematic mycoses. London: J. & A. Churchill Ltd., 1968.
16. Clark, B. M.: Unpublished observation.
17. Connole, M. D.: Equine phycomycosis. *Aust Vet J, 49*:214, 1973.
18. Coremans-Pelseneer, J.: Epidemiologie de la basidiobolomycose. *Ann Soc Belge Med Trop, 52*:315, 1972.
19. Coremans-Pelseneer, J.: Las phycomycetes pathogenes pour l'homme et les animaux in regions tropicales. Mem. Acad. Roy. Sci. Outremer, *Clin Sci Nat Med, 18*:3, 1972.
20. Couch, J. N.: A new *Conidiobolus* with sexual reproduction. *Am J Bot, 3*:119, 1939.
21. Destombes, P.: Histopathologie des mycoses et des fausses mycoses. *Arch Inst Pasteur Alger, 46*:5, 1968.

22. Destombes, P., Poirer, A., Nazimoff, O.: Mycoses profondes reconnues en 9 ans de pratique histopathologique a l'Institut du Cameroun. *Bull Soc Pathol Exot, 63*:310, 1970.
23. Destombes, P., Ravisse, P., Nazimoff, O.: Bilan des mycoses profondes establi en vingt annees d'histopathologie a l'Institut Pasteur de Brazzaville. *Bull Soc Pathol Exot, 63*:315, 1970.
24. Drechsler, C.: A *Basidiobolus* producing elongated secondary conidia and adhesive beaks. *Bull Torrey Bot Club, 74*:403, 1947.
25. Drechsler, C.: A southern *Basidiobolus* forming many sporangia from globose and from elongated adhesive conidia. *J Wash Acad Sci, 45*:49, 1955.
26. Eckert, H. L., Khoury, G. H., Pore, R. S., Gillbert, E. F., Gaskell, J. R.: Deep *Entomophthora* phycomycotic infection reported for the first time in the United States. *Chest, 61*:392, 1972.
27. Edington, G. M.: Phycomycosis in Ibadan, Western Nigeria. Two postmortem reports. *Trans R Soc Trop Med Hyg 58*:242, 1964.
28. Eidam, E.: *Basidiobolus* eine nue gattug der Entomophthoraceen. *Beit Biol Pfl, 4*:181, 1886.
29. Elebute, E. A., Okubadejo, O. A.: Subcutaneous phycomycosis in a Nigerian. *W Afr Med J, 11*:217, 1962.
30. El Hassan, A. M., Arbab, B., Mahgoub, E. S., Wahab, S.: Phycomycosis. *Trans Roy Soc Trop Med Hyg, 64*:134, 1970.
31. Emmons, C. W.: *In* Ciba Foundation symposium on systemic mycoses, London: J. & A. Churchill Ltd., 1968.
32. Emmons, C. W., Binford, C. H., Utz, J. P.: Medical Mycology (2nd ed.). Philadelphia: Lea & Febiger, 1970.
33. Emmons, C. W., Bridges, C. H.: *Entomophthora coronata* the etiologic agent of phycomycosis of horses. *Mycologia, 53*:307, 1961.
34. Fomufod, A. K., Anita, A. U.: Successful treatment of subcutaneous phycomycosis with trimethorpim-sulfamethoxazole (septrin). *Trop Geogr Med, 23*:208, 1971.
35. Frey, D.: Isolation of keratinophilic and other fungi from soils collected in Australia and New Guinea. *Mycologia, 57*:202, 1965.
36. Gamet, A., Brottes, H.: Processus pseudo-tumoral du a un phycomycete: *Basidiobolus ranarum*. *Bull Soc Pathol Exot, 56*:285, 1963.
37. Gatti, F., Renoirte, P., Nootens, J., Seynhaeve, V.: Premier cas de phycomycose sous-cutanee due a *Basidiobolus meristosporus* observe en Republique du Democratique du Congo. *Ann Soc Belge Med Trop, 48*:455, 1968.
38. Gilbert, E. F., Khoury, G. H., Pore, R. S.: Histopathological identification of *Entomophthora* phycomycosis, deep mycotic infection in an infant. *Arch Pathol, 90*:583, 1970.
39. Glasson, M., Dorman, D. C.: Personal communication. Dorman, D. C., 1973.
40. Greer, D. L.: Personal communication, 1973.

41. Greer, D. L., Friedman, L.: Studies on the genus *Basidiobolus* with reclassification of the species pathogenic for man. *Sabouraudia, 4*:231, 1966.
42. Grover, S., Agarwal, R. V.: Subcutaneous phycomycosis. *J Ind Med Assoc, 56*:315, 1971.
43. Grueber, H. L. E.: Subcutaneous phycomycosis in India. *J Christ Med Assoc India, 41*:284, 1966.
44. Gustafsson, M.: On the species of the genus *Entomophthora* Fries in Sweden. I. Classification and distribution. *Lantbr-Hogsk Annlr, 31*:103, 1965.
45. Hall, I. M., Dunn, P. H.: Entomophthorous fungi parasitic on the spotted alfalfa aphid. *Hilgardia, 27*:159, 1957.
46. Harman, R. R. M., Jackson, H., Willis, A. J. P.: Subcutaneous phycomycosis in Nigeria. *Br J Derm, 76*:408, 1964.
47. Hoo, T. T., Eng, N.-I. T., Joe, L. K.: Two new cases of subcutaneous found in Indonesia. *Dermatol Trop, 1*:23, 1962.
48. Hutchins, D. R., Johnston, K. G.: Phycomycosis in horses. *Aust Vet J, 48*:269, 1972.
49. Hutt, M. S. R.: In Ciba Foundation symposium on systemic mycoses. P. 193. London: J. & A. Churchill Ltd., 1968.
50. Hutt, M. S. R.: Personal communication, 1973.
51. Ive, F. A.: Subcutaneous phycomycosis—report of a case and assessment of treatment with amphotericin *B. Dermatol Int,* 5:203, 1966.
52. Jelliffe, D. B., Burkitt, D., O'Conor, G. T., Beaver, P. C.: Subcutaneous phycomycosis in an East African child. *J Pediatr,* 59:124, 1961.
53. Jelliffe, D. B., Wilson, A. M. M., Burkitt, D.: Subcutaneous phycomycosis responding to oral iodide therapy. *J Pediatr, 61*:448, 1962.
54. Joe, L. K., Eng, N.-I. T.: Subcutaneous phycomycosis: a new disease found in Indonesia. *Ann N Y Acad Sci, 89*:4, 1960.
55. Joe, L. K., Eng, N.-I. T.: Phycomycosis in tropical countries. *Med J Malaya, 16*:206, 1962.
56. Joe, L. K., Eng, N.-I. T., Pohan, A., Van Der Meulen, H., Emmons, C. W.: *Basidiobolus ranarum* as a cause of subcutaneous mycosis in Indonesia. *Arch Derm, 74*:378, 1956.
57. Joe, L. K., Harsono, T., Rukmono, Eng, N.-I. T.: Subcutaneous phycomycosis in man in Indonesia: description of three new cases. *J Trop Med Hyg, 65*:38, 1962.
58. Johnston, K. G.: Subcutaneous phycomycosis and swamp cancer in horses. *Aust Vet J, 47*:576, 1971.
59. Johnston, M. J., Sorensen, B., Saliba, A. M., Lacaz, C. Das, Neto, J. B., Cruz, J. M.: Ficomicse em muar. Isolamento da *Entomophthora coronata. Arch Inst Biol* (S. Paulo), *34*:51, 1967.
60. Kamlan, A.: Personal communication, 1973.

61. Kevorkian, A. G.: Studies in the Entomorphoraceae. I. Observations on the genus *Conidiobolus*. *J Agr Univ P Rico, 21*:191, 1937.
62. King, J. C., Dunphy, D.: Fatal phycomycosis without underlying disease. *J Iowa Med Soc, 62*:485, 1972.
63. Kjoller, A.: Microfungi isolated from tropical soils. With notes on *Trichoderma viride* and *Delacroixia coronata*. *Bot Tidsskr, 62*:323, 1967.
64. Klokke, A. H., Job, C. K., Warlow, P. F. M.: Subcutaneous phycomycosis in India. Report of four patients with a review of the disease. *Trop Geogr Med, 18*:20, 1966.
65. Koshi, G., Kurien, T., Sudursanam, D., Sei Vepandian, A. J., Mammen, K. E.: Subcutaneous phycomycosis caused by *Basidiobolus*. A report of three cases. *Sabouraudia, 10*:237, 1972.
66. Larribaud, J., Marcy, J., Dischamps, G., Pazat, R.: Un cas de rhinophycomycose. *Presse Med, 77*:1011, 1969.
67. Lasch, E. E., Luong N'G. T., Romani, J.: A propos d'un cas de phycomycose en Republique de Haute-Volta. *Med Trop, 25*:642, 1965.
68. Levisohn, I.: Beitrag zur entwicklungsgeschichte und biologie von *Basidiobolus ranarum* Eidam. *Jb wiss Bot, 66*:513, 1927.
69. Lowe, R. E., Rumbauch, R. B., Patterson, R. S.: *Entomophthora coronata* as a pathogen for mosquitoes. *J Invertebr Pathol, 11*, 5U6, 1968.
70. Lowenthal, W.: Beitrage zur kenntnis des *Basidiobolus lactertae* Eidam. *Arch Prostistenk, 2*:364, 1903.
71. Lucas, A. O.: *In* Ciba Foundation symposium on systemic mycoses. p. 201. London: J. & A. Churchill Ltd., 1968.
72. Lynch, J. B., Husband, A. D.: Subcutaneous phycomycosis. *J Clin Pathol, 15*:126, 1962.
73. Mankodi, R. C., Mohapatra, L. N.: Personal communication. Mohapatra, L. N., 1973.
74. Martinson, F. D.: Rhinophycomycosis. *J Laryngol Otol, 77*:691, 1963.
75. Martinson, F. D.: Clinical epidemiological and therapeutic aspects of entomophthoromycosis. *Ann Soc Belg Med Trop, 52*:329, 1972.
76. Martinson, F. D., Clark, B. M.: Rhinophycomycosis entomophthorae in Nigeria. *Am J Trop Med Hyg, 16*:40, 1967.
77. Mukerjee, S., Gore, S. B., Mansukhani, S. N., Kini, V. M.: Subcutaneous phycomycosis. *Ind J Child Hlth, 11*:502, 1962.
78. Nayak, N. C., Das, G. N.: Cited by Tunnell, N., Grueber, H. L. E., Samuel, I., 1968.
79. Neville, G., Miller, R.: Cited by Burkitt, D. P., Wilson, A. M. M., Jelliffe, D. B., 1964.
80. Peloux, Y., Foucard, H.: La phycomycose. *Med Trop 24*:447, 1964.

81. Rendirte, R., Vandepitte, J., Gatti, F., Werth, R.: Phycomycose naso-faciale (rhinophycomycose) due a *Entomophthora coronata*. *Bull Soc Pathol Exot, 58*:847, 1965.
82. Restrepo, M. A., Greer, D. L., Robledo, V. M., Diaz, G. C., Lopez, M. R., Bravo, R. C.: Subcutaneous phycomycosis: report of the first case observed in Colombia, South America. *A J Trop Med Hyg, 16*:34, 1967.
83. Restrepo, M. L. F., Morales, L. F., Robledo, V. M., Restrepo, M. A., Restrepo, S. G., Correa, R. I.: Rinoficomicosis por *Entomophthora coronata* en equinos. Informe sobre 15 cases. Antioquia Medical. In press.
84. Ridley, D. S., Wise, M.: Unusual disseminated infection with a Phycomycete. *J Pathol Bact, 90*:675, 1965.
85. Roy, A. D., Cameron, H. M.: Rhinophycomycosis entomophthorae occurring in a chimpanzee in the wild in East Africa. *Am J Trop Med Hyg, 21*:234, 1972.
86. Sirol, J., Delphy, P., Brottes, H., Guard, O.: Un cas de phycomycose observe au Tchad. *Bull Soc Pathol Exot, 64*:322, 1971.
87. Srinivasan, M. C., Thirumalachar, M. J.: *Basidiobolus* species pathogenic for man. *Sabouraudia, 4*:32, 1965.
88. Stockdale, P. M.: Personal communication, 1964.
89. Straatsma, B. R., Zimmerman, L. E., Gass, J. D. M.: Phycomycosis. A clinicopathologic study of fifty-one cases. *Lab Invest, 11*:963, 1962.
90. Stublier, R., Filaudeau, G., Ravisse, P.: Premier cas de phycomycose observe au Congo-Brazaville avec isolement de *Basidiobolus meristosporus*. *Bull Soc Pathol Exot, 63*:28, 1970.
91. Symmers, W. St. C.: Mucormycotic granuloma possibly due to *Basidiobolus ranarum*. *Br Med J, 1*:1331, 1960.
92. Symmers, W. St. C.: Further cases of exotic mycoses seen in Britain. Trans. *Roy Soc Trop Med Hyg, 55*:201, 1961.
93. Symmers, W. St. C.: Fungi in human and animal disease. *Proc R Soc Med, 57*:405, 1964.
94. Symmers, W. St. C.: Histopathology of phycomycosis. *Ann Soc Belge Med Trop, 52*:365, 1972.
95. Thasnakorn, P., Striboonma, V., Chantarakul, N., Bhadrakom, S.: Subcutaneous phycomycosis due to *Basidiobolus meristosporus*. Report of a case. *J Med Assoc Thailand, 52*:372, 1969.
96. Tio, H.: *In* Essays on tropical dermatology. Amsterdam: Excerpta Medica, 1972.
97. Tio, T. H., Djojopranoto, M., Joe, L. K.: Subcutaneous phycomycosis. *Arch Dermatol, 93*:550, 1966.
98. Tunnell, N., Grueber, H. L. E., Samuel, I.: Subcutaneous phycomycosis. *J Ind Med Assoc, 51*:355, 1968.

99. Ulehla, V., Moravek, V.: Uber die wirkung von sauren und salzen auf *Basidiobolus ranarum. Eid Ber Dt Bot Ges, 40*:8, 1922.
100. Vanbreuseghem, R.: *Guide Pratique de Mycologia Medicale et Veterinaire.* Paris, Masson et Cie. 1966.
101. Vanbreuseghem, R., Renoirte, A. M.: Evolution and treatment of a case of basidiobolomycosis. (Subcutaneous phycomycosis by *Basidiobolus meristosporus.)* Vth international congress of infectious diseases. Vienna. 1970.
102. Van Overeem, C.: Beitrage zur pilzflora von Niederlandisch Indian II. 10. Ueber ein merkwuerdiges vorkommen von *Basidiobolus ranarum* Eidam. *Bull Jard Bot Buitenz, 7*:423, 1925.
103. Villasco, J., Camain, R., Mazere, J., Orio, J., Segretain, G.: Description d'un deuxieme cas de phycomycose en Cote d'Ivoire avec isolement de la souche. *Bull Soc Pathol Exot, 59*:781, 1966.
104. Welchman, J. M.: Subcutaneous phycomycosis. *Br Med J, 2*:191, 1964.
105. Werth, R., Sabwe-Mubangu, J., Gatti, F., Bastin, J. P.: In *Deep Mycoses of the Tropics.* Antwerp, Prince Leopold Inst Trop Med, 1972.
106. Wilson, A. M. M.: Phycomycetes isolated from subcutaneous phycomycosis in Uganda. *Nature (London), 191*:612, 1961.
107. Yendol, W. G.: Factors affecting germination of *Entomophthora* conidia. *J. Invertebr Pathol, 10*:116, 1968.
108. Yendol, W. G., Paschke, J. D.: Pathology of an *Entomophthora* infection in the eastern subterranean termite *Reticulitermes flavipes* (Kollar). *J Invert Pathol, 7*:434, 1965.
109. Zimmerman, L. E.: Personal communciation, 1966.
110. Zylstra, W.: Personal communication, 1973.

Chapter 12

THE EPIDEMIOLOGY OF MUCORMYCOSIS

Roger Denio Baker

The disease was originally called mucormycosis by nineteenth century European pathologists and mycologists because *Mucor* had been isolated from cases (6, 13, 23). The first well-documented cases of this disease were reported by Gregory et al. in 1943 (14). This is a splendid clinicopathologic description of three postmortems of patients with acidotic diabetes mellitus who succumbed to mucormycosis in from two to five days. Today, we know that diabetes compromises the host, that is, makes him more susceptible to infection than a normal person. The diagnosis in these patients was made histopathologically by finding broad, nonseptate hyphae branching at right angles in the tissues. No fungi were grown. The authors used the term *mucormycosis* because the organisms in tissue sections looked like the organisms in previously reported cases of mucormycosis. It was generally believed that *Mucor* was the cause of mucormycosis. However, Bauer et al. recovered *Rhizopus oryzae,* from a patient with cerebral mucormycosis in 1955 (7); Harris, *R. arrhizus* from his case in 1955 (16); and Baker et al., *R. rhizopodiformis* in 1962 (5).

In the 1960's the term *phycomycosis* began to be used for infections with broad, nonseptate hyphae in tissues. Subcutane-

The opinions or assertions contained herein are the private views of the author and are not to be construed as official or as reflecting the views of the Department of the Army or the Department of Defense.

ous phycomycosis, described in Indonesia in 1956, belonged in this category histologically, but the disease was totally different from mucormycosis. Subcutaneous phycomycosis occurred in persons with no underlying condition. It was caused by *Basidiobolus haptosporus* and was chronic, lasted for about a year, and then disappeared spontaneously. Histopathologic examination revealed hyaline collars about the fungal hyphae, making diagnostic separation of this disease from mucormycosis simple. Another disease, entomophthoromycosis caused by *Entomophthora coronata,* was described in Africa and was similar to subcutaneous phycomycosis. In man there are three distinct diseases, three phycomycoses, rather than a single phycomycosis. The term *mucormycosis* should be retained for the acute, infarct-producing, opportunistic disease encountered in patients with neoplasia or diabetes.

The epidemiology of mucormycosis, like the epidemiology of other opportunistic infections, reflects decreased resistance to infection in the compromised host. The mold fungi that cause mucormycosis are ubiquitous, do not grow in healthy tissues, but are able to infect the compromised host. Mucormycosis is not a contagious disease. It is not spread from person to person and insects play no role as vectors.

THE MUCORACEAE CAUSING MUCORMYCOSIS

Among 255 cases of histopathologically diagnosed mucormycosis reported in the world literature up to mid-1968, Mucoraceae were grown from only forty-three subjects (3). The diagnosis of the disease was made by seeing the characteristic coenocytic (nonseptate), broad hyphae with right-angled branches in tissue sections. Although material for culture was planted on culture media in many cases, it was a common experience to obtain no growth of fungi.

Interestingly, Neame and Raynor were able to obtain cultures from many of their cases of gastrointestinal mucormycosis. They attributed their success to using culture medium enriched with ordinary white bread (22).

Forty-five cultures were obtained from forty-three cases reviewed by the author because three different species were obtained from one case (3). There were thirty-two *Rhizopus* cultures, ten *Mucor*, and two *Absidia*. The forty-fifth culture was described as a "fungus of the Mucorales order."

It was surprising to learn that the predominant organism in patients with mucormycosis was not *Mucor* but *Rhizopus*. Mucoraceae is the family of the Phycomycetes that includes all three of the causative genera of mucormycosis, namely *Rhizopus*, *Mucor*, and *Absidia*. The order Zygomycetales is characterized by zygote formation in the sexual stage and includes the family Mucoraceae.

The species were reported in some of the forty-five cultures obtained (Table 12-I). The genus *Rhizopus* is characterized by sporangiophores that arise singly or in clusters opposite rhizoids and bear spherical sporangia with spores between sporangial wall and columella (11, 12). *Rhizopus* grows rapidly and fills the Petri dish in four to five days with a cottony aerial mycelium that

TABLE 12-I

FUNGI CULTURED FROM 43 CASES OF MUCORMYCOSIS DIAGNOSED ON THE BASIS OF CHARACTERISTIC NONSEPTATE HYPHAE IN TISSUES, AS REPORTED IN THE LITERATURE UP TO MID-1968

Fungus Cultured	*Number of Cultures*
Rhizopus cultures	
R. oryzae	9
R. arrhizus	5
R. nigricans	5
R. rhizopodiformis	1
R. microsporus	4
Rhizopus	8
Mucor cultures	
M. corymbifer(a)	2
M. hiemalis	1
M. ramosissimus	1
Mucor	6
Absidia cultures	
A. lichtheimi	1
A. ramosa	1
Unspecified cultures	
Fungus belongs to Mucorales	1
Total	45*

*Three cultures were obtained from one case.

is white at first, then dark gray. The genus *Mucor* has a floccose aerial mycelium that is at first white, then dark gray. The rhizoids characteristic of *Rhizopus* are absent. The genus *Absidia* has rhizoids that resemble those of *Rhizopus* but come from the stolons between the sporangiophores, rather than opposite them, as is characteristic of *Rhizopus.*

The *Mucor ramosissimus* in Table 12-I should be ignored because it produced a chronic disease of the face and nose that was different from mucormycosis. On the other hand, *Mucor pusillus* should be added to the list of mucors causing mucormycosis (20). *Cunninghamella elegans* has been isolated from a case of mucormycosis (18). This species is not in the family of Mucoraceae.

THE PREVALENCE OF THE MUCORACEAE

In any infectious disease a prime epidemiologic consideration is the occurrence and prevalence of the causative organism in the environment of the susceptible person. For example, *Histoplasma capsulatum* must be present in the soil of a region if one is to contract histoplasmosis. There are zones of endemicity for histoplasmosis, and in these zones *H. capsulatum* is present in the soil; the disease is contracted by the inhalation of dust containing the mold form of the organism. The same conditions seem to apply to other mycotic diseases. Specific facts are meager concerning the prevalence of *Rhizopus, Mucor* and *Absidia* in soil, dust, and dwellings, and particularly in hospitals, where compromised patients contract mucormycosis.

In the literature, one reads that the Mucoraceae are ubiquitous. The fact that cases of mucormycosis have been reported from all continents indicates that Mucoraceae are present in the environment where the human cases develop. The Mucoraceae are troublesome contaminants in microbiology laboratories, and the medical mycologist is warned not to diagnose mucormycosis simply because *Rhizopus* is found growing in the culture medium of a slant or Petri dish inoculated with sputum or other material from a patient.

Some of the Mucoraceae are economically important because of the spoilage they cause in vegetables, bread and fruits, as in the liquefaction of strawberries. The growth of Mucoraceae may damage electronic components in missiles, aircraft and submarines (27). *Rhizopus nigricans*, the black mold on bread, is a household fungus that grows in the refrigerator and produces spoilage of many foods.

Mucor species are widely distributed in nature, growing saprophytically and parasitically. *Mucor* came into prominence in the early days of the orange juice industry because it seemed to produce a disease around the nail beds of the women processing oranges. *Absidia* is more restricted in its distribution (27).

In 1665 Robert Hooke, in his studies of plant tissue, observed and recorded the common terrestrial fungus *Mucor*. Michele, the father of mycology, who lived from 1679 to 1737, was the first biologist to cultivate fungi. He did this on natural media, such as squash, peas, melons and quince. *Mucor* was among the fungi he cultured.

Now that the species of *Rhizopus*, *Mucor*, and *Absidia* that cause mucormycosis are identified, it will be possible to determine the presence and frequency of these opportunistic pathogens in the environment of man in all parts of the world.

CASES OF MUCORMYCOSIS

The disease is reported from all continents, with a preponderance of cases from North America (3). Table 12-II gives geographic and anatomic distribution.

TABLE 12-II

GEOGRAPHIC DISTRIBUTION OF 255 CASES OF MUCORMYCOSIS CORRELATED WITH THE ANATOMIC FORMS OF THE DISEASE AS REPORTED IN THE LITERATURE UP TO MID-1968

Continent	*Cranial*	*Pulmonary*	*Digestive*	*Disseminated*	*Primary Cutaneous*	*Focal*	*Total*
N. America	79	34	12	31	6	4	166
S. America	4	0	4	0	1	0	9
Europe	10	10	4	3	1	2	30
Asia	8	2	4	2	0	0	16
Africa	2	0	27	0	0	0	29
Australia	4	0	0	1	0	0	5
Total cases	107	46	51	37	8	6	255

Mucormycosis is often a nosocomial, or hospital-acquired, infection. Patients being treated in the hospital for leukemia or renal disease or those immunosuppressed for organ transplantation may be infected with Mucoraceae from the hospital air or dust. The patient may have been a carrier of the fungus, and may have brought it into the hospital with him in a paranasal sinus or ear canal.

Diabetic patients who have mucormycosis usually develop it in their home environment and are brought to the hospital with the disease. The case of Harris, the first patient to recover from cranial mucormycosis, illustrates this sequence of events (16).

PREDISPOSING FACTORS

The epidemiology of mucormycosis is largely a matter of the presence of compromised hosts who are susceptible to these ubiquitous fungi. The formula is as follows: Compromised host *plus* lurking mucoraceous fungus *equals* mucormycosis. Compromised hosts tend to concentrate in cancer hospitals where cytotoxic drugs and corticosteroids are being used and where neutropenia develops in leukemic patients. The prevalence of diabetics also increases the prevalence of immunosuppressed patients.

The most frequent predisposing condition in the cranial form is diabetes. In the pulmonary and disseminated forms, blood dyscrasias, especially leukemias and cutaneous burns are underlying conditions. In the forms affecting the digestive tract the underlying condition is malnutrition.

Predisposing factors toward the development of mucormycosis include the acidosis and uremia of renal insufficiency, neutropenia, antibiotics, antileukemic drugs, corticosteroid drugs, splenectomy, total body irradiation and hypogammaglobulinemia (3). Table 12-III lists these in descending order of frequency.

Diabetes: Diabetes antedates mucormycosis in 70 percent of cranial infections and in a smaller proportion of infections at other sites. Some patients reported in the literature had been on an alcoholic binge and acidosis had been introduced by this indiscretion.

Animal experiments have suggested that acidosis is more important than hyperglycemia in predisposing the diabetic patient to mucormycosis (25).

Corticosteroids given therapeutically may cause a steroid-induced diabetes, which apparently acts like ordinary diabetes in making the patient more susceptible to the development of mucormycosis (18).

LEUKEMIA AND NEUTROPENIA: My studies on fatal mycoses complicating leukemia suggest that medicines are important factors (2). Corticosteroid and antileukemic drugs are more conducive to mucormycosis than bacterial antibiotics. A profound neutropenia in the course of leukemia is often coincident with the onset of the mucormycotic pulmonary infarction demonstrable in roentgenograms. Meyer et al. had patients with neutropenia treated with steroids who developed rhinocerebral mucormycosis (19, 21).

METABOLIC DISTURBANCES: Acidosis is important in the susceptibility of patients to mucormycosis. It accompanies diabetes, renal disease, vomiting, diarrhea and malnutrition. Uremia in renal and hepatic disease is a factor of predisposition to mucormycosis.

CORTICOSTEROID THERAPY: Corticosteroids reduce the effectiveness of the inflammatory response so necessary in combatting infection. The organisms of mucormycosis are too large to be phagocytized by polymorphonuclear neutrophils in the inflamed area.

Systemically administered corticosteroids favor the development of mucormycosis in experimental animals (1, 4), however, there have been human cases of mucormycosis in which corticosteroids were the only predisposing factor. Corticosteroids predispose to infection by stabilizing membranes and reducing the inflammatory response.

MALNUTRITION: Malnutrition acts through the mechanisms of acidosis, hypoproteinemia and reduced cell-mediated immunity.

HODGKIN'S DISEASE AND LYMPHOMA: These diseases may be

complicated by mucormycosis. The immune deficiency of Hodgkin's disease might be implicated.

Other blood dyscrasias: Neutropenia, pancytopenia, agranulocytosis and anemia belong here.

Cutaneous burns: Rabin et al. (24) reported in 1961 the first two patients with disseminated mucormycosis complicating burns. Bruck et al. (9) have recently reported more than a score of such cases. The fungus colonizes in the burn wound and invades surrounding tissues, often disseminating throughout the body. The severe protein loss and acidosis and uremia of the renal failure favor infection. If corticosteroids or intravenous catheters are used, they are also conducive to infection. Moreover, bacterial infections are controlled with antibiotics, which produce conditions in which mucormycosis has an opportunity to develop.

Heroin addiction and intravenous therapy: Chmel and Grieco (10) in 1973 reported the case of a twenty-three-year-old black man who used six bags of heroin daily. He had weakness and difficulty in speaking two days prior to admission to a New York hospital. There were needle tracks in his hands and arms. On the ninth day following the cerebral symptoms, fluid was aspirated from his brain through a burr hole in his skull, and the diagnosis of mucormycosis was made. The patient succumbed postoperatively, and mucormycosis of the brain, right lung, and right kidney was demonstrated at autopsy.

Baker et al. in 1962 reported the case of a seventy-nine-year-old diabetic patient who developed a swollen and reddened right forearm above a venous cannula (5). Material obtained from an unbroken vesicle on the swollen arm revealed *Rhizopus rhizopodiformis* and *Aerobacter aerogenes.* At autopsy the swollen arm showed microabscesses containing the broad hyphae of *Rhizopus.* This patient illustrates entry of the fungus into a compromised host through or around a venous cannula.

Immunosuppression for transplantation: Stinson et al. (26) report a patient with cardiac transplantation who developed rhinocerebral mucormycosis. The patient had been on large doses of prednisone (100 mg/day).

UNKNOWN: Very rarely, a case of mucormycosis is encountered in which there appears to be no predisposing factor.

TABLE 12-III

CONDITIONS PREDISPOSING TO MUCORMYCOSIS

	Predisposing Condition	*Order of Frequency*
1.	Diabetes	++++
2.	Leukemia and neutropenia	+++
3.	Metabolic disturbances	+++
4.	Corticosteroid therapy	++
5.	Malnutrition	++
6.	Hodgkin's disease and lymphoma	++
7.	Other blood dyscrasias	+
8.	Cutaneous burns	+
9.	Heroin addiction; intravenous therapy	+
10.	Immunosuppression for transplantation	+
11.	Unknown	+

DISCUSSION

Mucormycosis is a complication of diabetes mellitus and modern therapeutic regimens. It is drug induced in many instances (1).

In a study of fatal mycotic diseases complicating leukemia, the author reported that these infections at Duke University Hospital and the Veterans Administration Hospital in Durham, N. C., began to appear especially after the advent of the use of antileukemic drugs and corticosteroids (2). Bruck et al. reported complicating disseminated mucormycosis in twenty-two patients with burn wounds (9). Confronted with these data, one asks if there is not some connection between the modern therapy of burns and this unusually large number of infections.

Hale (15) collected data on mucormycosis of infants and children and gave as predisposing factors the following figures: diarrhea and vomiting—twenty-six; diabetes mellitus—three; burn —one; tonsillitis—one; unknown—four.

In explaining the increased incidence of opportunistic fungal infections, Hart et al. (17) reported that they were forced, by the very disease states that compromised their patients, to treat them with drugs that further depressed their ability to withstand infection. They thought that the more intensive employment of immunosuppressive drug therapy in recent years and the combination of this therapy with antibiotics were major causes of the increase in opportunistic infections in the compromised host. They believe that corticosteroids, cytotoxic drugs, antibiotics, irradiation, intravenous fluids and modern surgical procedures may all hamper the host's ability to resist fungal infection. Thus, attempts to prolong life simply allow the opportunistic organisms to cause fatal infections.

Meyer et al. (21) report on twenty-six fatal infections of mucormycosis at a cancer hospital during the ten-year period from 1962 through 1971. All developed in patients with leukemias and lymphomas. Leukopenia was common in patients with lymphomas. They thought that mucormycosis developed because of aggressive therapy of the underlying disease; supportive therapy, including platelet transfusions; and early antibiotic therapy. Patients survived bacterial infections but succumbed to mucormycosis.

Bennett et al. have recently pointed out that there is an upsurge in fungal infections (8). Patients without effective immune defenses are kept alive today by sophisticated chemotherapy and aggressive surgical techniques. These patients often fall prey to infection with opportunistic microorganisms, such as bacteria, viruses, parasites and fungi. Weakly pathogenic organisms, those causing mucormycosis, are able to infect these debilitated hosts. A typical sequence is that which is seen in a patient with a hematologic malignancy who is being treated with cytotoxic agents and corticosteroids; he develops a bacterial infection, perhaps two, and is successfully treated with anti-bacterial antibiotics. Then a shadow appears in the chest roentgenogram, and at autopsy pulmonary mucormycosis is discovered.

PREVENTION OF MUCORMYCOSIS

Mucormycosis could be prevented if the Mucoraceae were eliminated from the immediate environment of the compromised host. This might be accomplished in specialized rooms in hospitals by the use of sterilized bedding, aseptic techniques and filtration of air.

Increasing the resistance to infection in the susceptible person may be achieved by maintaining the diabetic patient in ideal control of his diabetes, by avoiding treatment with systemic corticosteroids, and by giving transfusions of neutrophils to neutropenic patients.

In summary, mucormycosis is an opportunistic fungus infection characterized by the invasion of fungi belonging to the Mucoraceae family of phycomycetes, most often by the genera *Rhizopus*, *Mucor*, or *Absidia*, in that order of frequency. *Rhizopus oryzae* is the species which has been most frequently cultivated from lesions of the disease.

These fungi are ubiquitous and grow rapidly in a Petri dish, at first white, then dark gray. *Rhizopus* and *Absidia* have rhizoids; *Mucor* has none. These fungi cause spoilage of fruits and contaminate laboratory cultures.

More than three hundred cases of human mucormycosis are described in the world literature from all the continents.

Diabetes, hematologic malignancy, especially leukemia, and malnutrition are common underlying diseases that compromise the host and make him susceptible to infection. Acidosis, neutropenia, and corticosteroids are the most important predisposing factors.

Mucormycosis is frequently a nosocomial, hospital-acquired, iatrogenic, drug-induced infection.

The prevention of mucormycosis is dependent upon keeping the Mucoraceae from contact with compromised patients, upon controlling diabetes, avoiding the use of corticosteroids and preventing the development of neutropenia.

REFERENCES

1. Baker, R. D.: Drug-induced mycosis. In: Drug-Induced Diseases. p. 50. Intern. Cong. Ser. No. 85. Excerpta Medica Foundation, Amsterdam, 1965.
2. Baker, R. D.: Leukopenia and therapy in leukemia as factors predisposing to fatal mycoses, mucormycosis, aspergillosis and cryptococcosis. *Am J Clin Pathol*, *37*:358, 1962.
3. Baker, R. D.: Mucormycosis (opportunistic phycomycosis). Chapter 21, p. 832, *in* Baker, R. D., (Ed.): *Human Infection with Fungi, Actinomycetes and Algae.* Springer Verlag, Berlin, Heidelberg, New York, 1970.

4. Baker, R. D., Linares, G.: Prednisolone-induced mucormycosis in rhesus monkeys. *Sabouraudia, 12*:75, 1974.
5. Baker, R. D., Seabury, J. H., Schneidau, J. D.: Subcutaneous and cutaneous phycomycosis. *Lab Invest, 11*:109, 1962.
6. Barthelat, G. J.: Les mucorinnes pathogenes et les mucormycoses chez les animaux et chez l'homme. *Arch Parasit, 7*:1, 1903.
7. Bauer, H., Ajello, L., Adams, E., Hernandez, D.: Cerebral mucormycosis. Pathogenesis of the disease. *Am J Med, 18*:822, 1955.
8. Bennett, J. E., Louria, D. B., Neu, H. C.: In consultation. Fighting the upsurge in fungal infections. *Med World News, 14*:28, 1973.
9. Bruck, H. M., Nash, G., Foley, F. D., Pruitt, B. A., Jr.: Opportunistic fungal infection of the burn wound with phycomycetes and *Aspergillus. Arch Surg, 102*:476, 1971.
10. Chmel, H., Grieco, M. H.: Cerebral mucormycosis and renal aspergillosis in heroin addicts without endocarditis. *Am J Med Sci, 266*:225, 1973.
11. Conant, N. F., Smith, D. T., Baker, R. D., Callaway, J. L.: *Manual of Clinical Mycology,* 3 ed. Philadelphia, Saunders, 1971.
12. Emmons, C. W., Binford, C. H., Utz., J. P.: *Medical Mycology,* 2 ed. Philadelphia, Lea & Febiger, 1970.
13. Furbringer, P.: Beobachtungen uber Lungenmycose beim Menschen. *Virchows Arch Pathol Anat, 66*:330, 1876.
14. Gregory, J. E., Golden, A., Haymaker, W.: Mucormycosis of the central nervous system. A report of three cases. *Bull Johns Hopkins Hosp, 73*:405, 1943.
15. Hale, L. M.: Orbital-cerebral phycomycosis. Report of a case and a review of the disease in infants. *Arch Ophthal, 83*:39, 1971.
16. Harris, J. S., Mucormycosis. Report of a case. *J Pediatr, 16*:857, 1955.
17. Hart, P. D., Russel, E., Jr., Remington, I. S.: The compromised host and infection. II. Deep fungal infections. *J Infect Dis, 120*:169, 1969.
18. Hutter, R. V. P.: Phycomycetous infection (mucormycosis) in cancer patients. A complication of therapy. *Cancer, 12*:330, 1959.
19. Meyer, R. D., Armstrong, D.: Mucormycosis—changing status. *CRC Crit Rev Clin Lab Sci, 421*, Dec., 1973.
20. Meyer, R. D., Kaplan, M. H., Ong, M., Armstrong, D.: Cutaneous lesions in disseminated mucormycosis. *JAMA, 225*:737, 1973.
21. Meyer, R. D., Rosen, P., Armstrong, D.: Phycomycosis complicating leukemia and lymphoma. *Ann Intern Med, 77*:871, 1972.
22. Neame, P., Raynor, D.: Mucormycosis. Report on twenty-two cases. *Arch Pathol, 70*:261, 1960.
23. Podack, M.: Zur Kenntnis des sog. Endothelkrebses der Pleura und die Mucormykosen in menschlichen Respirationsapparat. *Dtsch Arch Klin Med, 63*:1, 1899.

24. Rabin, E. R., Lundberg, G. D., Mitchell, E. T.: Mucormycosis in severely burned patients. Report of two cases with extensive destruction of face and nasal cavity. *N Engl J Med, 264*:1286, 1961.
25. Sheldon, W. H., Bauer, H.: The role of predisposing factors in experimental fungus infections. *Lab Invest, 11*:1184, 1962.
26. Stinson, E. B., Bieber, C. P., Griepp, R. B., Clark, D. A., Shumway, N. E., Remington, J. S.: Infectious complications after cardiac transplantation in man. *Ann Intern Med, 74*:22, 1971.
27. Swatek, F. E.: *Textbook of Microbiology*. St. Louis, Mosby, 1967.

Chapter 13

THE EPIDEMIOLOGY OF ASPERGILLOSIS

JAMES T. SINSKI

ASPERGILLOSIS IS DEFINED as any infection or colonization of tissues or cavities caused by a member of the genus *Aspergillus* (17). This genus includes 150 recognized species and varieties, of which only a small number are pathogenic (56).

Natural Habitat

Members of the genus *Aspergillus* are known to grow world wide. They can be isolated from a large number of natural substances including grains, leaves, and a variety of dry materials, dung, plant rhizophores and soil (56). The life cycle of a member of the genus *Aspergillus* is normally saprophytic and invasion of living tissues should be regarded as incidental to their normal life cycle (6). Many factors enter into the establishment of infection in man, but the fungal spore is considered the main external factor (6). Although all potentially pathogenic members of the genus *Aspergillis* have been found in the soil, they do not appear to constitute a hazard in this habitat (6).

Spores of members of the genus *Aspergillus* are well adapted for possible dispersal. They are lightweight, easily spread in the air, with thick walls and cell membranes resistant to dessication. As an example, the variability of the size and shape of the spores and the length of the conidiophores of *A. fumigatus* (the most frequently isolated from cases of aspergillosis) is much greater in the known pathogenic strains than in the strains that are saprophytic only (56). However, the relationship of these observations to the disease is unknown.

There have been over fifty reports of the isolation of *A. fumigatus* from the soil including one isolation from a zone of Sahara desert (5). In other reports *A. terreus* (42), *A. flavus* (36) and *A. nidulans* (67) have also been isolated. Optimum conditions for growth and sporulation in soil are not known (5), though *A. fumigatus* has been isolated from soil containing appreciable amounts of organic matter (50). Lesions on living plants caused by *A. fumigatus* have been found (5). Cultures made from molded grain left scattered in the field often yield *A. niger, A. glaucus, A. terreus* but rarely yield *A. fumigatus* (17).

Similarly, *Aspergillus* appears to be of world wide distribution and is one of the most frequently isolated fungi from the air (31, 35, 59). Because of a variety of factors influencing the capture and subsequent growth of the organism, comparisons of the results of different studies must be made with reservation. The spore counts given by investigators should not be regarded as absolute but as approximations or indications of trends. In the earlier investigations, settling or gravity plates were used. This is an inefficient method of air sampling compared to the aerosol sampling devices used at the present. In addition to the sampling method and other factors such as the media used and the incubation temperature, it was found that the number of the fungal spores collected (colonies) are affected by a variety of natural factors, namely locality, season, humidity, rain, wind, sunshine, time of day, vegetation, altitude, etc. (5, 10, 31, 35, 48, 54).

Relationships of the Fungus to Host

For infections in man the inhalation of spores is considered a common mode of entry. An active man could inhale 5.7×10^7 spores of all types daily, but *Aspergillus* spores would comprise less than 8 percent of the total. A man working three hours during the peak work time in a barn with hay or grasses would inhale a calculated 8.4×10^7 spores of which 82 percent might be *Aspergillus* and *Mucor* type (5). Because of the size of the *A. fumigatus* spore (2.0 to 3.5 μ) a high portion of such single spores would be expected to be retained deep enough in the lung to escape removal by bronchial ciliary action. Though the levels of spore intake for man that would lead to infection are not known, it must be assumed that the majority of human beings can inhale high doses of *Aspergillus* spores without getting an infection. Though considerable numbers of *Aspergillus* spores were encountered in an isolated community of individuals at the south pole, no individuals developed precipitins during a one-year period though the men supposedly had high respiratory exposure (43). In experimental infections in mice following intravenous injection of viable spores, infection was never observed microscopically in the lungs of these animals (21). It may be that the lungs of normal human beings are equally as efficient in clearing themselves of inhaled spores of *Aspergillus*.

Members of the genus *Aspergillus* have been shown to have strain differences in regard to virulence, metabolic rate and growth rate. Years ago (27) it was reported that many strains of *A. fumigatus* from the air showed no virulence, whereas strains of *A. fumigatus* isolated from spontaneous infections exhibited a surprising degree of virulence. Such differences were found recently in isolates of *A. terreus* (60). Also the human strain grew slower at 25 degrees C, while the soil isolate was found to have a lower metabolic rate. In the more pathogenic strains of *A. terreus*, an increased metabolic rate was accompanied by an increase in virulence and a conversion to thick walled budding yeast in an area of highest concentration of cysteine on these plates.

Aspergillus fumigatus has generally been reported to be the most pathogenic species in man. In a survey of twenty-six patients with pulmonary aspergillosis, none were found to have liver disease before death and no evidence was found of aflatoxins or metabolic products affecting the liver (10). However, necrotic substances can diffuse from *A. fumigatus*, and sparse but definite penetration of mycelium into normal pulmonary tissue has been observed (10). A necrotizing pneumonia may be the result of colonization of pulmonary infarcts (70). In one case of rapidly fatal pulmonary aspergillosis the patient developed a toxic epidermal necrolysis (62).

Types of Infection

The following are recognized as types of infection in aspergillosis. These are pulmonary, disseminated, ocular and cutaneous aspergillosis. Further, aspergilli may cause onychomycosis, otomycosis, endocarditis and mycetoma.

Pulmonary aspergillosis is certainly one of the most important forms of infection with this genus. No figures appear available to allow for accurate comparison with other types of aspergillosis, however, a number of reviews of the world literature, as well as summaries of cases in specific continents, countries and hospitals or clinics are available (3, 10, 20, 24, 28, 30, 33, 34, 40, 41, 46, 50, 53, 54, 58, 66, 71, 74). Pulmonary aspergillosis was considered a rare disease in 1930 (27) and considerably important in 1973. In one clinical center from 1964 to 1969 to 1971 a doubling and quadrupling of the number of cases have been reported (40).

There have been a number of attempts to classify the types of pulmonary aspergillosis. And at present the most often used classification of forms of pulmonary aspergillosis is as follows: (1) infection with or without allergic sensitization to the fungus, (2) intracavitary aspergilloma (fungus ball) and (3) infection associated with necrosis (70).

Though the largest number of cases of pulmonary aspergillosis is found in patients with some other disease, making the infection with *Aspergillus* secondary or opportunistic, there are some reports of primary, pulmonary aspergillosis in which no predisposing conditions could be detected (1, 8, 10, 24, 36, 72).

In this type are found *A. fumigatus*, *A. flavus*, *A. nidulans*, *A. niger*, *A. terreus*, *A. versicolor*, *A. candidus*, *A. amstelodami* and *A. niveus* (1, 2, 10, 13, 15, 36, 50, 54, 65). There have been some dual and triple infections with more than one species of *Aspergillus* (54).

In review of disseminated aspergillosis twenty-two cases were found in the world literature (71). In a more recent report including the period of 1964 to 1971 a total of twenty-three cases of disseminated aspergillosis was reported from two medical units alone in New York (40). These twenty-three cases of disseminated aspergillosis were found in ninety-three cases of aspergillosis, ninety of which had pulmonary involvement. This does indicate that the incidence of disseminated aspergillosis is truly on the increase.

Most authors agree that the primary site of infection in disseminated aspergillosis is usually the lungs (7, 40, 65, 71). Other primary sites possible are the buccal mucous membranes and the accessory nasal sinuses (65). Of the 136 cases of disseminated aspergillosis in which the lungs were infected the following sites were also involved: brain (28), heart (17), pericardium (7), myocardium (4), endocardium (8), intestines (20), liver (16), thyroid gland (13), spleen (14), trachea, bone, diaphragm, lymph nodes, central nervous system, skin, adrenal glands, larynx, pulmonary artery, sinuses, orbit, mediastinum, blood vessels, pancreas, psoa muscle, bladder, blood, genito-urinary, stomach, gall bladder, arteries, uterus and aortic aneurysm (7, 11, 15, 16, 20, 29, 30, 40, 41, 65, 71).

Generalized dissemination in children following pulmonary infection has been reported in three instances. In two of these cases the organism was identified as *A. fumigatus* and third as *Aspergillus* species. The organs involved were liver, spleen, bowel, bronchial lymph nodes, bones and cerebellum (1). Two cases of generalized aspergillosis in adults have been reported caused by *A. fumigatus* with a large number of organs involved (25).

A number of infections in the brain have been reported to be the result of dissemination from the lungs. Others have resulted from dissemination from the sinuses. And one report of a primary infection by *A. oryzae* with no predisposing conditions has also been reported (83).

Only seven species of *Aspergillus* have been reported to be the causal agent in disseminated disease. Listed in order from the most frequently isolated: *A. fumigatus, A. flavus, A. nidulans, A. sydowi, A. niveus, A. terreus* and *A. restrictus* (11, 15, 16, 17, 20, 65, 71).

Most investigators agree that onychomycosis caused by *Aspergillus* is a fairly uncommon disease (73). In a survey of materials sent in for diagnosis out of a total of 373 patients, thirty-six had infected toenails and five had infected fingernails caused by nondermatophytes. Of this group infected by nondermatophytes various species of *Aspergillus* caused toenail infections in thirteen patients and fingernail infections in one patient. In an effort to find what the incidence was in a less select population, all the toenails of patients attending the dermatological clinics were examined. Of the 200 persons examined, seventy-two had diseased nails with five cases of onychomycosis caused by species of *Aspergillus.* Though there may be no valid interpretation of a comparison of these results it was noted that none of the five patients from the later general survey that had infections caused by species of *Aspergillus* complained of abnormal toenails (75). In a survey of 120 patients hospitalized for a variety of reasons 8 percent were found to have white opaque areas on the surface of the toenails. In another survey of twenty patients with this form of onychomycosis, one was found to have the pathology caused by *A. terreus* (80). In a survey of diseased nails in a diabetic clinic in Boston, the most often isolated causal agent including dermatophytes was *Aspergillus* (61). The disease in general, without reference to causative agents, was reported more frequently found in women, forty to fifty years of age; the first toe most often involved and the right hand more often infected than the left (68). Other authors have reported the disease was more often found in men rather than women (68).

The following species of *Aspergillus* have been reported to be the cause of onychomycosis: *A. flavus, A. nidulans, A. terricola, A. candidus, A. terreus, A. sydowi, A. ustus, A. versicolor, A. fumigatus, A. unguis, A. oryzae, A. glaucus, A. gratioti, A. diplocystis* and *A. onychophylus* (8, 42, 75, 80).

Infections of the outer ear (otomycosis) may be caused by a wide variety of microorganisms. In those infections that are caused by fungi, about 90 percent of these are caused by members of the genus *Aspergillus* (52, 78, 79). Various countries of the world have been mentioned to have greater frequency of otomycosis (27, 77). This may be due to the climate as a predisposing factor to be mentioned later. The disease is found in all age groups but the number of infections in young adults appears to be greater.

The fungus causing otomycosis grows on cerumm, epithelial scales and detritus deep in the external canal. A plug is formed.

There may be superficial erosion of the membranes but without deep penetration (17). In a survey of two hundred cases of infections of the external ear, relation of the species of *Aspergillus* as a causative agent to the main signs and symptoms has been made. Lesions produced by different fungi, in the earlier literature (77), have been reported to be clinically similar.

The most complete listing of causal organisms for otomycosis is given by Wolf (78). He lists eighteen species of *Aspergillus.* Only one more species, *A. flavines,* has been added to this list (69): *A. niger, A. fumigatus, A. flavus, A. glaucus, A. flavescens, A. nidulans, A. terreus, A. candidus, A sydowi, A. oryzae, A. montevidensis, A. repens, A. versicolor, A. ochraceus, A. wentii, A. fischeri, A. phoenicis* and *A. Macfiei.*

The first reported case of ocular aspergillosis was published in 1879 (44). From 1879 to 1916, reaching a peak in 1910 to 1915, there were forty-two cases reported (12). From 1951 to 1962 there were eighty-four cases reported (12) and in another review extending to 1970 a total of 109 cases of keratomycosis were reported of which thirty-eight were caused by various species of *Aspergillus* (44). This later review obviously did not include some of the cases previously reported. It has been stated that of all the cases of ocular mycosis reported, one-half have been recorded in the ten-year period from 1960 to 1970 (44). Members of the genus *Aspergillus* are the most common cause of ocular mycosis in San Francisco (57) and the second most common cause of this disease in Great Britain (32) and Florida (57).

The most often observed type of aspergillosis of the eye is the exogenous type due to the accidental or surgical penetration of the eye (12, 19). There are also hematogenous infections and isolated occurrences of endogenous intraocular infections (19). Chronic orbital aspergillosis has also been reported (70).

Aspergillus fumigatus has been the most frequent species isolated from ocular mycoses (12, 32, 44). Of seventy-six cases in one review fifty-seven were caused by *A. fumigatus.* There appears to be differences in incidence of infection in relation to geography and season. The most common cause of ocular mycoses in San Francisco is *A. fumigatus.* However, *A. fumigatus* is the second most common cause of ocular mycoses in Florida

(57). The other species causing ocular mycoses are *A. flavus, A. nidulans, A. niger, A. glaucus, A. flavescens, A. niveus, A. ochraceus, A. versicolor* and *A. terreus* (32, 44).

Cutaneous aspergillosis has been reported where the organism was growing saprophytically as well as parasitically between the toes in very superficial lesions (18) and under the dressing following a surgical wound (22). The organism invaded the skin to produce an extensive infection which gave the appearance of leprosy (9). A similar case of subcutaneous dissemination has been reported (51). Granulomas (22), ulcers on the hand (45), chronic suppurations of the skin back of the ear with grains in the pus discharge (27) have also been reported.

Not all cutaneous infections by members of the genus *Aspergillus* have been reported to have predisposing conditions. In the superficial infection of the skin between the toes the possible predisposing factors suggested were soaking in mustard baths, crowded toes, sweaty feet and erythrasma. In the infection under the surgical dressing the organism could have been growing on the serum discharged from the incision that did not dry. When the dressing was removed and topically cleaned the organism disappeared within one day (22). The deep seated growth of the organism in other tissues served as the predisposing condition for other dermatologic complications (9). The cutaneous infection that produced the leprosy-like appearance was stated definitely to be primary without any predisposing factors.

The causal organisms isolated from cutaneous aspergillosis are *A. niger* (9, 18, 22, 51), *A. nidulans* (27), *A. terreus* (45) and *A. flavus* (70).

Before 1950 only two cases of endocarditis caused by members of the genus *Aspergillus* were reported (82). Since that time fungal endocarditis has increased. This increase has been stated to coincide with the advances in cardiac surgery. In a review of thirty-one cases of fungal endocarditis made in 1958 four cases were caused by *Aspergillus* (38).

The disease appears to result from hematogenous dissemination from foci of chronic pulmonary infection. Other than the direct access to the heart during surgery, as already mentioned, there are a number of other predisposing conditions for this disease. These conditions can be possible chronic open skin lesions, frequent administration of intravenous infusions, septic amputations, interistitial pneumonia, "collagen disease," chronic lymphocytic leukemia, general debilitating disease, prolonged antibiotic therapy, corticotrophic hormones, leukopenia and chronic intestinal inflammation (38, 76, 82).

The species of *Aspergillus* reported to cause endocarditis are *A. fumigatus* (38) and *A. flavus* (38, 76). Other reports do not identify the species (82).

Mycetoma caused by members of the genus *Aspergillus* is rare (67). The disease appears to have been first described in 1906 as caused by *A. bouffardi.* This is no longer a valid species. Several other cases involving the feet, face, and arms caused by *A. nidulans* have been described (17). Mycetoma of the extremities as caused by *A. oryzae* has been reported from Guatemala (37). The granules produced in all of these infections have varied in color from white, to yellow, to red, to dark brown, to black. The black granules were described as produced by *A. bouffardi;* the red granules by an unidentified *Aspergillus* species, and the white to black granules by *A. nidulans.*

Sex

Though investigators disagree whether males are truly more susceptible than females to aspergillosis, some experimentation supports the view that a hormonal influence is possible. Stimulation of the reticuloendothelial system and subsequent increase in phagocytic activity is best accomplished by estrogens. When administered alone testosterone had no effect on the RE system (47). Progesterone and testosterone had no apparent effect on the growth of *Aspergillus in vitro*; there was a marked susceptibility of *Aspergillus* to naturally occurring estrogen.

Predisposing Factors

Most of the various forms of aspergillosis in man are considered to be opportunistic diseases. In recent years with the use of various therapeutic agents the incidence of aspergillosis has increased (40). In an effort to determine the underlying reasons for this increase the effect of cortisone treatment, one of the predisposing factors, has been studied in laboratory animals. A significant enhancement in mortality and tissue invasion due to cortisone treatment in mice was observed using various species of *Aspergillus* (64). Normal mice were found quite resistant to species of *Aspergillus* by inhalation. The exception was *A. fumigatus*. When alveolar macrophages from experimentally infected mice are microscopically examined the fungus spores are phagocytized in the control and the steroid treated animals within fifteen to thirty minutes (39). Spores phagocytized by macrophages of control animals did not show signs of germination or pregermination, however the spores phagocytized in the experimental group showed evidence of both pregermination and germination. In the early germination stage germ tubes were formed. In the control animals there was an aggregation of lysosomes about the newly formed vacuoles containing the fungal spores. In the experimental group, neither aggregation of lysosomes about the vacuoles nor fusion between lysosomes and phagocytic membranes occurred to a specific degree (39). In a study of the enhancement of aspergillosis in leukemic chickens, the diminished number of mature, normal leukocytes may be a factor in the increased invasiveness of the fungus. Lesions in these animals were more widespread with greater visceral involvement and hyphal proliferation than in the control chickens.

In approximately the past twenty years a long list of predisposing conditions or diseases have been reported associated with pulmonary aspergillosis. Among these predisposing conditions listed with the most frequently mentioned in the literature first are tuberculosis, leukemia, carcinoma, bronchiectasis, use of steroids, sarcoidosis, various antibiotics, pneumonia, abscesses, bronchitis, anemia of various types, asthma, diabetes, lymphoma, various bacterial diseases, cysts, various forms of surgery, Hodgkins, leukopenia, malnutrition, cytotoxic agents, leupus erythematosis, empymea, candidiasis, previous cases of aspergillosis, phycomycosis, blastomycosis, *Allescheria boydii*, histoplasmosis, nocardiosis, emphysema, Marie Strumpell disease, sickle cell disease, alcoholism, rheumatoid arthritis, radiation, trauma, obstruction in lung, panmyelophthesis, marrow aplasia, pneumoconiosis, paneytopenia, debilitation, splenectomy, preexisting lung cavity, silicosis, cirrhosis of the liver, infancy, ulcerative colitis, chronic obstructive pulmonary disease, pulmonary embolism, rheumatic mitral stenosis, polycythemia vera, Wegener's ganulomatosis, renal failure, cystic fibrosis, tetralogy of Fallot, gun shot wound, asbestosis, amoebic abscess of the liver, use of sulfas, viral hepatitis, pancreatitis, occupational backgrounds, sarcoma of various types and Boeck's sarcoid (2, 3, 4, 7, 10, 11, 13, 20, 23, 24, 28, 30, 33, 34, 40, 41, 46, 49, 50, 53, 54, 55, 58, 63, 65, 74, 81).

In the case of disseminated aspergillosis the predisposing factors have been stressed by a number of authors (7, 40, 65, 82) as a combination of (1) a general lowering of resistance by a debilitating disease usually leukemia or malignant lymphoma, (2) a local point of entry for the fungus, and (3) the use of antibiotics and steroids causing suppression of the normal bacterial flora and inflammatory responses (71). Among the diseases reported to be associated with disseminated aspergillosis are those listed in Table 13-I (7, 16, 30, 40, 65, 71).

In eleven of twenty-nine cases of otomycosis no predisposing factors were discovered (69). But in other cases eczema, chronic suppurative otitis media, antibiotic powders and general use of antibiotics have been described as predisposing factors. There has been an increase in the incidence of otomycosis possibly due to the use of antibiotics. In the same hospital in Canada a report in 1904 listed only two cases during the entire experience of the physicians while during thirty months from 1952 to 1954 there were twenty-nine cases reported by another team of physicians (69). Experimental evidence supports the view that trauma plays a part in establishing the infection (26). Heat and moisture have also been listed as contributing factors for the disease (14). The seasons of spring, late summer and autumn in tropical and subtropical countries are associated with increased incidence (79). Ear wax was reported to favor germination of fungus spores (27) but other workers have reported the protective effect, even a fungicidal or fungistatic effect, of ear wax on fungi (79). Swimming in infected pools has been mentioned as a source of infection but with little supporting evidence (77).

Since approximately one-half—sixty-two cases—of the reported cases of fungal infections of the eye occurred before the availability of antibiotics and steroids, that is from 1879 to 1962, trauma and/or concomitant bacterial infections were stated to be the paramount predisposing factor(s) (12). But several authors reporting from 1962 to 1970 (19, 32, 44) state that the indiscriminate use of corticosteroid drugs and antibacterial antibiotics, especially tetracyclines and aureomycin, are the major predisposing factors for ocular aspergillosis now. Organisms may enter the eye during surgical procedures, i.e. removal of a foreign body,

TABLE 13-I

DISEASES ASSOCIATED WITH DISSEMINATED ASPERGILLOSIS

Disease	*No. Cases*
Leukemia	15
Lymphocytic leukemia	5
Myelogenous leukemia	6
Myelobastic leukemia	1
Myelcytic leukemia	1
Lymphosarcoma	3
Reticulum cell sarcoma	3
Hodgkin's disease	5
Breast carcinoma	4
Pneumonia	2
Pancytopenia	2
Hepatitis	2
Anemia	2
Carcinoma of the bladder	1
Hepatoma	1
Hepatic transplant	2
Leg amputation	1
Thigh abscess	1
Agonulocytosis	1
Ascariasis	1
Prematurity	2
Hemolytic anemia	1
Leukopenia	1
Menorrhagia	1
Erythroblastosis	1
Thrombocytopenia	1
Diarrhea	1
Boeck's sarcoid	1
Malnutrition	1
Pancreas carcinoma	1
Leprosy	1
Pancreatitis	1

relief of glaucoma or cataract extraction (19). Ocular mycosis has been found in association with corneal ulcers (32). Also ocular grafts have been infected. The location of the inoculum may be more important than the amount of inoculum.

In summary, although spores of species of *Aspergillus* are found world wide and human beings come in contact with large numbers of spores few people acquire aspergillosis. There are a wide variety of tissues, organs and systems in man that can be invaded by this organism growing parasitically or saprophytically. The disease is said to be opportunistic, for the most part, with a large number of possible predisposing factors. Recently some basic information on the early cellular level concerning infection has been determined. It is hopeful that with cooperation of many investigative disciplines that the prevention, acquisition and treatment of this disease will be determined in the reasonably near future.

REFERENCES

1. Allan, G. W., Andersen, D. H.: Generalized aspergillosis in an infant eighteen days of age. *Pediatrics, 26*:432, 1960.
2. Argen, R. J., Leslie, E. V., Leslie, M. B.: Intracavitary fungus ball-pulmonary aspergillosis. *JAMA, 179*:106, 1962.
3. Aslam, P. A., Eastridge, C. E., Hughes, F. A.: Aspergillosis of the lung —an eighteen-year experience. *Chest, 59*:28, 1971.
4. Asper, S. P., Heffernan, A. G.: Insidious fungal disease. Trans. *Am Clin Climat Assoc, 76*:99, 1964.
5. Austwick, P. K. C.: Ecology of *Aspergillus fumigatus* and the pathogenic phycomycetes. *Recent Prog in Microb, 8*:644, 1962.
6. Austwick, P. K. C.: Pathogenicity. *In* Raper, K. B. and Fennell, D. I. (Eds.): *The Genus Aspergillus,* Baltimore, Williams & Wilkins, 1965.
7. Baker, R. D.: Leukopenia and therapy in leukemia as factors predisposing to fatal mycoses. *Am J Clin Pathol, 37*:358, 1962.
8. Bereston, E. S., Waring, W. S.: Onychomycosis and dermatomycosis caused by *Trichophyton rubrum* and *Aspergillus nidulans. Arch Dermatol Syph,* 52:162, 1945.
9. Cahill, K. M., El Mofty, A. M., Kawaguchi, T. P.: Primary cutaneous aspergillosis. *Arch Dermatol, 96*:545, 1967.
10. Campbell, M. J., Clayton, Y. M.: Bronchopulmonary aspergillosis. *Am Rev Respir Dis, 89*:186, 1964.
11. Cawley, E. P.: Aspergillosis and the aspergilli. *Arch Intern Med, 80*:423, 1947.

12. Chick, E. W., Conant, N. F.: Mycotic ulcerative keratitis: A review of 148 cases from the literature. *Invest Ophthmol, 1*:419, 1962.
13. Coleman, R. M., Kaufman, L.: Use of the immunodiffusion test in the serodiagnosis of aspergillosis. *App Microb, 23*:301, 1972.
14. Conant, N. F., Smith, D. T., Baker, R. D., Callaway, J. L.: *Manual of Clinical Mycology* (3rd ed.). Philadelphia, Saunders, 1971.
15. Davies, R. R.: Iatrogenic fungal infection. *In* Proc. 5th Con. Int. Soc. Human and Animal Mycol. Louis-Jean, Paris. 1971.
16. Destombes, P., Ravisse, P., Nazimoff, O.: Bilan des mycoses profondes etabli en vingt annees d'histopathologie a l'institut Pasteur de Brazzaville. *Bull Soc Path Exot, 63*:315, 1970.
17. Emmons, C. W., Binford, C. H., Utz, J. P.: *Medical Mycology*, (2nd ed.). Philadelphia, Lea & Febiger, 1970.
18. English, M. P.: Invasion of the skin by filamentous non-dermatophyte fungi. *Br J Dermatol, 80*:282, 1968.
19. Fine, B. S.: Intraocular mycotic infections. *Lab Invest, 11*:1161, 1962.
20. Finegold, S. M., Will, D., Murray, J. F.: Aspergillosis, a review and report of twelve cases. *Am J Med, 27*:463, 1959.
21. Ford, S., Friedman, L.: Experimental study of the pathogenicity of aspergilli for mice. *J Bact, 94*:928, 1967.
22. Frank, L., Alton, O. M.: Aspergillosis: A case of post operative skin infection. *JAMA, 100*:25, 1933.
23. Gonzalez-Mendoza, A.: Opportunistic mycosis. In *International Symposium on Mycoses*, PAHO Sci. Pub. No. 205: Washington, D. C., 1970.
24. Grcevic, N., Matthews, W. F.: Pathologic changes in acute disseminated aspergillosis. *Am J Clin Pathol, 32*:536, 1959.
25. Grekin, R. H., Cawley, E. P., Zheutlin, B.: Generalized aspergillosis. *Arch Pathol, 49*:387, 1950.
26. Haley, L. D.: Etiology of otomycosis III. *Arch Otolaryngol, 52*:214, 1950.
27. Henrici, A. T.: *Molds, Yeasts and Actinomycetes.* New York: John Wiley & Sons, Inc., 1930.
28. Hinson, K. F. W., Moon, A. J., Plummer, N. S.: Bronchopulmonary aspergillosis, a review and a report of eight new cases. *Thorax*, 7:317, 1952.
29. Hunt, W., III, Broders, A. C., Jr., Stinson, J. C., Carabasi, R. J.: Primary pulmonary aspergillosis with invasion of the mediastinal contents and lymph nodes. *Am Rev Respir Dis, 83*:886, 1961.
30. Hutter, R. V. P., Collins, H. S.: The occurrence of opportunistic fungus infections in a cancer hospital. *Lab Invest, 11*:1035, 1962.
31. Jillson, O. F., Adami, M.: Allergic dermatitis produced by inhalant molds. *Arch Dermatol, 72*:411, 1955.
32. Jones, B. R., Richards, A. B., Morgan, G.: Direct fungal infection of the eye in Britain. *Trans Ophthal Soc U K, 89*:727, 1970.

33. Keye, J. D., Magee, W. E.: Fungal diseases in a general hospital, a study of 88 patients. *Am J Clin Pathol, 26*:1235, 1956.
34. Macpherson, P.: Pulmonary aspergillosis in *Argyll Br J Dis Chest, 59*:148, 1965.
35. Madson, R. A.: The incidence of airborne fungi in the Tucson area, thesis, University of Arizona Graduate School, Tucson, 1967.
36. Mahgoub, E. S.: Aspergillosis in Sudan. In Proc. 5th Cong. Int. Soc. for Human and Animal Mycol. Louis-Jean, Paris, 1971.
37. Mayorga, R.: Prevalence of subcutaneous mycosis in Latin America. *In* Int. Symp. Mycoses. PAHO Sci. Pub. No. 205, Washington, D. C., 1970.
38. Merchant, R. K., Louria, D. B., Geisler, P. H., Edgcomb, J. H., Utz, J. P.: Fungal endocarditis: review of the literature and report of three cases. *Ann Intern Med, 48*:242, 1958.
39. Merkow, L. P., Epstein, S. M., Sidransky, H., Verney, E., Pardo, M.: The pathogenesis of experimental pulmonary aspergillosis. *Am J Pathol, 62*:57, 1971.
40. Meyer, R. D., Young, L. S., Armstrong, D., Yu, B.: Aspergillosis complicating neoplastic disease. *Am J Med, 54*:6, 1973.
41. Mirsky, H. S., Cuttner, J.: Fungal infection in acute leukemia. *Cancer, 30*:348, 1972.
42. Moore, M., Weiss, R. S.: Onychomycosis caused by *Aspergillus terreus. J Invest Dermatol, 11*:215, 1948.
43. Muchmore, H. G., Scott, E. N., Tatem, B. A.: Precipitins to aspergillus antigens in serums of personnel wintering over at the South Pole. *In* Abst. of Ann. Meeting Am. Soc. Microb., 1973.
44. Munro, S.: Ocular aspergillosis. Trans. *Ophthal Soc U K, 89*:743, 1970.
45. Myers, J. T., *Aspergillus* infection of the hand. *JAMA, 95*:794, 1930.
46. Naji, A. F.: Bronchopulmonary aspergillosis. *Arch Pathol, 68*:282, 1959.
47. Nicol, T., Vernon-Roberts, R., Quantock, D. C.: The influence of various hormones on the reticuloendothelial system: endocrine control of body defense. *J Endocrinol, 33*:365, 1965.
48. Noble, W. C., Clayton, Y. M.: Fungi in the air of hospital wards. *J Gen Microb, 32*:397, 1963.
49. Okudaira, M., Schwarz, J.: Tracheobronchopulmonary mycoses caused by opportunistic fungi, with particular reference to aspergillosis. *Lab Invest, 2*:1053, 1962.
50. Orie, N. G. M., De Vries, G. A., Kikstra, A.: Growth of *Aspergillus* in the human lung. *Am Rev Respir Dis, 82*:649, 1960.
51. Paldrok, H.: Report of a case of subcutaneous dissemination of *Aspergillus niger* type *awamore. Acta Dermatol Venerol, 45*:275, 1965.
52. Papavassiliou, J., Stylianea, A.: On the etiology of mycotic infections of the external ear. *Zentralbl Bakt* (orig), *209*:412, 1969.

53. Parker, J., Sarosi, G., Doto, I., Tosh, F.: Pulmonary aspergillosis in sanatoriums in the South Central United States. *Am Rev Respir Dis, 101*:551, 1970.
54. Pepys, J., Riddell, R. W., Citron, K. M., Clayton, Y. M., Short, E. I.: Clinical and immunologic significance of *Aspergillus fumigatus* in the sputum. *Am Rev Respir Dis, 80*:167, 1959.
55. Procknow, J. J., Loewen, D. F.: Pulmonary aspergillosis with cavitation secondary to histoplasmosis. *Am Rev Respir Dis, 82*:101, 1960.
56. Raper, K. B., Fennell, D. I.: *The Genus Aspergillus*. Baltimore, Williams & Wilkins, 1965.
57. Rebell, G.: Ocular mycosis. Read before the Arcane and esoteric mycoses seminar 73rd Ann. Meet. Am. Soc. Microb., Miami Beach, Fla., May 7, 1973.
58. Reddy, P. A., Christianson, C. S., Brasher, C. A., Larsh, H., Sutaria, M.: Comparison of treated and untreated pulmonary aspergilloma, an analysis of sixteen cases. *Am Rev Respir Dis, 101*:928, 1970.
59. Rincon, G. C.: Contribucion al estudio de *Aspergillus* y aspergilosis. Proc. 5th Cong. Int. Soc. Human and Animal Mycol. Louis-Jean, Paris, 1971.
60. Rippon, J. W., Soo Hoo, M.: Aspergillosis: Comparative virulence, metabolic rate, growth rate and ubiquinone content of soil and human isolates of *Aspergillus terreus*. *In* Abst. Ann. Meet. Am. Soc. Microb., Miami, Fla., 1973.
61. Rockwood, E. M.: A study of fungus-infected nails. *Arch Dermatol Syph, 22*:395, 1930.
62. Rowell, N. R., Thompson, H.: Toxic epidermal necrolysis in a patient with pulmonary aspergillosis. *Br J Dermatol, 73*:278, 1961.
63. Salfelder, K., De Mendelovici, M., Schwarz, J.: Multiple deep mycoses. Proc. 5th Cong. Int. Soc. Human and Animal Mycol. Louis-Jean, Paris, 1970.
64. Sandhu, D. K., Sandhu, R. S., Damodaran, V. N., Randhawa, H. S.: Effect of cortisone on bronchopulmonary aspergillosis in mice exposed to spores of various *Aspergillus* species. *Sabouraudia, 8*:32, 1970.
65. Seabury, J. H., Samuels, M.: The pathogenetic spectrum of aspergillosis. *Am J Clin Pathol, 40*:21, 1963.
66. Segretain, G.: Pulmonary aspergillosis. *Lab Invest, 11*:1046, 1962.
67. Segretain, G., Mariat, F.: Recherche sur l'ecologie des agents de mycetomes fongiques au Senegal. Proc. 5th Cong. Int. Soc. Human and Animal Mycol. Louis-Jean, Paris, 1971.
68. Stefanovic, M., Krstic, A.: Onychomycosis in our country. In Sowinski, W. (Ed.), Proc. 2nd Int. Symp. Med. Mycol., Poland, 1967.
69. Stuart, E. A., Blank, F.: Aspergillosis of the ear, a report of twenty-nine cases. *Can Med Assoc J, 72*:334, 1955.

70. Symmer, W. S. C.: Histopathologic aspects of the pathogenesis of some opportunistic fungal infections, as exemplified in the pathology of aspergillosis and the phycomycetoses. *Lab Invest 11*:1073, 1962.
71. Tan, K. K., Kenji, S., Tan, K. L.: Disseminated aspergillosis, case report and review of the world literature. *Am J Clin Pathol, 45*:697, 1966.
72. Vedder, J. S., Schorr, W. F.: Primary disseminated pulmonary aspergillosis with metastatic skin nodules, successful treatment with inhalation nystatin therapy. *JAMA, 209*:1191, 1969.
73. Vilanova, X., Casanovas, M., Francino, J.: Onychomycosis, an experimental study. *J Invest Dermatol, 27*:77, 1956.
74. Villar, T. G., Pimentel, J. C., Avila, R.: Some aspects of pulmonary aspergilloma in Portugal. *Dis Chest, 51*:402, 1967.
75. Walshe, M. M., English, M. P.: Fungi in nails. *Br J Dermatol, 78*:198, 1966.
76. Welsh, R. A., Buchness, J. M.: *Aspergillus* endocarditis, myocarditis and lung abscesses. *Am J Clin Pathol, 25*:782, 1955.
77. Whalen, E. J.: Fungous infections of the external ear. *JAMA, 111*:502, 1958.
78. Wolf, F. T.: Relation of various fungi to otomycosis. *Arch Otolaryngol, 46*:361, 1947.
79. Youssef, Y. A., Abdou, M. H.: Studies of fungus infection of the external ear. I. Mycological and clinical observations. *J Laryngol Otol, 81*:401, 1967.
80. Zaias, N.: Onychomycosis. *Arch Dermat, 105*:263, 1972.
81. Zatzkin, H. R., Johnson, L., Abrahams, I.: Pulmonary intracavitary aspergilloma fungus ball. Report of three cases. *J Thorac Cardiovasc Surg, 61*:619, 1971.
82. Zimmerman, L. E.: *Candida* and *Aspergillus* endocarditis with comments on the role of antibiotics in dissemination of fungus disease. *Arch Pathol, 50*:591, 1950.
83. Ziskind, J., Pizzolato, P., Buff, E. E.: Aspergillosis of the brain. Report of a case. *Am J Clin Pathol, 29*:554, 1958.

Chapter 14

THE EPIDEMIOLOGY OF SPOROTRICHOSIS

Glenn D. Roberts

Sporotrichosis, caused by *Sporothrix schenckii*, commonly presents as a chronic ulcerative lesion of the skin with lymphadenopathy extending from the initial lesion to the regional lymph nodes. This sequence develops as a result of trauma at the site of the primary inoculation followed by abscess development and subsequently by the appearance of subcutaneous nodules along the lymphatics. (These nodules later ulcerate.) They may resemble cutaneous tuberculosis, staphylococcal lesions, or tularemia if the infection is left untreated; this sometimes presents a serious diagnostic problem.

Primary pulmonary sporotrichosis is being reported with increasing frequency, although in the past it had been considered a rare infection. The manifestations include pulmonary infiltration possibly with cavitation, and there may be lymphadenopathy of the tracheobronchial lymph nodes in some cases.

Osseous sporotrichosis is a chronic bone infection which may arise as a result of dissemination or may be a localized lesion. Many of the patients have skin lesions, local edema, and tenderness of the involved bone or joint; X-ray examination shows bone destruction. The occurrence of this type of infection is uncommon.

Mycology

S. *schenckii* is a dimorphic fungus that grows on most artificial media at room temperature as a characteristic moist, creamy white, yeast-like colony that becomes dry, wrinkled and leathery, and cream to tan, brown, or black with age.

Microscopic examination of the filamentous form reveals small, delicate, septate hyphae, with conidiophores producing, at their apices, small, hyaline or lightly pigmented, oval to pyriform conidia arranged in clusters resembling a flowerette. The colonies of the yeast form of the organism are bacterial in appearance, creamy, and grayish white. Microscopic examination reveals small yeast cells that are oval to elongate and have single or multiple buds.

Source of Infection

Classically, the most common method of infection has been through trauma to the skin by a prick from a thorn or a piece of any one of a variety of trees or bushes, or hay. This is confirmed by the fact that S. *schenckii* has been cultured directly from plant material.

The organism survives in nature as a saprobe and can be found on most substrates. An early study by de Beurmann and Gougerot (9) showed the fungus to be present on wood, bark, thorns, leaves, straw, soil, and several types of insects. Benham and Kesten (3) grew the organism on carnations and barberry bushes.

Gastineau et al. (14) found sphagnum moss to be the most common source of contamination for six cases of sporotrichosis. Crevasse and Ellner (5) reported an outbreak of sporotrichosis in a nursery, and Hayes (17) described five cases; in both series, sphagnum moss was suspected but was not cultured. In an outbreak of fourteen cases at a state nursery in Vermont, described by D'Alessio et al. (7), the organism was isolated from samples of moss that was in contact with all patients. In another case of sporotrichosis (29), subsequently the organism was isolated from a barn owned by the patient as well as from roses stored in moss in the barn.

Hay has been found to be a source of infection for epidemics in children. In one instance, nine children were infected while playing in prairie hay (6), and Powell and Hodges (33) reported two additional cases related to prairie hay. Recently, a case was found, at the Missouri State Chest Hospital in Mount Vernon, in a five-year-old boy who had previously played in prairie hay. An additional six cases related to handling of hay were described by Sanders (39); bricks stored in contaminated hay had been handled in a bucket-brigade fashion by several college students. During an alcohol-induced melee the bricks landed on bare skin, resulting in sporotrichosis in several of these students.

In another instance Kedes et al. (22) reported sporotrichosis in a rose gardener who often subdued the day's problems by drinking wine while he tended the rose bushes. Often he fell asleep while working and he subsequently came down with sporotrichosis and was described as the first to be afflicted with "the syndrome of the alcoholic rose gardener." This brings to mind the verse by Vaisrub (43):

When drinking wine amongst the roses
Or guzzling beer while throwing bricks
Or playing games in bales of hay
Where lurks the tricky sporothrix,
Beware, the price you pay for play
When you get struck by dread mycoses.

Alcohol has not yet been proved to be a cause of sporotrichosis; however, it may produce an underlying condition which predisposes one to the infection.

Several other plants have been implicated, including cactus (37) and corn (40), but it seems that rose bushes are the most common source of contamination. The largest epidemic of sporotrichosis reported was directly related to the growth of *Sporothrix* on timbers in a mine (18), and this directly shows the relationship of plant material as a source of infection.

Bites of insects and animals have been mentioned (2) as a source of transmission of sporotrichosis. In all of the cases related to bites, there is no definite proof that the vector harbored the fungus, but the number of reported cases suggests more than a coincidence.

A review of the cases of sporotrichosis seen at the Mayo Clinic during the last twenty years (Table 14-I) confirms the most common sources of infection. The source of infection becomes much more difficult to define in cases of pulmonary and osseous sporotrichosis. This is illustrated by the fact that all of the seven cases in Table 14-I listed as from an undetermined source were the pulmonary or osseous form. It is logical that inhalation of the organism would be the mode of infection for pulmonary sporotrichosis and possibly the initial site for an eventual disseminating process that could lead to articular involvement. This is speculation with no studies to substantiate it.

TABLE 14-I

SOURCE OF INFECTION IN 31 CASES OF SPOROTRICHOSIS SEEN AT MAYO CLINIC, 1953 TO 1973

Source	*Cases*
Rose bush	12
Corn husks	2
Japanese shrub	1
Raspberry bush	1
Evergreen	1
Sphagnum moss	1
Splinter	2
Insect bite	2
Cat bite	1
Unknown etiology	7
Unknown vegetation	1

Geographical Distribution

Sporotrichosis was first described in France by de Beurmann and Gougerot (9). Reports of cases throughout the world followed, illustrating its cosmopolitan distribution. It is, however, found primarily in the warm temperate zones where the fungus can grow readily.

Numerous cases have been reported throughout North America and in virtually every part of the United States. Previously it was thought that sporotrichosis was more prevalent in the Missouri Valley and in the Mississippi Valley (14, 42). The cases seen at the Mayo Clinic show a distribution primarily limited to the Midwest (Table 14-II); however, this is the area from which most of its patients come.

In Central and South America the infection is very prevalent. In Mexico City it is second to mycetoma in importance (23) and

TABLE 14-II

GEOGRAPHIC DISTRIBUTION OF CASES OF SPOROTRICHOSIS SEEN AT MAYO CLINIC, 1953 TO 1973

Location	*Cases*
Minnesota	8
Illinois	4
Iowa	4
Nebraska	4
Indiana	2
Michigan	2
Missouri	2
North Dakota	1
Wisconsin	1
Colorado	1
Tennessee	1
Kansas	1

is the most important of the mycoses in Guadalajara (1). Cases have been reported in Brazil (38), Colombia (16), and Argentina (34).

The largest single epidemic, reported by Dangerfield and Gear (8) and Helm and Berman (18), involved approximately 3,000 cases in the mines of South Africa. Mariat (27) mentioned that there is no sporotrichosis in South Africa other than in the mines; shortly thereafter, Findlay (11) reported a number of cases seen outside of that area.

A small number of cases seen in Australia were reviewed by Frey and Durie (13). Jovicic and Jovicic (21) reported sporotrichosis in Yugoslavia, and cases have been described in Russia (41).

It appears that the number of reports of sporotrichosis in Europe has decreased, and the reason for this is not clear. However, about one hundred cases in France were described by de Beurmann and Ramond (10). Some cases have been seen in England (36), Germany (20), and Norway (30). Other reports have appeared from countries where sporotrichosis is uncommon.

Age Incidence

Orr and Riley (31) mentioned that sporotrichosis is an uncommon infection and that it rarely occurs in children, but Lynch and Botero (25) found thirty-six reported cases of childhood sporotrichosis and contributed an additional eleven cases seen at the University of Michigan Hospital. Chandler et al. (4) presented four childhood cases and Park et al. (32) described an additional two. In 1972 an outbreak of sporotrichosis occurred in Mooreland, Oklahoma, where eleven children became infected after playing in prairie hay (35). In Brazil approximately one of every five patients is a child less than ten years old (34). Findlay (11) reported that 17 percent of his cases occurred in children less than ten years old, and Sampaio and da Silva Lacaz (38) reported 22 percent under ten years. These combined reports include a total of 452 cases of sporotrichosis. It appears that childhood infection is more common than previously thought. A random sampling of the literature together with cases made available personally gives an idea of the true age incidence (Table 14-III).

Sex Incidence

From data in the literature, Mariat (27) calculated that in a total of 219 cases the distribution was 55 percent males and 45 percent females. When Ramos e Silva's (34) cases are included, the percentages change to 46 and 54 percent for males and females, respectively. The 541 previously mentioned cases (Table 14-III) show a sex distribution of 71 percent males and 29 percent females.

Occupation

Foerster (12) described sporotrichosis as an occupational dermatosis and said that most cases occurred among manual

TABLE 14-III

AGE INCIDENCE OF SPOROTRICHOSIS IN 541 CASES SELECTED AT RANDOM

Age (yr.)	*Incidence (Percent)*
0-10	18.8
11-20	19.2
21-30	9.6
31-40	13.7
41-50	15.1
51-60	11.6
>60	11.8

workers such as farmers and horticulturists. This was later demonstrated by Gastineau et al. (14) in a study of 146 cases which gave the percentages of cases associated with the most common occupations as follows: farmers, 32 percent; gardeners and nurserymen, 14 percent; laborers, 17 percent; and housewives, 12 percent. Gonzalez Ochoa (15) reported the occupational incidence as follows: school children and students, 26 percent; peasants, 24 percent; and housewives, 24 percent. Mariat (27) calculated the distribution of 310 cases as farmers, 29 percent; domestic workers and housewives, 20 percent; and school children and students, 14 percent. Table 14-IV shows the occupational distribution of patients with sporotrichosis seen at the Mayo Clinic.

It is evident that the incidence of sporotrichosis is higher in persons whose occupations require outdoor exposure. The preponderance of infections in males is probably due to more intense exposure during their occupational requirements. The increased incidence among housewives is directly related to their increased exposure during horticultural activities. The prevalence of cases among children is not discussed among occupations; however, it is due to the exposure to hay and various plants during play.

Contributing Factors

The environmental growth factors for the organism are important. MacKinnon (26) reported that sporotrichosis has a seasonal distribution in Uruguay and occurs more frequently during autumn and winter. He thought that this was related to the saprobic growth in nature and was not a feature of the ambient temperature of the skin of man. Londero et al. (24) showed that

TABLE 14-IV

OCCUPATIONAL DISTRIBUTION OF SPOROTRICHOSIS SEEN AT MAYO CLINIC, 1953 TO 1973

Occupation	*Cases (Percent)*
Farmers and laborers	23
Gardeners and horticulturists	27
Housewives	31
Students	<1
Other	19

a temperature of 15 degrees C or more and a relative humidity above 90 percent are favorable for the growth of the organism. Mariat et al. (28) pointed out that a high relative humidity is not necessary because in Mexico the increased incidence is not during the rainy season. Gonzalez Ochoa (15) described the seasonal incidence as follows: Autumn, 34 percent; winter, 37 percent; spring, 12 percent; and summer, 15 percent. Natural land differences may explain these discrepancies with regard to humidity and temperature.

S. *schenckii* is found in nature and most of the isolates are slightly pathogenic (12), and no definite physiologic or antigenic differences have been seen (19). The question of why some persons are infected after contact with the organism while others are not is still unresolved for sporotrichosis and other mycotic infections. Perhaps with the immunologic research now being done, it might be found that some defect in the humoral or cellular immune system is necessary for the development of sporotrichosis in man.

REFERENCES

1. Aceves Ortega, R., Aquirre Castillo, R., Sosta Peralta, F.: Esporotricosis analisis de 70 casos estudiados en la ciudad de Guadalajaro. *Bol Dermatol Mex, 1*:5, 1961.
2. Baker, R. D.: *Human Infection With Fungi, Actinomycetes and Algae*, ed. 1. New York, Springer-Verlag, Inc., 1971.
3. Benham, R. W., Kesten, B.: Sporotrichosis: its transmission to plants and animals. *J Infec Dis, 50*:437, 1932.
4. Chandler, J. W., Jr., Kriel, R. L., Tosh, F. E.: Childhood sporotrichosis. *Am J Dis Child, 115*:368, 1968.
5. Crevasse, L., Ellner, P. D.: An outbreak of sporotrichosis in Florida. *JAMA, 173*:29, 1960.
6. Dahl, B. A., Silberfarb, P. M., Sarosi, G. A., Weeks, R. J., Tosh, F. E.: Sporotrichosis in children: Report of an epidemic. *JAMA, 215*:1980, 1971.
7. D'Alessio, D. J., Leavens, L. J., Strumpf, G. B., Smith, C. D.: An outbreak of sporotrichosis in Vermont associated with sphagnum moss as the source of infection. *N Engl J Med, 272*:1054, 1965.
8. Dangerfield, L. F., Gear, J.: Sporotrichosis among miners on the Witwatersrand gold mines. *S Afr Med J, 15*:128, 1941.
9. De Beurmann, L., Gougerot, H.: Etiologie et pathogenie de la sporotrichose. *Trib Med Paris, 40*:693, 1907.

10. De Beurmann, L., Ramond, J.: Abces sous-cutanes multiples d'origine mycosique. *Ann Dermatol Syphiligr (Paris), 4*:678, 1903.
11. Findlay, G. H.: The epidemiology of sporotrichosis in the Transvaal. *Sabouraudia, 7*:231, 1970.
12. Foerster, H. R.: Sporotrichosis, an occupational dermatosis. *JAMA, 87*:1605, 1926.
13. Frey, D., Durie, E. B.: Deep mycoses reported from Australia and New Guinea during the years 1956 to 1969. *Med J Aust, 2*:1117, 1970.
14. Gastineau, F. M., Spolyar, L. W., Haynes, E.: Sporotrichosis: Report of six cases among florists. *JAMA, 117*:1074, 1941.
15. Gonzalez Ochoa, A.: Contribuciones recientes al conocimiento de la esporotricosis. *Gac Med Mex, 95*:463, 1965.
16. Gonzalo Calle, V., Angela Restrepo, M.: Esporotricosis. *Antioquia Med, 11*:4444, 1961.
17. Hayes, W. N.: Sporotrichosis in employees of a tree nursery. *GP, 22*:114, 1960.
18. Helm, M. A. F., Berman, C.: The clinical, therapeutic and epidemiological features of the sporotrichosis infection on the mines. *In* Transvaal Mine Medical Officers' Association: Sporotrichosis infection on mines of the Witwatersrand. A symposium. Johannesburg: The Transvaal Chamber of Mines, 1947.
19. Howard, D. H., Orr, G. F.: Comparison of strains of *Sporotrichum schenckii* isolated from nature. *J Bact, 85*:816, 1963.
20. Itani, Z., Die sporotrichose. *Hautarzt, 22*:110, 1971.
21. Jovicic, B., Jovicic, A.: O epidemiologiji i klinici Sporotrichosis schenckii. *Med Pregl, 25*:119, 1972.
22. Kedes, L. H., Siemienski, J., Braude, A. I.: The syndrome of the alcoholic rose gardener: sporotrichosis of the radial tendon sheath; report of a case cured with amphotericin B. *Ann Int Med, 61*:1139, 1964.
23. Latapi, F.: La sporotrichose au Mexique. *Laval Med, 34*:732, 1963.
24. Londero, A. T., Fischman, O., Ramos, C. D.: Sporotrichosis in Rio Grande do Sul: Observations in the interior of the state (observacoes nu interior desse estado). *Hospital (Rio), 63*:1441, 1963.
25. Lynch, P. J., Botero, F.: Sporotrichosis in children. *Am J Dis Child, 122*:325, 1971.
26. MacKinnon, J. E.: The dependence on the weather of the incidency of sporotrichosis. *Mycopath, 4*:367, 1949.
27. Mariat, F.: The epidemiology of the mycosis: Some comments in relation to a particular case of sporotrichosis. *In* Systemic mycoses: A Ciba Foundation symposium. Edited by G. E. W. Wolstenholme and R. Porter. Boston: Little, Brown & Company, 1968.
28. Mariat, F., Lavalle, P., Destombes, P.: Recherches sur la sporotrichose:

Etude mycologique et pourvoir pathogene de souches Mexicaines de *Sporotrichum schenckii*. *Sabouraudia, 2*:60, 1962.

29. McDonough, E. S., Lewis, A. L., Meister, M.: *Sporothrix (Sporotrichum) schenckii* in a nursery barn containing spagnum. *Pub Hlth Rep, 85*:579, 1970.
30. Norden, A.: Interna svampsjukdomar. *Nord Med, 47*:271, 1952.
31. Orr, E. R., Riley, H. D., Jr.: Sporotrichosis in childhood: Report of ten cases. *J Pediatr, 78*:951, 1971.
32. Park, C. H., Greer, C. L., Cook, C. B.: Cutaneous sporotrichosis: Recent appearance in northern Virginia. *Am J Clin Pathol, 57*:23, 1972.
33. Powell, K. E., Hodges, B. E.: Epidemic sporotrichosis (letter to the editor). *JAMA, 217*:340, 1971.
34. Ramos e Silva, J.: La sporotrichose au Bresil. *Laval Med, 34*:739, 1963.
35. Rhodes, J. C.: Personal communciation.
36. Riddell, R. W.: Survey of fungus diseases in Britain. *Br Med Bull, 7*:197, 1951.
37. Riordan, T. J.: Sporotrichosis. *Arch Dermat, 60*:979, 1949.
38. Sampaio, S. A. P., da Silva Lacaz, C.: Klinische und statistische untersuchungen uber Sporotrichose in Sao Paulo (Brazilien), *Hautarzt, 10*:490, 1959.
39. Sanders, E.: Cutaneous sporotrichosis: Beer, bricks, and bumps. *Arch Int Med, 127*:482, 1971.
40. Sartory, A.: Presence du *Sporotrichum beurmanni* de Beurm. et Goug. sur un epide ble. *C R Soc Biol (Paris), 78*:740, 1915.
41. Stepanishtcheva, Z. G., Arievitch, A. M., Minsker, O. B., Sooteyeva, T. B.: Investigation of deep mycoses in the U.S.S.R. *Int J Dermatol, 11*:181, 1972.
42. Sutton, R. L.: Sporotrichosis in the Mississippi basin. *JAMA, 63*:1153, 1914.
43. Vaisrub, S.: Beware, the sporothrix (editorial). *JAMA, 215*:1976, 1971.

Chapter 15

THE EPIDEMIOLOGY OF CHROMOMYCOSIS

YOUSEF AL-DOORY

CHROMOMYCOSIS IS a noncontagious, chronic, mycotic disease. As in the other subcutaneous and systemic mycoses, this disease does not transfer from man to man. Rather, it is a disease of nature, with an exogenous type infection. The fungal agent is transmitted to humans through actual implantation from reservoirs in soil, plants or debris.

Chromomycosis is suppurative and proliferative granulomatous in appearance, and usually characterized by extensive warty, crusted and ulcerated lesions. Irregular surfaces are apparent on the lesions, simulating a cauliflower-like appearance.

Human factors which appear to play the most significant roles in susceptibility to this disease are sex, age and race. There are, however, certain structural variables which must be taken into consideration with any explanation of existing records.

Cases have been reported from all races, including Orientals, Negroes and American Indians. Caucasian individuals, however, have made up the majority of reports. Most cases have been reported in males, without consideration as to locality or occupation. Also, most cases reported occurred in persons twenty to sixty years of age, although a case has been reported in an eighty-four-year-old man (37) and in a three-year-old child (40).

Situational variables to be considered include the prominence

---

Our thanks is extended to Mountain Press Publishing Company for allowing us to use Tables 15-I to 15-IV.

of fungal causative agents, exposure to these agents and the physiological parameters of susceptibility/resistance to the agents of chromomycosis.

In certain occupations individuals are more frequently exposed to accidental trauma involving vegetable debris, soil particles and other natural fragments; examples are agriculture workers, laborers and mine workers, especially in those cases where individuals work without the protection of shoes. Such persons are more likely to be exposed to the etiologic agents of chromomycosis; thus, they make up a high percentage of reported cases.

However, while it is true that frequent contact with etiologic agents, involving accidental trauma, must be a major factor in the establishment of the disease, it is apparently not the necessary condition for involvement, else there would be many more cases among the millions of farmers, laborers and mine workers of the world. The general belief among most medical mycologists is that factors such as personal habits and nutritional and metabolic conditions predispose the individual toward the establishment of the disease.

Source of Infection

Although there is much disagreement regarding the nomenclature of the causative agents of chromomycosis, it is agreed that they are a group of genetically related dematiaceous fungi. These may be classed into two groups: 1) organisms moldy in appearance, which produce an abundance of dry aerial hyphae on culture media such as, *Fonsecaea pedrosoi, F. compactum, Phialaphora verrucosa, Cladosporium carrionii, Torula poikilospora* and *Hormodendrum* sp.; 2) those which primarily have soft, dark, moist colonies that undergo what appears to be a yeast-like phase in the course of their development such as, *F. dermatitidis* and black *Candida*-like species.

Four other fungi belonging to the dermatiaceous group were reported in 1968, from patients with chromomycosis or various types of granulomas and subcutaneous infections. These were *P. gougerotii* (32), *P. richardsiae* (33), *P. spinifera* (27) and *Chmelia slovaka* (6). The latter was isolated from a chromomycotic patient in Czechoslovakia.

The etiological agents under discussion can survive without a specific type of soil or certain organic composition in nature. However, they do appear to favor other environmental variables, i.e. certain ecological life zones of moist and wet tropical and lower montaine, wet and rain forest environments.

The mean annual biotemperature in such areas usually ranges from 12 degrees to 24 degrees C and the mean rainfall is from 2,000 to 4,000 mm. It has been theorized that the fungi involved here are parasitic in nature, on certain plants which grow in these ecological environments.

Through experimentation on these fungi by inoculating various plant specimens with certain strains obtained from human cases, Montero-Gei (26) found that temperature and humidity were more important factors for growth than the substrate itself.

It would appear that the sufficient condition for developing a chromomycotic infection is actual implantation of the pathogen within host tissues; therefore, the presence of these fungi in nature, i.e. in soil, plant debris or wood fragments, should be a key factor in tracing incidence for a particular locality.

As previously mentioned, climatic conditions greatly influence the growth of these particular fungi, and probably play a role in the species which will predominate in any given area. Furthermore, it is expected that a species from this group will undergo a process of adaptation, upon passing from the natural habitat to a human host. Some species must possess a greater potential for adaptation than others.

Thus the factors which appear influential in determining the locale or prominence of the specific fungal agents involved, are climate and adaptability of fungi. Both are expected to work together in producing the occasion for incidences of chromomycosis.

As a very good example of this association, in 1960 Drygoo and Segretain established that cases of chromomycosis were caused in Madagascar by *C. carrionii* in areas with little rain (500 to 600 mm per year), while *F. pedrosoi* was the etiologic agent in cases from rainy areas (2,200 to 3,000 mm per year)(7).

F. pedrosoi is the most common etiologic agent reported for chromomycosis. The widespread distribution of chromomycotic patients infected with *F. pedrosoi* indicates its ubiquity.

This species appears to favor warmer, wet localities. In a survey by Carrion (10), 83 percent of isolates from ten chromomycotic cases were *F. pedrosoi,* where patients appeared to have contracted the disease in tropical or subtropical climates. Only 17 percent from this survey were from temperate zones.

Paradoxically, this fungal agent has been infrequently isolated from nature. Ruiz obtained *F. pedrosoi* from Costa Rican soils. Isolates were obtained by slowly agitating various herbs of the area over coconut milk agar, from a height of about twenty centimeters.

In a report by Montero-Gei (26), Trejos proved by autoinoculation that a strain of *F. pedrosoi* isolated from soil was pathogenic for man. Salfelder, et al (30) sampled soil and wood fragments, and from 336 specimens produced isolates for intratesticular and intravenous inoculation in guinea pigs and in mice, respectively. *F. pedrosoi* was isolated from six samples.

Nissassorakarn (45) reported *F. pedrosoi* isolated from the air in a survey for aerial fungi in Thailand. No cases were reported by the author. In a report by Mackinnon (45), *F. pedrosoi* was isolated from samples of branches, bark, tree trunks, rotten palm tree trunks, soil and other materials, in Uruguay. The richness of this climate for two prominent chromomycotic agents was demonstrated by the isolation, also, of *P. verrucosa* from the 339 natural samples. About sixty-three strains of the two fungi were reported upon by this author.

Interestingly enough, in the survey by Carrion (10) mentioned previously, it appeared that of the existing isolates of *P. verrucosa,* five out of six were from patients coming from colder climates.

P. verrucosa was also documented by Martin (23). Isolated from wood pulp, this agent had been previously misidentified as *Cadaphora americana* (39).

In a search for chromomycotic agents in nature, Ridley (28) obtained 109 isolates of *Cladosporium* species from 387 specimens of soil, leaves, bark, grasses, and other materials. Two isolates proved to be *C. carrionii.*

Since Conant first provided evidence in 1937 (14) that the fungal agents of chromomycosis may be found in nature, there have been numerous attempts to document the isolation of these etiologic agents from various natural substances, under varying conditions, worldwide. The examples given are not inclusive, but were chosen to illustrate the range of materials chosen for study, as well as the relationship of climatic conditions to the incidence of the disease in certain localities.

The relationship of the natural environment, including substrate, climate and potential adaptability of species, is important to an understanding of the dissemination of chromomycotic infection within human subjects.

In most reported cases, for example, it is sufficient to assume that the disease originated by primary inoculation of the causative fungi through skin trauma and wounds contaminated by soil. This explanation is feasible for cases involving feet, legs, hands or other exposed areas of the body. It is not fully satisfactory, however, in cases where body surfaces are covered by clothes, as in those cases involving buttocks, abdominal areas, etc. Neither is it explanatory in those instances where internal organs, including the lungs, heart and brain, are affected. Thus, in some instances, infection has been hypothesized to come through aerial inoculation.

It has been suggested (44) that some cases of chromomycosis may occur in the same manner in which chronic cutaneous blastomycosis is disseminated, i.e. from a previously unrecognized primary focus in the lungs, rather than by primary cutaneous inoculation. As partial support of this belief, it is offered that Baquero was unable to locate pulmonary lesions in early cases of cutaneous chromomycosis by X-ray studies of Cuban patients.

Geographic Distribution and Incidence

Although chromomycosis is a disease with worldwide distribution, it is considered rare in some areas and countries, and even absent in others; present reports tend to picture a high incidence of this disease in zones lying between 30 degrees North and 30 degrees South, within which most tropical and subtropical regions are located. Such regions should present optimal conditions for growth of the etiologic agents involved.

Experience tells us, however, that another important factor in the tracing of the incidence of any disease is knowledge of, and interest in, the disease by practitioners. Thus the incidence of any disease is usually higher in areas where physicians keep the disease in mind during differential diagnosis.

The best two examples of physician interest in a disease are 1) the finding of nine new cases of chromomycosis during a two-year period in a small area of Louisiana (20), and 2) the finding of 36 new cases in the Dominican Republic (43). In each case a particular group was aware of the disease. It would be well to keep this factor in mind in ascertaining the accuracy of any epidemiological study.

The purpose of a recent survey by the author was to gather together a working history of reported and, to that date, unreported cases to give an indication of the spread of chromomycosis worldwide. In some instances the personal impression of the author that the disease is chromomycosis was accepted. In others, inference that the isolated fungus "appeared to be similar to" the chromomycotic fungi, or that the fungal isolate was found to be *P. jeanselmei* or *Hormodendrum*-like species was considered. Such diagnostic approaches cannot be considered definitive due to the lack of observation of the typical chestnut-brown, spherical, sclerotic cells of the etiologic agent in the direct mount, biopsy material or tissue sections, nor the identification of the isolated fungal agent.

Scientifically, however, failure of exactitude could be explained on the basis of misdiagnosis, lack of facilities, lack of knowledge, complicated chromomycotic cases with or without another disease, or a combination of any of these factors. Therefore, there is the chance that some of those cases of chromomycosis might be legitimate. In that the aim of the author, in this survey, was to gather all available data on the incidence of chromomycosis and etiologic agents involved, all reports were included, leaving judgment up to the individual investigator. Duplication of reports was eliminated, however, which was a task difficult to achieve.

To give a general overview of that survey, the following reported cases are noted, either for their interest as to locale, or as to specific details of the case.

SPAIN: Miguens reported that he did not find any case of chromomycosis among the 6,000 mycotic cases studied in his clinic. However, Spanish literature, he claims, lists two such reports (4, 34).

BULGARIA: A case was investigated by Balabanov, from which *F. pedrosoi* was isolated, from a multi-lesion on the left leg of a man.

CHILI: Although this country was previously reported upon as being without chromomycosis (10, 11), Prunes and Frey reported a case in 1941 (45), however, this was without isolation of the etiologic agent.

MALAYA: A month after the author had been informed that there was no chromomycosis in this country, Jobling wrote from London regarding a male patient in their dermatology clinic. This chromomycotic patient was from Malaya. There were no details on the history of the infection, but there remains the possibility that the disease was initiated in Malaya.

BOLIVIA: Until this survey, Bolivia was one of few Latin American locales considered free of chromomycosis. Perez reported three cases, two women, one man, ages thirty-two, forty and twenty, respectively. *F. pedrosoi* was isolated from one of the female cases, while *F. compactum* was isolated from the other two patients.

DOMINICAN REPUBLIC: Up to receipt of a report from Weber, the author had accumulated through the literature fifty cases from this country. However, Weber reported observation of one hundred chromomycotic cases over a period of five years, raising the count to one hundred and fifty cases. Weber also stated his belief that there are at least 1,500 to 2,000 cases of chromomycosis in this country alone. (43, 45).

PARAGUAY: This country was reported upon by Bader who observed ten cases in the last ten years, including the three previously reported upon by Maas. One isolate of *F. compactum* and nine of *F. pedrosoi* were taken from these cases. Bader expresses the same impression as Weber and others, that there must be many more unreported cases over the world (45).

ARGENTINA: Chromomycosis is uncommon in this country. Negroni confirmed only four publications on the disease appearing during the years 1932 through 1969. *F. pedrosoi* was found to be the etiologic agent (45).

URUGUAY: Three cases were reported from this country, one unpublished. All three cases occurred in the upper limbs. Also, Mackinnon remarks that both *F. pedrosoi* and *P. verrucosa* have been isolated from nature (45).

AFRICA: Eleven cases, all occurring in males, were reported upon by Gatti. Localized lesions on the extremeties were apparent in ten cases, while the eleventh case had lesions on arms, legs and trunk. *F. pedrosoi* was the etiologic agent.

NIGERIA: In addition to the two cases already published in this country, Clark and her colleagues reported two new cases. One was a forty-six-year-old farmer with an infection of two years duration. The clinical picture revealed a multifocal warty growth on left foot and leg, with lesions rough, some hypopigmented, others hyperpigmented. A lesion of similar appearance was located on the lateral aspect of the knee, triangular in shape and about three inches wide. The second case was a forty-five-year-old rubber tapper with ulcerated lesions over the entire leg; the lesions were patch, scabby and hyperkeratotic. The infection had been observed two years earlier as a maculo-lesion with serpiginous border, resembling ringworm. *F. pedrosoi* was isolated from both cases (45).

INDIA: A case of chromomycosis on the face of a fourteen-year-old boy from which *P. jeanselmei* was reported as having been isolated, was cited by Grueber in the "Mycoses Newsletter" (19). Further details on the case were not forthcoming, however.

INDONESIA: Five new cases were reported upon from this country, by Soeprihatin; in addition, he cites five published reports (1928 through 1937). One of the new cases (1964 through 1971) was reported as occurring on the right foot and lower leg of a fifty-year-old man. *F. pedrosoi* was the etiologic agent (45).

Among other unpublished new cases, the author was informed of the following: seven cases from South Africa; five cases from Papua, New Guinea; one case each from Solomon Islands, East Germany, Uruguay, England and the Dominican Republic. At the same time, at least one native medical mycologist reported that chromomycosis is not known in these countries: Ireland, North Ireland, Italy, Norway, Sweden, Hungary, Poland, Denmark, Greece, Turkey, countries of the Arab Peninsula, Iran, Pakistan, Afghanistan, Egypt, Libya, Sudan, Tunisia and Ethiopia (45).

The total number of reported cases of chromomycosis worldwide has steadily increased. Carrion and Silva reported 151 authentic cases in 1947 (11); this was increased to 159 in 1950 (1) and to 197 in 1953 (29). These cases were thoroughly documented. If the new cases reported to this author in the survey under discussion are legitimate, their number increases the worldwide figure by an appreciable amount. Table 15-I lists the number of cases from each country, arranged alphabetically.

Brazil predominates with 505 cases, then Madagascar, Costa Rica, Dominican Republic, Australia, Cuba and Japan. By actual count, the number of cases totals 1,790, the highest figure recorded over the last few years. Although some cases appear without sufficient documentation to our mind, it is clear that the number of total cases is on the increase, for the figure of 1,790 is doubtless much less than the actual existing number of cases.

Epidemiological value of numbers of cases for any disease is calculated according to inhabitants per case. That is the base, therefore, for the breakdown of geographic distribution of chromomycosis in the various countries.

Adopted from Romero and Trejos (29), Table 15-II shows the ratio of chromomycosis in the twelve countries with the greatest incidence of the disease in 1953, using population figures from the same year (29). This is compared to figures from the present survey, using 1972 population figures.

This clearly indicates that Costa Rica is the highest in incidence of chromomycosis (1 case per 12,000 inhabitants). The

TABLE 15-I

DISTRIBUTION OF CASE REPORTS OF CHROMOMYCOSIS IN THE WORLD*

Country	*No. of Cases*	*Year Reported*
Algeria	2	1927-1963
Argentina	6	1937-1970
Australia	102	1936-1958
Brazil	505	1914-1967
Bulgaria	2	1967-1968
Burma	1	1957
Cameroun	6	1947-1963
Canada	3	1945-1950
Canal Zone	1	1956
Central Africa	2	1961-1963
Ceylon	14	1960-1962
China	3	1951-1966
Colombia	59	1961-1971
Costa Rica	157	1953-1971
Cuba	90	1941-1962
Czechoslovakia	6	1963-1969
Dominican Republic	150	1938-1972
Dutch Indies	5	1937-1968
East Germany	1	1964
Ecuador	9	1962
El Salvador	2	1956-1971
England	12	1960-1968
Finland	19	1959-1970
France	4	1967
French Congo	1	1963
Fr. Equatorial Africa	2	1958-1968
Guadaloupe	1	1964
Guatemala	16	1941-1970
Guyana	5	1962-1969
Honduras	27	1956-1970
India	27	1953-1971
Indonesia	10	1928-1970
Jamaica	5	1952-1954
Japan	74	1961-1971
Kenya	3	1965
Madagascar	179	1957-1967
Mexico	56	1958-1970
Morocco	1	1946
New Zealand	1	1953
Nicaragua	1	1968

TABLE 15-I—Continued

DISTRIBUTION OF CASE REPORTS OF CHROMOMYCOSIS IN THE WORLD*

Country	*No. of Cases*	*Year Reported*
Nigeria	4	1966-1972
Panama	6	1946-1971
Papua New Guinea	5	1970
Paraguay	30	1964-1972
Peru	3	1970
Philippines	3	1939-1955
Poland	1	1937
Puerto Rico	16	1933-1959
Reunion	2	1964
Rhodesia	1	1941
Russia	17	1940-1968
Rwanda	1	1970
South Africa	33	1943-1971
Sumatra	1	1938
Tanzania	2	1967
United States	24	1915-1968
Uruguay	4	1933-1972
Venezuela	57	1953-1958
Zaire	11	1951-1972

*Adapted from Y. Al-Doory, *Chromomycosis* (Montana, Mountain Press, 1972).

U. S. shows the lowest incidence (1 case per 8,625,000 inhabitants). Comparing the two survey years, 1953 and 1972, the Dominican Republic's incidence in this disease has increased almost seventy-seven times. Others with large increases were Japan (64 times), Australia (30 times), and Mexico (25 times).

In regard to incidence on continents, Costa Rica has the highest rate on the American continent, Finland in Europe, Japan in Asia and Madagascar in Africa. In 1960 Brygoo and Segretain reported that one region in Madagascar, Antandroy, had a case of chromomycosis for every 6,819 inhabitants. At the time, this was considered the highest incidence rate in the world.

In addition to total numbers, other interesting statistics gleaned from the survey were on race, age, sex, occupation, site and duration of lesion and etiologic agent involved.

TABLE 15-II

INCIDENCE OF CHROMOMYCOSIS IN 12 COUNTRIES IN 1953 AND 1972 SURVEYS ACCORDING TO NUMBER OF INHABITANTS PER CASE FOR EACH COUNTRY*

Country	*1953*	*1972*
Brazil	1/970,000	1/196,000
Madagascar	1/170,000	1/38,000
Costa Rica	1/24,000	1/12,000
Dominican Republic	1/2,151,000	1/28,000
Australia	1/3,791,000	1/127,000
Cuba	1/118,000	1/95,000
Japan	1/26,739,000	1/416,000
Colombia	(Not reported)	1/374,000
Venezuela	1/489,000	1/196,000
Mexico	1/23,434,000	1/940,000
South Africa	1/967,000	1/652,000
United States	1/16,004,000	1/8,625,000

*Table adapted from Y. Al-Doory, *Chromomycosis* (Montana, Mountain Press, 1972).

Race

From 124 clinical histories, Carrion (10) found 60 percent Caucasian, 30 percent Negro and 10 percent of other races. In a review of 202 cases chosen at random from all listed countries, this author found 50 percent Caucasian, 37 percent Negro and 13 percent of other races. Thus, it would appear that Caucasians are more susceptibleto chromomycosis.

Age

The majority of reports cites occurrences of this disease during middle age. The range twenty to sixty years of age has been reported by most sources to be optimum for the disease (10, 11). But of 751 cases it was found that both periods twenty-one to thirty and sixty-one to seventy produced the same percentage of incidence, i.e., 11.5 and 11.2 percent incidence, respectively (Table 15-III).

Although the optimum age span could be considered twenty to seventy at 90 percent or thirty to sixty at 67.1 percent, it is the belief of this investigator, in agreement with others (8), that twenty to seventy should be optimum.

TABLE 15-III

AGE DISTRIBUTION AMONG 751 CASES OF CHROMOMYCOSIS

Years	*No. Cases*	*Percent*
0-10	15	2.0
11-20	25	3.3
21-30	86	11.5
31-40	209	27.8
41-50	141	18.8
51-60	153	20.3
61-70	84	11.2
71-80	32	4.3
81 & above	6	0.8

*Table adapted from Y. Al-Doory, *Chromomycosis* (Montana Mountain Press, 1972).

Sex

This factor plays a major role in the incidence of chromomycosis. In averaging the data from six reports (10, 12, 25, 29, 36, 44), it was found that cases occurring in one female for every twenty males. This ratio is higher than that obtained from surveying 717 clinical cases (Table 15-I), where 83 percent of the patients were males, approximately four males to one female.

Ridley was able to demonstrate that a lesion produced on a man's arm lasted longer and was more similar to the natural infection than those appearing on a woman's arm (28).

Occupation

In a survey of 247 clinical cases, 173 were farmers or related fields, yielding 73 percent of the total. Laborers comprised 24 percent, while office workers and professions were three percent. Carrion had found that, from a survey of seventy-two cases, 82 percent were farmers (10).

Site and Duration

In reviewing 439 clinical cases in the literature, it was found that lesions of ten years duration or less formed 72 percent of total cases. It was not unusual, however, to find cases with lesions of forty years duration. The site of infection is expected to be on the exposed parts of the body, mainly on lower extremities. There are cases, however, which do not follow this typical route.

In surveying 613 clinical cases of localized chromomycosis, the following percentage distribution was found: hand, 62; arm, 76; hand and arm, 13; face, 16; buttock, 15; and others, 13 percent. This shows 68 percent in lower limbs, 25 percent in upper limbs and 7 percent on other parts of the body (Table 15-IV).

TABLE 15-IV

DURATION—YEARS

	0-5	*6-10*	*11-15*	*16-20*	*Over 21*
No. Cases	223	93	66	30	27
Percent	51	21	15	7	6

*Table adapted from Y. Al-Doory, *Chromomycosis* (Montana, Mountain Press, 1972).

The most common causative agent for chromomycosis was found to be *F. pedrosoi* (60% in all cases surveyed). However, *C. carrionii* appears to be concentrated in certain areas. Five percent of forty-eight cases from Queensland, Australia, were caused by *F. pedrosoi*, the rest by *C. carrionii* (15, 24). Brygoo and Segretain reported twenty-four isolates of *C. carrionii* in twenty-nine cases of chromomycosis from Madagascar (21). *F. dermatitidis* is frequently found in Japan (41).

Chromomycosis is rarely associated with a deep mycosis; rather, it is usually associated with viral, bacterial or even some physiological disorders. It has been detected in patients with leprosy (13), leishmaniasis (38), echinococcosis (42) and with carcinoma (9). Combinations with other mycotic diseases has been observed with paracoccidioidomycosis (12), histoplasmosis (3), paracoccidioidomycosis and sporotrichosis (17), with candidosis and staphylococcosis (5).

Such combinations of double or triple infection may be much greater in number; but it is expected that the symptoms of one disease, or for that matter, its etiologic agent, may mask the others.

Among the many cases reported upon, some were of special interest due to clinical circumstances. The first record of a case of endocarditis, caused by *F. dermatitidis*, was reported by Engelman et al. (16). The infection occurred on the prosthetical homograft valves of a forty-seven-year-old woman. She was operated upon and the aortic mitral valves were replaced. Recuperating normally for about two months, she suddenly developed a low-grade fever. Although oral penicillin was administered, the temperature elevated to between 103 and 104 degrees within the next four months. The patient was readmitted to the hospital with a right-sided headache and mental confusion (7 months following the initial operation). Blood cultures were negative.

Sternotomy was performed, aortic and mitral valves removed and replaced by new ones, due to the presence of abundant, thick, black vegetation on the interior and superior surfaces of the valves. Heart surfaces were slightly involved. Amphotericin B was administered during and after the operation. *F. dermatitidis* was isolated from the vegetation growth. The patient died within three days after replacement of the valves.

Kakotti and Dey (22) reported upon an unusual case out of India. A female, thirty-four years of age, married, with four children and with an occupation which combined agriculture and house service, was complaining of nodular growth of two years duration over the vulva, with slight discomfort, heaviness and occasional itching. Verrucous lesions were apparent upon examination, over the labia major and adjoining skin. The vulva was oedematous, the skin over it thick and firm. Lightly violaceous in color, the nodules were small, discrete and firm, with thin scales on the surface. Inguinal lymph nodes on both sides were enlarged and firm. There was a slight whitish discharge from the vagina. The vaginal canal and cervix were without lesions. The fungal agent was *F. compactum*.

From Japan, Sasano et al. (31) presented a case in 1961, where a 3½-year-old boy began to chew tobacco at one year of age. He began smoking cigarettes in the amount of ten a day. He complained of a stomach ache. When he was admitted to the hospital, he had a fever of approximately 101 degrees F and experienced nightsweats. Antibiotics did not reduce the fever nor improve his condition.

The patient developed general tonic spasm, right-sided paralysis, suffered loss of consciousness, and died two weeks from date of admission. Although clinical diagnosis was cancer of the liver, with metastasis to the brain, pathological diagnosis revealed dark-brown granuloma of "fowl-egg" size, mostly in the liver. Granulomas appeared in the brain, the lymph nodes of the mesentrium, around the stomach and in the posterior abdomen. Caecal mucosa revealed smaller-sized granulomas, while microscopic granulomas appeared in the right kidney.

Spontaneous Infection in Animals

A variety of experimental animals have revealed susceptibility to chromomyosis: mice, rats, guinea pigs, dogs, rabbits and monkeys number among them. But spontaneous infection of this disease in animals is yet to be documented, although it is reported upon. The typical, dark chestnut-brown, round sclerotic cells in biopsy materials or the isolation of a known etiologic agent has been lacking in such reports.

Akun (1) described a mycotic infection in a horse. There were myxomatoid amber-yellow granulations, with brownish granules observed in the fresh-cut surfaces of the nasal mucous membrane. According to Akun the granuloma in tissue sections was similar to that of actinomycosis.

Simpson (35) described biopsy material obtained from a draining lesion in the neck of a horse, 1 to 2 cm in diameter. A granulomatous lesion consisting of masses of chronic and acute inflammatory cells, hemorrhage and necrosis, surrounded by a stroma of mature fibrous connective tissues was revealed by histopathology. Brown septate hyphae and budding cells were identified within the cellular aggregations, and *Hormodendrum* species was isolated.

Simpson cited a report where chromomycosis was supposedly found in a dog (In "Canine Medicine"—Vet. Publ., Santa Barbara, Calif., 1959).

Frank (18) identified an amphibian as a carrier for *F. dermatitidis*. Dawkins included *verrucose dermatitis* as one of the foot diseases in cattle, in his 1969 report. His description included enlarged papillae, sensitivity, free bleeding. He reported that these lesions usually appeared on the lateral aspect of the pastern, and they always appeared to be associated with the lateral digit. The lesions responded to treatment with penicillin.

There is no reason to believe that chromomycosis cannot infect animals as it does man, as do most other mycotic diseases. However, no report within the purview of this author appears authentic, due to the obvious lack of clinical, histopathological or mycological evidence to confirm the diagnosis.

In conclusion, it is obvious that many factors control the incidence of chromomycosis. These include personal habits, nutritional states, accidental trauma, sex, age, occupation, etc. However, it is the belief of this writer that the hormones of the body play a corresponding role in dictating susceptibility or resistency to the disease.

Such hormones vary in substance as well as quantity from male to female, with more variations appearing in adulthood. It is the theory, here, that hormones play a role during the early stages of the host-parasite relationship, immediately after implantation of the fungal agent within the host's tissues (or following inhalation of fungal particles).

The effects of hormones may be apparent in the various stages of the disease process; they also may be a factor in the development of cerebral or generalized cases. Experimental studies in human beings of opposite sex, and of various ages, might help in providing support for this hypothesis. However, it goes without saying that we are firmly opposed to human experimentation to prove a point of scientific inquiry. An animal model, however, from among the subhuman primates would undoubtedly satisfy the need for such an investigation.

REFERENCES

1. Akun, R.: Eine chromoblastomykosiseahnliche Pilzkrankeit beim Pferde. *Zbl Allg Pathol Jena, 90*:294, 1953.

2. Al-Doory, Y.: *Chromomycosis.* Missoula, Mont., Mountain Press, 1972.
3. Almeida, F., Silva Lacaz, C.: Cogumelo do genero *Histoplasma* isolado de lesoes de cromomicose. Associacao de fungos nas lesoes. *Folia Clin Biol, 11*:65, 1939.
4. Baez Marrero, Hernandez, Garcia Padron, Vivancos Gallego: Segundo caso de cromomicosis en Canarias. VII Conf. Hisp. Portugues de Dermat. Med. Quirurgica. Granada, p. 22, 1969.
5. Balabanov, von V. A., Jovev, S.: A case of Chromoblastomycosis in Bulgaria in combination with other parasitosis and against a predisposing background. *Dermatol Vener, 6*:232, 1967.
6. Bojanovska, A., Kochova, I.: Histological picture of a new causative agent of chromomycosis "Chmelia slovaca" in the human skin. *Bratisl Lek Listy, 49*:346, 1968.
7. Brygoo, E. R., Segretain, G.: Clinical, epidemiological and mycological study of chromoblastomycosis in Madagascar. *Bull Soc Pathol Exot, 53*:443, 1960.
8. Campins, H.: Sintesis de las investigaciones micologicas realizadas en Venezuela durante los anos 1946-1956. *Mycopath Mycol Appl, 9*:152, 1958.
9. Caplan, R. M.: Epidermoid carcinoma arising in extensive chromoblastomycosis. *Arch Dermatol, 97*:38, 1968.
10. Carrion, A. L.: Chromoblastomycosis. *Ann N Y Acad Sci, 50*:1255, 1950.
11. Carrion, A. L., Silva, M.: Chromoblastomycosis and its etiologic fungi. *Ann Cryptogamici Phytopathol, 6*:20, 1947.
12. Cespedes, F. R.: Chromoblastomycosis. In *Chromomycosis in Human Infection with Fungi, Actinomycetes and Algae* by R. D. Baker, et al. Springer-Verlag, N. Y., 1971.
13. Coelho, J. T.: Considerations on the incidence of mycosis and leprosy in the same patient. *An Brasil Dermatol, 41*:229, 1966.
14. Conant, N. F., Martin, D. S.: The morphologic and serologic relationships of the various fungi causing dermatitis verrucosa (chromoblastomycosis). *Am Jour Trop Med, 17*:553, 1937.
15. Durie, E. B.: A critical survey of mycological research and literature for the years 1946-1956 in Australia. *Mycopath Mycol Appl, 9*:80, 1958.
16. Engleman, R. M., Chase, R. M., Spencer, F. C., Benjamin, M. V., Rosenthal, S. A.: Mycotic infections on prosthetic and homograft heart valves: Report of the first case of endocarditis caused by *Hormodendrum dermatitidis. Ann Surg, 173*:455, 1971.
17. Fernandez-Baquero, G.: Generalized chromoblastomycosis, report of the first case observed in Cuba. *Rev Cuba Med, 1*:53, 1962.
18. Frank, W., Roester, U.: Amphibia as carriers of *Hormiscium (Hormodendrum dermatitidis* Kano, 1937, a causative agent of chromo-

blastomycosis (chromomycosis) in man. *Z Tropenmed Parasit, 21*:93, 1970.
19. Grueber, H. L. F.: Mycoses Newsletter No. 20, 1971.
20. Howles, J. K., Kennedy, C. B., Garvin, W. H., Brueck, J. W., Buddingh, G. J.: Chromoblastomycosis. Report of nine cases from a single area in Louisiana. *A M A Arch Derm, 69*:83, 1954.
21. Janaud, Mm Roux, Fissarou, M., Saint-Gaudens, M. B.: Un cas de chromoblastomycose au debut. *Bull Soc Francaise Dermatol Syph, 74*:655, 1967.
22. Kakoti, L. M., Dey, N. C.: Chromoblastomycosis in India. *J Ind Med Assoc, 28*:351, 1957.
23. Martin, D. S.: Antigenic similarity of fungus *Cadophora americana* isolated from wood pulp to *Phialophora verrucosa* isolated from patients with dermatitis verrucosa (chromoblastomycosis), *Am J Trop Med, 18*:421, 1938.
24. Mead, M., Ridley, M. F.: Sporotrichosis and chromoblastmoycosis in Queensland. *Med J Aust, 44*:192, 1957.
25. Montero-Gei, F.: Aspectos clinicos y etiologica de la cromomicosis en Costa Rica. In Resumenes, IV Cong. Latino-amer. Microbiol., 204-205, 1967.
26. Montero-Gei, F.: Ecology and epidemiology of chromomycosis. In Proc. Intern, Symp. Mycoses, PAHO, 182-184, 1970.
27. Nielsen, H. S., Jr., Conant, N. F.: A new human pathogenic Phialophora. *Sabouraudia, 6*:228, 1968.
28. Ridley, M. F.: The natural habitat of *Cladosporium carrionii*, a case of chromoblastomycosis in man. *Aust J Derm, 4*:23, 1957.
29. Romero, A., Trejos, A.: La cromoblastomicosis en Costa Rica. *Rev Biol Trop, 1*:95, 1953.
30. Salfalder, K., Schwarz, J., Romero, A., Liscano, T. R., Zambrano, Z., Diaz, I.: Habitat de *Nocardia asteroides, Phialaphora pedrosoi* y *Cryptococcus neoformans* en Venezuela. *Mycopath Mycol Appl, 34*:144, 1968.
31. Sasano, N., Okamoto, T., Takahashi, T., Suzuki, S.: An autopsy case of primary chromoblastomycosis arising from the internal organs. Dark-brown granulomas in the liver and the brain without skin symptoms, observed in a smoking child three years old. *Tohoku J Exp Med, 73*:180, 1961.
32. Salvo, A. F., Chew, W. H.: *Phialophora gougerotii*—An opportunistic fungus in a patient treated with steroids. *Sabouraudia, 6*:241, 1968.
33. Schwartz, I., Emmons, C. W.: Subcutaneous cystic granuloma caused by a fungus of wood pulp (*Phialophora richardsiae*). *Am J Clin Pathol, 49*:500, 1968.
34. Simon, A., Pena Yanez, J.: Primera observacion espanola de cromomicosis. *Med Cut, 1*:121, 1966.

35. Simpson, J. G.: A case of chromoblastomycosis in a horse. *Vet Med, 61*:1207, 1966.
36. Solane, E. A.: Cromomicosis. *Acta Med Costa Rica, 9*:77, 1966.
37. Sonck, C. E.: Chromoblastomycosis: Five cases from Finland. *Acta Dermatol (Stockholm), 39*:300, 1959.
38. Terra, F., Torres, M., Fonseca, O. Da, Area Leao, A. E.: Novo typo de dermatite verrucosa, mycose por Acrotheca, com associacao de leishmaniosa. *Brasil-Medico, 36*:363, 1922.
39. Tsai, C. Y., Lu, Y. C., Dang, L. T., Hsu, T. L., Sung, J. L.: Systemic chromoblastomycosis due to *Hormodendrum dermatitidis* (Kano) Conant. Report of the first case in Taiwan. *Am J Clin Pathol, 46*:103, 1966.
40. Tschernajawski, J.: Chromoblastomycosis. *Arch Derm Syph, 157*:196, 1936.
41. Utz, J. P.: Recognition and current management of the systemic mycoses. *Med Clin N Am, 51*:519, 1967.
42. Vanbreuseghem, R., Vandepitte, J., Thys, A., Windey, W:. Premier cas de chromoblastomycose par *Phialophora pedrosoi* chez un indigene au Congo Belge. *Ann Soc Belg Med Trop, 21*:495, 1951.
43. Weber, A. G. C.: Contribucion al estudio de la chromoblastomicosis en la Republica Dominicana. *Rev Domin Derm, 2*:3, 1968.
44. Wilson, L. A., Sexton, R. R., Ahern, D.: Keratochromomycosis. *Arch Ophthal (Chicago), 76*:811, 1966.
45. Personal communications, 1971-1972.

Chapter 16

THE EPIDEMIOLOGY OF MYCETOMA

ERNESTO MACOTELA-RUIZ AND RUBEN LOPEZ-MARTINEZ

MYCETOMAS ARE chronic tumoral lesions located primarily in the subcutaneous tissue with fistulas that excrete pus generally containing granules made up of saprophytic colonies of *Actinomycetes* or true fungi. This definition excludes as mycetomic lesions those subcutaneous tumoral processes or abscesses produced by fungi or *Actinomycetes* in which the parasite does not have the tendency to form more or less structured colonies (granules).

Eight aerobic species of *Actinomycetes have* been isolated as pathogenic agents of Actinomycotic mycetomas: *Nocardia brasiliensis, N. asteroides, N. caviae, N. pelleteri, N. madurae, Streptomyces somaliensis,* S. *albus* and S. *paraguayensis* (21, 23, 27).

The species of true fungi that have been found to produce eumycotic mycetomas are *Madurella mycetomi, M. grisea* (22), *Allesheria boydi (Monosporium apiospermum), Monosporium sclerotiale, Cephalosporium recifei* (20), *C. falciforme, C. granulomatis, C. madurae, C. infestans, Phialophora jeanselmei, Leptosphaeria senegalensis* (37), *Pyrenochaeta romeroi* (10), *Neotestudina rosati* (38), *Curvularia lunata, Glenosporella* sp., *Aspergillus fumigatus* (4), *A. coryzae, A. nidulans* (5), *Geotrichum candidum, Corynespora casiicola* (26), *Botryodiplodia* sp., *Penicillium* sp. and *Fusarium* sp.

There are some subcutaneous forms of actinomycosis, for example the cervicofacial type, that should also be considered mycetomas. The pathogenic agent is anaerobic *Actinomyces israelii.*

Special note should be taken of the fact that actinomycotic mycetomas are only the tumoral lesions that have just been defined. Nocardiasis is the term used for subcutaneous or infections in which *N. asteroides* is present in its filament form but does not form granules.

Frequency and Distribution

There are several reports on the frequency and distribution of mycetomas (1, 7, 19, 34). However, the authors consider Mariat's report (28) as the most extensive and precise international survey on this subject to date. The geographical distribution and etiological types of the 854 cases studied by him are summarized in Table 16-I. It is noteworthy that 57 percent of the total were actinomycotic mycetomas.

TABLE 16-I

SURVEY OF MYCETOMA

Origin	*Actinomycotic*	*Eumycotic*	*Unclassified*	*Total*
United States	9	8	5	22
West Indies	1	3	—	4
Mexico	202	4	—	206
South America	49	58	1	108
Africa	196	249	19	464
Asia	25	5	—	30
Australia and New Zealand	2	—	4	6
Europe	3	11	—	14

An interesting finding of the survey is that *Nocardia brasiliensis* is the most common agent of mycetomas in Mexico. This fact has been confirmed by other studies, such as that of Gonzalez-Ochoa (11), who found that 94 percent of the mycetomas observed at the Institute of Tropical Diseases were produced by this aerobic *Actinomycete.* On the other hand, in Africa the most commonly observed mycetomas are of the eumycotic type (29).

The ecological environment surely determines the presence of the different etiologic agents. For instance, Rey pointed out that in the African strip between 10 degrees and 20 degrees north latitude, particularly in Mauritania and Senegal, the rain conditions, the flora and the soil determine different climatological zones which correlate with frequencies of different fungi causing mycetoma. In the arid septentrional region the common fungus is S. *somaliensis*, in the intermediate part of the country *M. mycetomi* and *L. senegaliensis* predominates and in the humid meridional part *N. pelletieri* (35) is most common. On the other hand, there are some species with a wide geographic distribution as *M. grisea* which has been found in several American countries (29), including the United States (9, 16), as well as in Africa (35) and eastern countries (18). *Nocardia brasiliensis*, which is the most frequent etiological agent causing mycetoma, is also a wide spread species mainly in tropical and subtropical American countries (17, 29). Although the geographical distribution of the species most frequently isolated (Table 16-II) is varied (28), there is a certain general pattern.

TABLE 16-II

MYCETOMA: GEOGRAPHICAL DISTRIBUTION OF THE MOST COMMON SPECIES

Species	*Geographical Distribution*
N. brasiliensis	Universal; predominates in Central America and Mexico.
N. asteroides	Universal.
S. madurae	Universal.
S. somaliensis	Predominates in Africa.
S. pelletieri	Predominates in Africa.
S. paraguayensis	Predominates in South America.
M. mycetomi	Universal.
M. grisea	South America, Africa.
L. senegalensis	Africa.
P. romeroi	South America, Africa.
C. lunata	Africa.
M. apiospermum	Universal; predominates in the Americas.
Cephalosporium sp.	Universal.
N. rosatii	Africa.
Aspergillus sp.	Europe.
Penicillium sp.	Europe.

The reported frequency of mycetomas depends to some extent on the location and type of mycological study centers. However, there does seem to be a tendency toward endemic zones within a particular region, as has been found in Morelos, Mexico (2).

During the last eight years, 13,386 patients in whom mycotic infection has been suspected were seen at the Division of Dermatology and Medical Mycology, National Medical Center, Mexico City, with 2,753 cases confirmed by laboratory studies. The mycetomas were second in frequency (Candidosis was first) with forty-three cases diagnosed (33 *N. brasiliensis*, 2 *N. asteroides*, 2 *S. madurae*, 1 *M. apiospermum*, 1 *M. mycetomi* and 4 in whom it was not possible to identify the responsible *Actinomycete*).

The Host

Mycetomas are more commonly found in males. Race does not seem to be a factor. The disease is most often present in young rural workers. However, there are some exceptions of affected persons who have lived exclusively in urban areas.

In our recent series of forty-three mycetomas, thirty-seven were observed in males, and the average age at onset was seventeen years. A total of thirty-eight patients came from rural areas, while five had always lived in Mexico City. Their professions were varied but all who came from the rural areas were involved in some way with farming. Of the five urban dwelling patients, one was an engineer, one was an auto repair specialist, one was a housewife and one was a mason. With one exception, the socioeconomic level was relatively low. It is interesting to note that thirteen cases produced by *N. brasiliensis* came from the endemic sugar cane region of Morelos State. None of the patients showed any general disease that could favor opportunistic infection.

Antecedents of multiple and frequent trauma were present in all the cases, and in 81 percent of them the mycotic tumor was located at the site of a previous wound. Inadequate habits of dress, in particular, use of scant footwear or none at all, were very common among the patients. It is believed that these factors together account for the frequency distribution in the localization of mycetomas (13) which in descending order is lower limbs, trunk, upper limbs, neck and face (Figs. 16-1, 16-2).

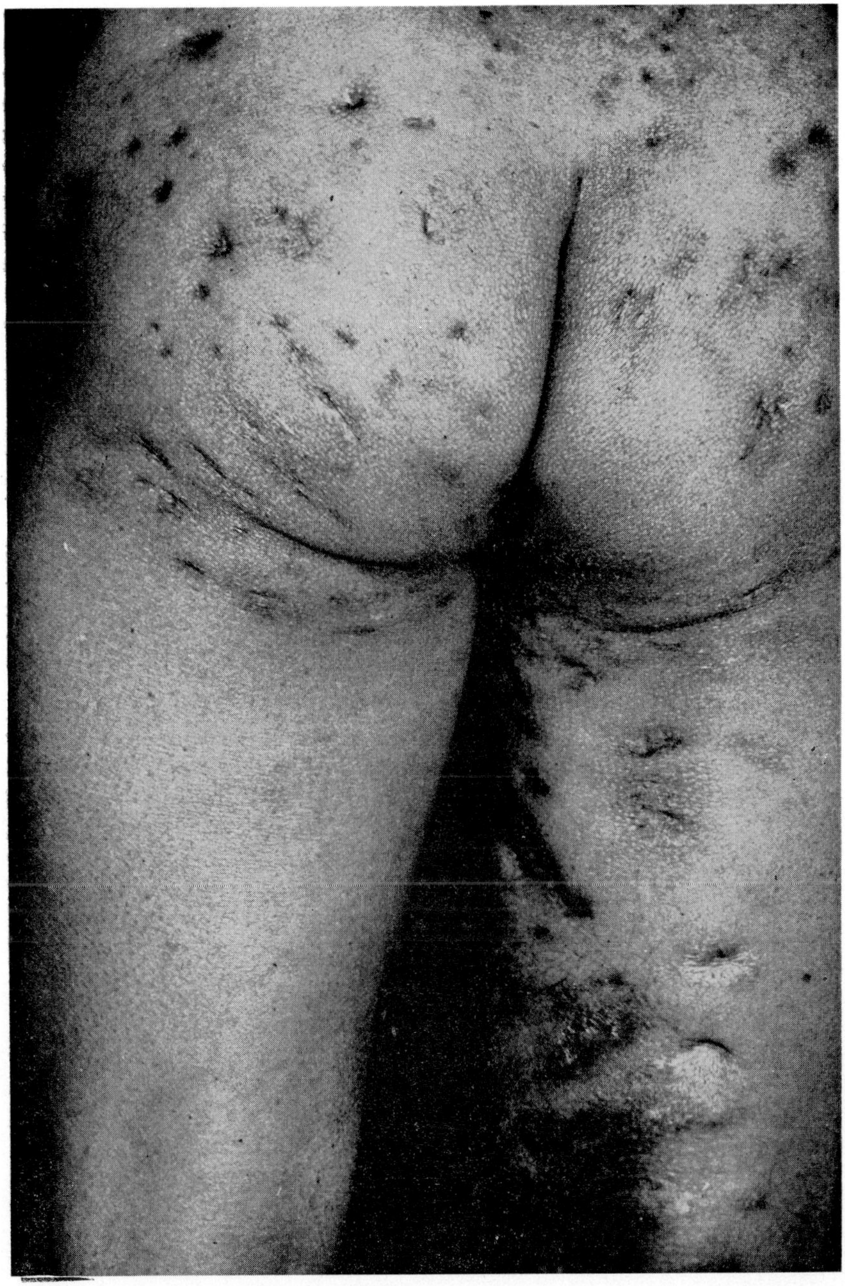

Figure 16-1. Disseminated actinomycotic mycetoma in a fabril worker.

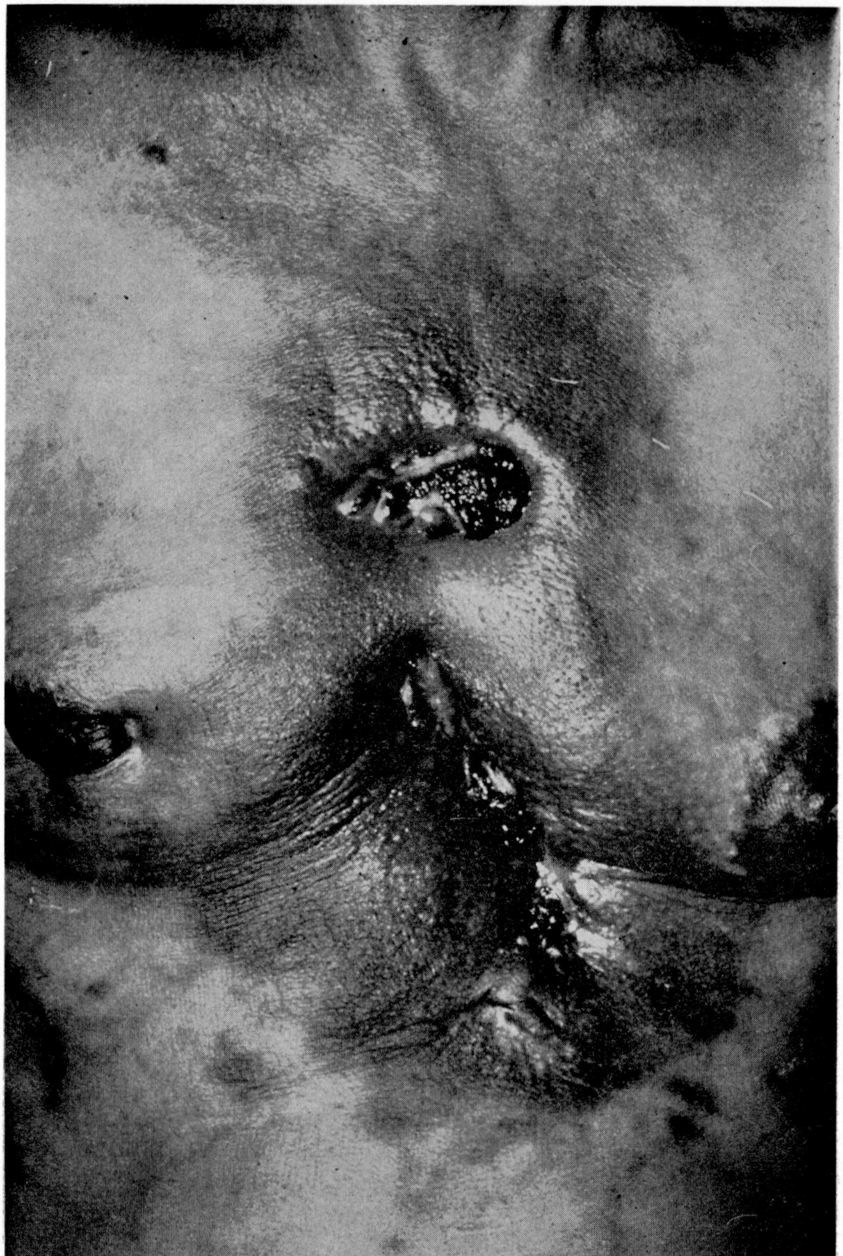

Figure 16-2. Maduromycotic mycetoma by *Madurella mycetomi* in a rural worker woman.

The characteristics of traumatism are variable, but in general it is a question of inadequately treated wounds, as pointed out by Mackinnon (21).

A history of previous surgical procedures of multiple microtraumas in the gums has been seen in cervicofacial actinomycosis, while in some aerobic mycetomas it is possible to identify the exact traumatic agent, such as the thorn shown in Figure 16-3 with the periferial granule (8).

Gonzalez-Ochoa and Baranda (12) described a cutaneous-specific test using polysaccharides from *N. brasiliensis* for the diagnosis of mycetoma. Protein fraction of *N. brasiliensis* produced 9 to 47 percent positive reaction in a normal population (36). Recent studies with a purified cytoplasmatic extract from *N. brasiliensis* and *N. asteroides* (32, 33) have shown a high specificity in the delayed hypersensitivity reactions in patients with mycetoma (*N. brasiliensis*), tuberculosis, leprae, as well as healthy people living in endemic areas for mycetoma. The same antigen introduced intradermally in patients with mycetoma produced a positive reaction with the homologous agent (Table 16-III).

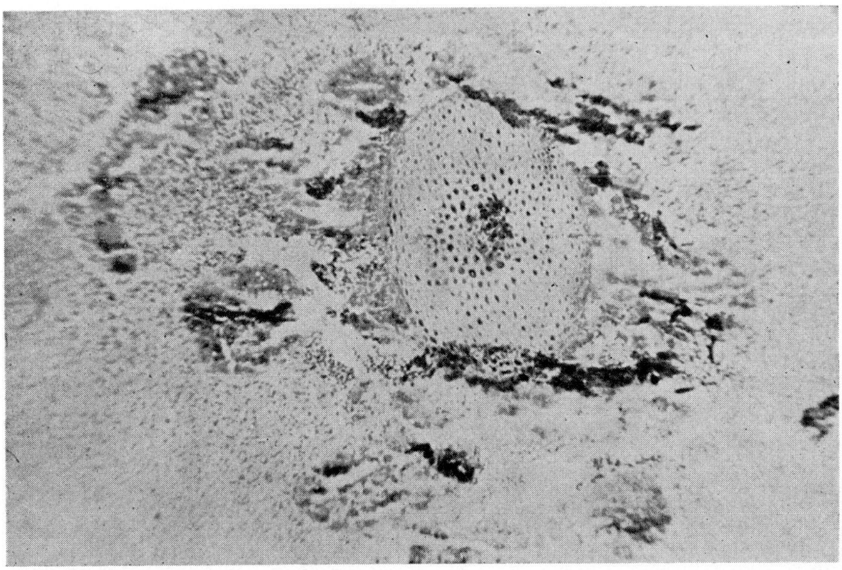

Figure 16-3. Granule of *Madurella mycetomi* around a thorn. (Courtesy of Dr. O. Welch).

TABLE 16-III

DELAYED HYPERSENSITIVITY OF ANTIGEN OF *N. BRASILIENSIS* AND *N. ASTEROIDES* IN PATIENTS WITH ACTINOMYCOTIC MYCETOMA

Agent	*PCE-Nb** *N. brasiliensis*	*PCE-Na** *N. asteroides*	*PPD* *(Control)*
N. brasiliensis	+	—	+
N. brasiliensis	+	—	+
N. brasiliensis	+	—	+
N. brasiliensis	+	+	+
N. asteroides	—	+	+
S. madurae	—	+	+
Non-identified Actinomycetes	—	+	+

*From Dr. Bojalil, University of Mexico School of Medicine.

The Parasite

Aerobic *Actinomycetes* and true fungi have been isolated from soil and vegetable material in various parts of the world (3, 6, 14, 15). In the host, the parasites group together forming granules (colonies) whose macro and microscopic morphology is generally constant (10) (Table 16-IV). (Figs. 16-4, 16-5).

TABLE 16-IV

MYCETOMA: CHARACTERISTICS OF GRANULE ACCORDING TO CAUSATIVE AGENT

Species	*Color*	*Size*	*Clubs*
A. israelii	Yellow	500μ	+
N. brasiliensis	Yellow	100μ	+
N. asteroides	Yellow	100μ	+
S. madurae	White, pink	1 mm	+
S. somaliensis	Yellow	2 mm	—
S. pelletieri	Red	500μ	—
S. paraguayensis	Black	500μ	+
M. mycetomi	Black	1 mm	—
M. grisea	Black	1 mm	—
P. romeroi	Black	0.5-1 mm	—
M. apiospermum	White	500μ	—
N. rosatii	White	500μ	—
Cephalosporum sp.	White	500μ	—

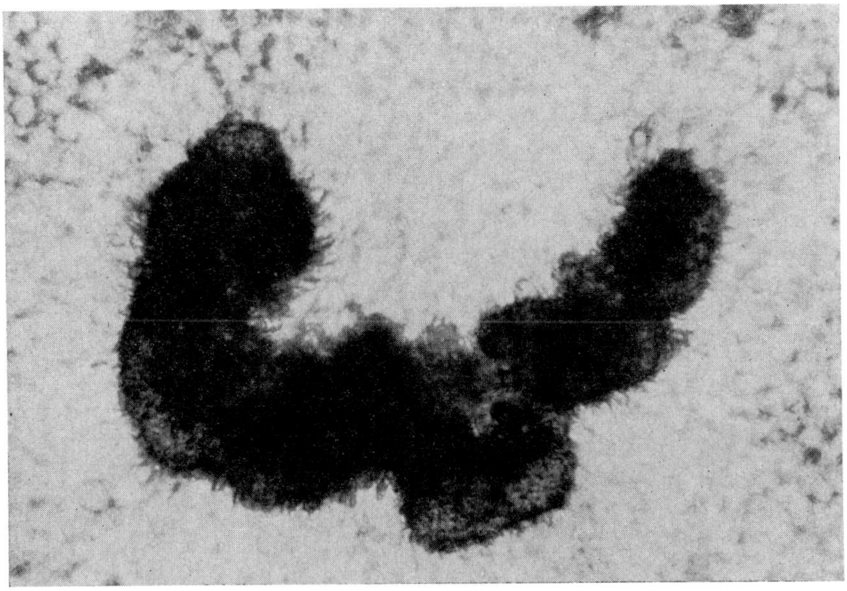

Figure 16-4. Granule of *Nocardia brasiliensis* in purulent exudate, showing the peripheral clubs.

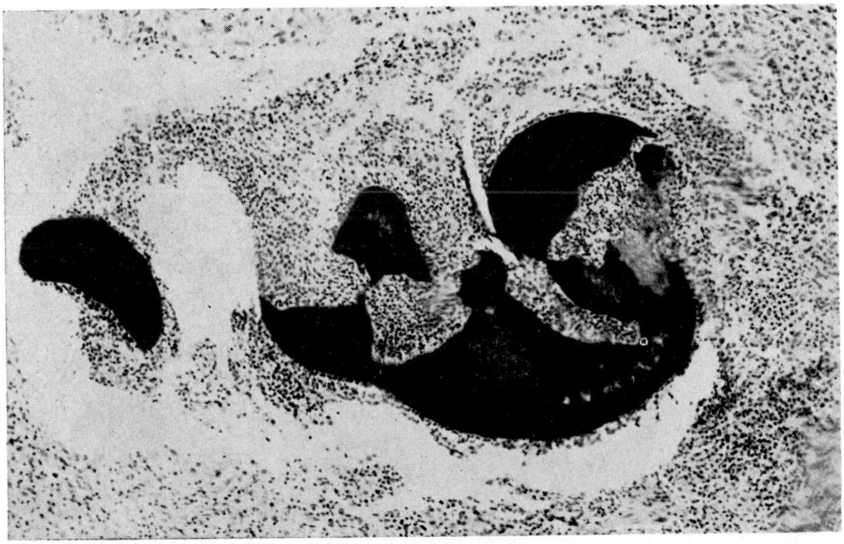

Figure 16-5. Granule of *Nocardia pelletieri* in tissue. Note the typical fragmentation. (H & E stain).

As in some cases of superficial and deep mycoses, mycetomas can be produced by more than one species. Nino (31) reported the finding of *Madurella mycetomi* and *M. grisea* in a black granule in a case of mycetoma of the foot.

Microscopically, it is easy to differentiate actinomycotic from eumycotic granules by the appearance and the width of the mycelial filaments in the granules (Fig. 16-6). Further, the size, presence of clubs and cement, and staining properties aid in the identification of the species, which can be confirmed only by culture.

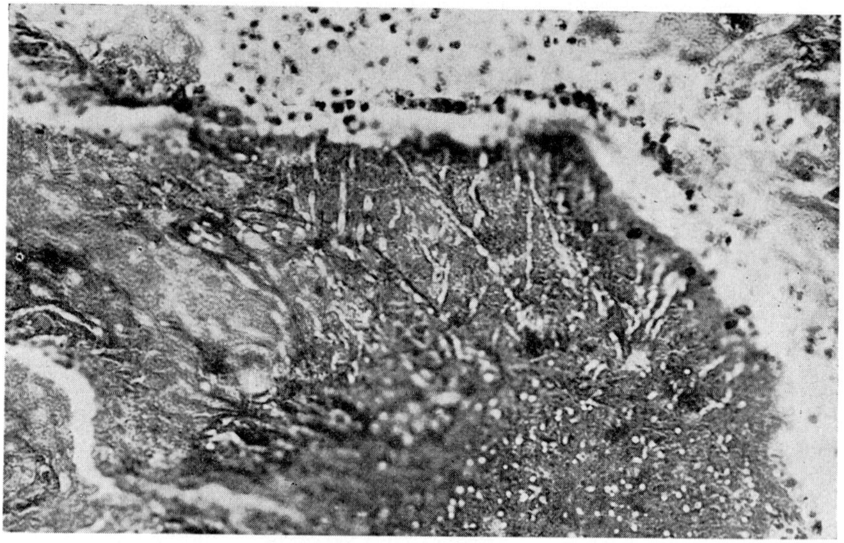

Figure 16-6. Granule of *Madurella mycetomic,* note the coarse filaments (4 μ width), vesicles and interfilamentous cement. (H & E stain).

The Mechanism of Infection

Most authors agree that the microorganisms are introduced by local trauma (28), although some have suggested that a previous pulmonary infection is related to the process (38). Murray et al. (30) found that using multiple peritoneal inoculations of mice with *M. mycetomi* increased the number of granules when the fungus was inoculated in association with dead cultures of *Mycobacterium tuberculosis.*

Macotela and Mariat (25) working with three different kinds of laboratory animals, succeeded in producing peritoneal granules or mycetomas by intraperitoneal or subcutaneous inoculations of *N. brasiliensis* or *N. asteroides*. Some of the animals were previously sensitized with dead cultures of homologous *Nocardia*. The proportion developing intraperitoneal granules of mycetomas varied.

The experimental subcutaneous lesions showed two kinds of histopathological patterns: abscesses and granulomas. Both of these contained the typical granules.

The growth of the lesions did not seem to be influenced by the sex of the animal or by previous sensitization with dead homologous organisms. This finding was later confirmed by Gonzalez-Ochoa (11) who produced mycetomas on the footpads of mice without previous sensitization. It is interesting to note that when performing a series of biopsies on these animals it is possible to follow the development of the typical granules.

The interior of the actinomycotic granules does not contain any other kind of bacteria, and they have too clearly defined areas that are easily distinguishable with an electron microscope (24). Nevertheless, in cultures from human lesions it is possible to isolate various forms of bacterial flora in which *Staphylococcus aureus* is always present (11). *Staphylococcus aureus* was isolated in twenty of twenty-three recent human cases of mycetoma caused by *N. brasiliensis*, and a *Salmonella typhi* in a case of mycetoma due to *M. mycetomi*.

In conclusion, the following are the important points in the epidemiology of mycetomas:

1. Their distribution is universal, with the greatest frequencies occurring in tropical and subtropical developing regions.
2. The pathogenic agents normally live in the soil.
3. Although these organisms grow in the host and produce varied histopathological reactions unquestionably related to immunological and bacteriological conditions that have not yet been completely studied, it is currently believed that a previous sensitization is probably not necessary.

4. Conditions related to the precipitating trauma are of great importance.
5. The further evolution of mycetomas depends on the species of the parasite, its sensitivity to chemotherapeutic agents, and the availability of medical care.

REFERENCES

1. Abbott, P. H.: *Mycetoma: Clinical and Epidemiological Study.* Cambridge Univ. Press, 1954.
2. Adan, C. M. C.: Los Micetomas en el Estado de Morelos. In press, 1973.
3. Ajello, L.: The isolation of *Allescheria boydii*, an etiologic agent of mycetomas, from soil. *Am J Trop Med, 1*:227, 1952.
4. Avram, A.: Quelques particularities concernant les mycetomes d'une contree a climat tempere: La Roumanie. *Dermatol, 139*:390, 1969.
5. Baylet, R., Camain, R., Chabal, J., Izarn, R.: Nouvelle contribution a l'etude des mycetomes au Senegal. Neotestudina rosatii-Pyrenochaeta romeroi-Aspergillus nidulans. *Bull Soc Med Afr Noire Lgu fr, 13*:311, 1968.
6. Baylet, R., Camain, R., Rey, M.: Champignons de mycetomes isoles des epineux au Senegal. *Bull Soc Med Afr Noire Lgue fr, 6*:317, 1961.
7. Bocarro, J. E.: An analysis of 100 cases of mycetoma. *Lancet, 1*:797, 1893.
8. Borelli, D.: *Pyrenochaeta romeroi*, n. sp. *Rev Derm Venez, 1*:325, 1959.
9. Butz, W. C., Ajello, L.: Black grain mycetoma. A case due to *Madurella grisea. Arch Dermatol, 104*:197, 1971.
10. Destombes, P.: Structure histologique des mycetomes. *Ann Soc Belg Med Trop, 44*:897, 1964.
11. Gonzalez Ochoa, A.: Micetoma por *Nocardia brasiliensis.* Mem. I Reunion Mex-Centroamer. *Dermatologia* Mexico, D. F., 1966.
12. Gonzalez Ochoa, A., Baranda, F.: Una prueba cutanea para el diagnostico del micetoma actinomicotico por Nocardia brasiliensis. *Rev Inst Salub Enf Trop (Mex), 13*:189, 1953.
13. Gonzalez Ochoa, A., Gonzalez Mendoza, A.: La micologia medica en Mexico. *Mycopathologia, 13*:56, 1960.
14. Gonzalez Ochoa, A., Sandoval, M. A.: Aislamiento de *Nocardia brasiliensis* y *N. asteroides* a partir de suelos. *Rev Inst Salub Enf Trop (Mex), 20*:147, 1960.
15. Gordon, R. E., Hagan, W. A.: A study of some acid-fast actinomycetes from soil, with special reference to pathogenicity for animals. *J Infect Dis, 59*:200, 1936.

16. Gould, W. M.: Black grain mycetoma originating in northern California. *Arch Dermatol, 99*:426, 1969.
17. Green, W. O., Adams, T. E.: Mycetoma in the United States. A review and report of seven additional cases. *Am J Clin Pathol, 42*:75, 1964.
18. Klokke, A. H., Swamidasan, T., Anguli, R.: The causal agents of mycetoma in South India. *Trans Roy Soc Trop Med Hyg, 62*:509, 1968.
19. Latapi, F., Ortiz, Y.: Los micetomas en Mexico; datos nuevos clinicos y epidemiologicos relativos a 197 casos. Mem. I Cong. Mex. Derm. Mexico, D. F., 1961.
20. Mackinnon, J. E.: A contribution to the study of the causal organisms of maduromycosis. *Trans Roy Soc Trop Med Hyg, 48*:470, 1954.
21. Mackinnon, J. E.: Mycetomas as opportunistic wound infections. *Lab Invest, 11*:1124, 1962.
22. Mackinnon, J. E., Ferrada-Urzua, L. V., Monte-Mayor, L.: *Madurella grisea n. sp. Mycopathologia, 4*:384, 1949.
23. Macotela-Ruiz, E.: Caracteristicas immunologicas de los actinomycetes patogenos para el hombre. I Sus relaciones serologicas segun la tecnica de anticuerpos fluorescentes. *Dermatol Trop, 1*:175, 1963.
24. Macotela-Ruiz, E., Gonzalez-Angulo, A.: Electron microscopic studies on granules of *Nocardia brasiliensis* in man. *Sabouraudia*, 5:92, 1966.
25. Macotela-Ruiz, E., Mariat, F.: Sur la production de mycetomes experimentaux par *Nocardia brasiliensis* et *Nocardia asteroides. Bull Soc Pathol Exot, 56*:46, 1963.
26. Mahgoub, E. S., *Corynespora casiicola*, a new agent of maduromycetoma. *J Trop Med Hyg*, 72:218, 1969.
27. Mariat, F.: Criteres de determination des principales especes d'actinomycetes aerobies pathogenes. *Ann Soc Belg Med Trop, 4*:651, 1962.
28. Mariat, F.: Notes epidemiologiques a propos des mycetomes. In *Recent Progress in Microbiology*. Toronto, Univ., Toronto Press. 1967.
29. Mariat, F.: Sur la distribution Geographique et la Repartition des agents de Mycetomes. *Bull Soc Pathol Exot, 56*:35, 1963.
30. Murray, I. G., Spooner, E. T. C., Walker, J.: Experimental infection of mice with *Madurella mycetomi. Trans Roy Soc Trop Med Hyg, 54*:335, 1960.
31. Nino, F. L.: Coexistencia de *Madurella mycetomi* y de *M. grisea* en una misma observacion de maduromicosis podal negra. *Mycopathologia, 16*:323, 1962.
32. Ortiz-Ortiz, L., Bojalil, L. F.: Delayed skin reactions to cytoplasmic extracts of *Nocardia* organisms as a means of diagnosis and epidemiological study of *Nocardia* infection. *Clin Exp Immunol, 12*: 225, 1972.

33. Ortiz-Ortiz, L., Contreras, M. F., Bojalil, L. F.: The assay of delayed hypersensitivity to ribosomal proteins from *Nocardia*. *Sabouraudia, 10*:147, 1972.
34. Rey, M.: *Les Mycetomes dans l'Ouest Africain*. Paris, Foulon, 1962.
35. Rey, M., Baylet, R., Camain, R.: Donnees actuelles sur les mycetomes a propos de 214 cas africains. *Ann Dermatol, 89*:511, 1962.
36. Rodriguez Millan, A.: Resultados de una encuesta con nocardina en escolares y en habitantes de Acambaro, Gto. Tesis Escuela Nacional de Medicina, Mexico, D. F., 1964.
37. Segretain, G., Baylet, H., Darasse, H., Camain, R.: Leptosphaeria senegalensis n. sp. Agent de mycetomes a grains noirs. *C R Acad Sci (D), 248*:3730, 1959.
38. Segretain, G., Destombes, P.: Description d'un nouvel agent de maduromycose *Neotestudina rosatii* n. gen. n. sp. isole en Afrique. *C R Acad Sci (D), 253*:2577, 1961.

Chapter 17

THE EPIDEMIOLOGY OF THE DERMATOPHYTOSES

LIBERO AJELLO

THE DERMATOPHYTES ARE a group of moulds that have the highly specialized ability to invade and destroy the keratinaceous tissues of animals. As a result of their capability they cause diseases of the skin, hair and nails of humans. Collectively these diseases are referred to as the dermatophytoses. Specific names are given to infections in reference to their topographical location on the body. Hence, we have such useful names as tinea-capitis for infections of the scalp, tinea pedis for foot infections (more commonly known as athlete's foot) and tinea unguium for mycotic infections of the nails.

The dermatophyte species, in their imperfect states, are classified in three genera on the basis of the types of asexual spores that they produce. The three genera are *Epidermophyton, Microsporum* and *Trichophyton. Epidermophyton* is a monotypic genus. Its single species *E. floccosum* produces only smooth-walled macroconidia. Currently fourteen species of fungi are classified in the genus *Microsporum.* These species produce both micro- and macroconidia. The large spores have an echinulate or rough wall. The twenty-two species of *Trichophyton* also produce both micro- and macroconidia, but their macroconidia are smooth-walled (2, 3).

The epidemiology of the dermatophytoses is intimately linked with the natural habitats of the dermatophytes. Ecological studies have shown that the members of the genera *Epidermophyton, Microsporum* and *Trichophyton* are of three basic types:

1. Anthropophilic species—parasites of man not known to exist as saprophytes in soil and seldom found to infect lower animals.
2. Zoophilic species—basically parasites of lower animals that do not exist as saprophytes in nature, and that, depending on the species, rarely or frequently infect humans.
3. Geophilic species—parasites found free-living in nature, with or without the ability to infect either lower animals or humans, or both.

The anthropophilic dermatophytes (Table 17-I) are believed to live exclusively on the skin and its appendages. Infections by these species, in their clinical expression, range from relatively inactive, asymptomatic forms to active and symptomatic forms. Individuals with low grade inapparent infections serve as carriers of the anthropophilic species of *Epidermophyton, Microsporum* and *Trichophyton* (14). When infections flare up, the dermatophytes are disseminated into the environment on shed bits of infected skin, hair or nails (16). Tinea pedis is frequently acquired by individuals who walk barefooted on contaminated floors in their homes or in public places such as gymnasia and bathing areas (9). Tinea capitis may be acquired from contact with unsterilized barbershop instruments or from the backs of theatre seats that have cushioned the heads of patrons with scalp ringworm. Intimate personal contacts between individuals may also serve to directly transmit infections from one individual to

TABLE 17-I

ANTHROPOPHILIC DERMATOPHYTES

Epidermophyton	*T. gourvilii*
E. floccosum	*T. megninii*
Microsporum	*T. mentagrophytes var. interdigitale*
M. audouinii	*T. rubrum*
M. ferrugineum	*T. schoenleinii*
M. praecox	*T. soudanense*
Trichophyton	*T. tonsurans*
T. concentricum	*T. violaceum*

another (10). The exchange of hats by children and close body contacts at play also serve to transmit and spread tinea capitis in a school or a community. Epidemics of *M. audouinii* infections in the urban areas probably develop through such activity.

T. schoenleinii and *T. violaceum* infections are perpetuated within families from one generation to another for centuries (23). The carrier is generally a mother with a smoldering low-grade infection of the scalp (7, 12). In our country the pockets of *T. schoenleinii* infections that exist in Appalachia and the Ozarks probably had their origin in the British Isles, the ancestral home of the infected settlers who migrated to the states of Arkansas, Georgia, Kentucky, Missouri, North and South Carolina, West Virginia and Tennessee (6, 8, 15).

Occasionally lower animals such as cattle and dogs are found to be infected by *E. floccosum* and *T. rubrum*. It has been postulated that these dermatophyte infections are acquired through contact with infected humans (1).

TABLE 17-II

ZOOPHILIC DERMATOPHYTES

Microsporum	*Trichophyton*
M. amazonicum	*T. equinum*
M. canis	*T. erinaceae*
M. distortum	*T. flavescens*
	T. gallinae
	T. mentagrophytes var. mentagrophytes
	T. verrucosum

TABLE 17-III

GEOPHILIC MICROSPORUM AND TRICHOPHYTON SPECIES

Microsporum	*Trichophyton*
M. boullardii	*T. ajelloi*
M. cookei	*T. georgiae*
M. fulvum	*T. gloriae*
M. gypseum	*T. longifusus*
M. nanum	*T. phaseoliforme*
M. persicolor	*T. simii*
M. racemosum	*T. terrestre*
M. vanbreuseghemii	*T. vanbreuseghemii*

T. mentagrophytes merits special mention since there are two basic varieties of this species: *T. mentagrophytes* var. *interdigitale* and *T. mentagrophytes* var. *mentagrophytes*. The *interdigitale* variety is anthropophilic and is one of the most common agents of tinea pedis. It also causes tinea capitis, tinea corporis and tinea unguinam in susceptible individuals. In contrast the *mentagrophytes* or granular variety is a common parasite of a host of lower animals (1). Animals infected by this pigmented and granular form of *T. mentagrophytes* may transmit their fungus to humans by contacts or indirectly through their shed infected hairs.

Neither of these two forms of *T. mentagrophytes* is known to be geophilic. On occasion this species is isolated from soil specimens but the author considers this to be the result of a temporary contamination of a circumscribed site with infected material rather than the result of saprophytic growth in nature.

Despite their close affinity for man, the anthropophilic dermatophytes are not equally distributed around the world. Some species are cosmopolitan and are found wherever humans have settled. Others, for undefined ecological reasons, are limited to restricted regions of the world (Table 17-IV).

In the course of their evolution, the zoophilic dermatophytes (Tables 17-II, 17-V), like the anthropophilic ones, apparently lost the ability to withstand the competition of free living microorganisms in soil. They became adapted to live primarily on the keratinaceous tissues of lower animals. The majority of these species can also infect humans. In some regions of the world one species, *M. canis*, is the dominant etiological agent of skin and hair infections in the general population.

Humans generally become infected by these animal-borne moulds by coming in direct contact with their various hosts. Farmers, members of their families, and others who handle cattle infected by *T. verrucosum* frequently acquire the disease. Similarly, individuals who work with horses are apt to become infected by *T. equinum*. Human infections caused by *T. gallinae* are apparently infrequent, probably because avian infections by this dermatophyte are rare. In contrast, as mentioned previously, *M. canis* infections are commonly acquired by inhabitants of both rural and urban areas. This is the direct result of man's intimate and long association with cats and dogs, the principal carriers and transmitters of *M. canis*.

TABLE 17-IV

GEOGRAPHIC DISTRIBUTION OF ANTHROPOPHILIC DERMATOPHYTES

Species	*Endemic Areas*
Epidermophyton	
E. floccosum	World wide
Microsporum	
M. audouinii	World wide
M. ferrugineum	Africa, Asia, Europe*
M. praecox	France†
Trichophyton	
T. concentricum	Asia, Latin America, Oceania
T. gourvilli	Africa
T. megninii	Europe
T. mentagrophytes	World wide
T. schoenleinii	Africa, Asia, Europe‡
T. soudanense	Africa (may be spreading to rest of world)
T. tonsurans	World wide
T. violaceum	Africa, Asia, Europe‡

*Endemic foci exist in several European countries, notably Bulgaria, Czechoslovakia and Yugoslavia. These may have been established long ago by Mongol invaders who introduced the fungus.

†Known only from a single isolate. It may be conspecific with *M. gypseum*.

‡Endemic foci in New World; introduced by European settlers and African slaves

TABLE 17-V

GEOGRAPHIC DISTRIBUTION OF ZOOPHILIC DERMATOPHYTES

Species	*Endemic Areas*
Microsporum	
M. amazonicum	Brazil
M. canis	World wide
M. distortum	Australia, New Zealand, United States
Trichophyton	
T. equinum	World wide
T. erinaceae	France, Great Britain, New Zealand
T. flavescens	Australia
T. gallinae	World wide
T. mentagrophytes mentagrophytes	World wide

Little is known about the epidemiology of the infections that the other two zoophilic *Microsporum* species cause. In a few cases. *M. distortum* infections in humans have been traced to contact with animals. However, in other instances no such connection has been demonstrated (24).

The description of *M. amazonicum* is based on two isolates from wild rats captured near Manaus in Brazil. The hosts were free of lesions which indicates that eventually this fungus will be found to be geophilic (17).

T. flavescens has yet to be incriminated as an agent of human disease. Up to the present it has been isolated only from the feathers of three different species of Australian birds (19, 22). Since lesions were not evident on these birds, it may eventually be found that *T. flavescens* is a geophilic fungus.

T. erinaceae is basically a parasite of the European hedgehog (*Erinaceus europaeus*), but infections in humans have been diagnosed in New Zealand, Great Britian and France. In these instances infection was transmitted by either direct or indirect contact with infected animals or with their nests (11).

The zoophilic form of *T. mentagrophytes* is a common pathogen of individuals who came into contact with the large variety of hosts of this fungus.

Among the sixteen species of geophilic *Microsporum* and *Trichophyton* species (Tables 17-III, 17-VI), nine have yet to be implicitly found to infect man or lower animals. These species are *M. boullardii, M. racemosum, T. ajelloi, T. georgiae, T. gloriae, T. longifusus, T. phaseoliforme, T. terrestre* and *T. vanbreuseghemii*. On occasion they have been isolated from the pelts of lower animals and even from humans. However, an infectious role was not established for those isolates. Their presence must be assumed to have resulted from soil contamination (3).

M. cookei, a not uncommon soil mould throughout the world, has been found to cause infections in an African baboon and humans in Australia and Europe.

Infections among humans as well as animals by members of the *M. fulvum* and *M. gypseum* complex are quite frequent. Both species are rather common soil inhabitants throughout the world.

M. nanum is a geophilic mould that has a predilection for pigs.

It is the most common cause of ringworm among swine. Infections in humans not always traceable to contact with infected animals, have been documented in Australia, New Zealand, Cuba, Europe and the Americas (4).

Recent studies have revealed not only that *M. persicolor* is geophilic but that it is not confined to Europe. This species, once considered to be a variety of *T. mentagrophytes*, has been isolated from soil in Bulgaria, India and South Africa. Non-European infections have been diagnosed in Africa, Asia, Australia and North and South America (20, 21).

M. vanbreuseghemii is a little known dermatophyte. To date it has been recovered from soil in India and Mozambique. Human infections were first described in the United States and then in Hungary. The only other isolations of this dermatophyte have been from a dog and a captive Malabar squirrel in the United States (3).

TABLE 17-VI

GEOGRAPHIC DISTRIBUTION OF GEOPHILIC DERMATOPHYTES

Species	*Endemic Areas*
Microsporum	
M. boullardii	Guinea
M. cookei	World wide
M. fulvum	World wide
M. gypseum	World wide
M. nanum	Africa, Asia, Australia, Europe, New Zealand, North America
M. persicolor	Africa, Australia, Europe, New World
M. racemosum	Brazil, Rumania, Venezuela
M. vanbreuseghemii	Hungary, India, Mozambique, United States
Trichophyton	
T. ajelloi	World wide
T. georgiae	Australia, Europe, South America, United States
T. gloriae	United States
T. longifusus	Hungary
T. phaseoliformis	Poland, Switzerland, Venezuela
T. simii	Brazil, Guinea, India
T. terrestre	World wide
T. vanbreuseghemii	Canada, Germany, Rumania, Tunisia

The geophilic nature of *T. simii* was established by the repeated isolation of this versatile dermatophyte from soil in India. Infections have been recorded in humans as well as a variety of domesticated and wild animals (13, 18).

Although medical mycology has come a long way, since Remak's 1837 discovery that fungi can cause human disease, much remains to be learned about the dermatophytes (5). The evolutionary factors that led to their differentiation into geophilic, zoophilic and anthropophilic species remain unknown. Nor do we understand the genetical, physiological and biochemical basis for the gamut of pathogenicity possessed by the various dermatophytes and the related species of *Microsporum* and *Trichophyton.* The members of the genera *Epidermophyton, Microsporum,* and *Trichophyton* offer a fertile field for study by microbiologists of all persuasions.

REFERENCES

1. Ainsworth, G. C., Austwick, P. K. C.: *Fungal Diseases of Animals,* 2nd ed. Commonwealth Agricultural Bureau, Farnham Royal, Slough, England, 1973.
2. Ajello, L.: A taxonomic review of the dermatophytes and related species. *Sabouraudia, 6*:147-159, 1968.
3. Ajello, L.: Natural history of the dermatophytes and related fungi. *Mycopath Mycol Appl, 53*:93-110, 1974.
4. Ajello, L., Varsavsky, E., Ginther, O. J., Bubash, G.: The natural history of *Microsporum nanum. Mycologia, 56*:873-884, 1964.
5. Alkiewicz, J. A.: On the discovery of *Trichophyton schoenleinii (Achorion schoenleinii). Mycopath Mycol Appl, 33*:28-32, 1967.
6. Barrett, C. C.: Endemic favus. *South Med J, 43*:685-689, 1950.
7. Carslaw, R. W.: Favus of the scalp. Observations on the manner of spread. *Br J Dermatol, 67*:392-396, 1955.
8. Dobes, W. L.: Favus: Occurrence in Georgia. *Urol Cutaneous Rev, 52*:729-734, 1948.
9. Drouhet, M. E., Marcel, M., Labonde, J.: Flore dermatophytique des piscines. *Bull Soc Fran Dermatol Syph, 74*:719-724, 1967.
10. English, M. P.: *Trichophyton rubrum* infection in families. *Br J Med, 5021*:744-746, 1957.
11. English, M. P., Morris, P.: *Trichophyton mentagrophytes* var. *erinacei* in hedgehog nests. *Sabouraudia, 7*:118-121, 1969.
12. Grin, E. I.: Principles of mass treatment of tinea capitis. *Mycopath Mycol Appl, 24*:243-249, 1964.

13. Gupta, P. K., Singh, R. P., Singh, I. P.: Dermatophytes from man, dogs and pigs with special reference to *Trichophyton simii* and *Microsporum nanum*. *Ind J Anim Hlth*, *7*:247-253, 1968.

14. Ive, F. A.: The carrier stage of tinea capitis in Nigeria. *Br J Med*, *78*: 219-221, 1966.

15. Lorenc, E., Woolridge, W. E.: An endemic focus of favus in South Central Missouri. *Missouri Med*, *59*:860-862, 1962.

16. Midgley, Gillian, Clayton, Yvonne M.: Distribution of dermatophytes and Candida spores in the environment. *Br J Dermatol*, *86*:69-77, 1972.

17. Moraes, M., Borelli, D., Feo, Mildred: *Microsporum amazonicum* nova species. *Med Cut*, *2*:281-286, 1967.

18. Padhye, A. A., Thirumalachar, M. J.: Isolation of *Trichophyton simii* and *Cryptococcus neoformans* from soil in India. *Hindustan Antibiot Bull*, *9*:155-157, 1967.

19. Padhye, A. A., Carmichael, J. W.: The genus *Arthroderma* Berkelev. *Can J Bot*, *9*:155-157, 1967.

20. Padhye, A. A., Blank, F., Koblenzer, P. J., Spatz, S., Ajello, L.: *Microsporum persicolor* infection in the United States. *Arch Dermatol*, *108*:561-562, 1973.

21. Padhye, A. A., Ajello, L.: The natural history of *Microsporum persicolor*. *Int J Dermatol*, in press.

22. Rees, R. G.: *Arthroderma flavescens* sp. nov. *Sabouraudia*, *5*:206-208, 1967.

23. Sabouraud, R.: Evolution et moeurs du favus. Nouvelle Derm. Vol. 2, pp. 120-121, Masson et Cie, Paris, 1936.

24. Smith, J. M. B.: *Microsporum distortum* ringworm in New Zealand. *Aust J Dermatol*, *11*:131-138, 1970.

Chapter 18

THE EPIDEMIOLOGY OF OTHER MYCOTIC DISEASES

RONALD F. SPROUSE

REVIEW OF THE voluminous literature suggests a variety of mycotic diseases either limited in occurrence or insignificant in pathology to warrant extensive discussion. However, one would be remiss to not at least update existing reviews or make mention of some of the more common of these diseases.

A few other diseases are either of recent report or questionable fungal etiology which should also receive mention. These include Cladosporiosis, Cercosporamycosis, Onychoialperonychomycosis, Protothecosis, Pneumocysticosis, Trichomycosis Axillaris and Erythrasma. *Cladosporium trichoides* and other species in the genus have been isolated from pulmonary meningeal and cerebral lesions (37). There are numerous reports of onychomycosis and peronychial lesions caused by species in the genus *Scopulariopsis,* especially *S. brevicaulis* (6). Subcutaneous lesions produced an isolate of *Cercospora apii* (18) and the achloric algae, *Prototheca segbwema* (*Arch. Derm., 1046*:490, 1971; *Trans. St. Johns Hosp. Derm. Soc., 58*:38, 1972) and pulmonary lesions caused by *Pneumocystis carinii* (*Ann. Thor. Surg., 14*:335 and 445, 1972) also have been reported. Trichomycosis axillaris and erythrasma are relatively common diseases of limited pathologic consequence (14, 44). The former is characterized by invasion of pubic hair by either *Corynebacterium tenuis* (yellow nodule), *Micrococcus castellani* (red nodule) or *M. nigresiens* (black nodule). The latter erythrasma is characterized by maculo-papular lesion on the epidermis caused by the Gram positive filamentous bacterium *Corynebacterium minutissimum.*

Torulopsis

Torulopsis is an infrequent disease usually exhibiting itself as an acute or subacute post-operative infection. The single-budding ovoid yeast originally was isolated from human feces and named *Cryptococcus glabratea* (3). Berlese in 1895 introduced the generic name *Torulopsis* which presently contains some 36 species, including *T. colliculosa,* the type species for the genus, and *T. glabrata,* the only species reported as pathogenic for man (30). The frequency with which the microorganism is isolated from urine and feces would suggest an endogenous etiology (49).

A fatal case of septicema was reported (16), as well as a patient with meningoencephalitis which was successfully treated with 5-fluorocytosine (55). Previous complicating factors were evident in both cases. Undoubtedly the microorganism is opportunistic, similar to the *Candida species* (49). Its normal role probably is that of an inhabitant of the gastrointestinal tract and it assumes a pathogenic role only under extraordinary circumstances such as concomitant disease, prolonged antibiotic therapy, or immunosuppression.

Geotrichosis

Geotrichosis is an infrequent infection which usually exhibits itself as a bronchopulmonary syndrome or, less frequently, an infection of the epithelial lining of the buccal cavity or intestinal mucosa. The etiologic agent *Geotrichum candidum,* like *Candida* species, more than likely is a normal or transitional inhabitant of the gastrointestinal tract, and invades tissue only under extenuating circumstances. Schnoor (45) examined faecal specimens from 319 individuals with no apparent lesions and isolated *G. candidum* from 29 percent of the subjects. Examination of 1,147 patients indicated *G. candidum* was a common inhabitant of bronchial secretions (40). Similar observations indicated past or present contact with *G. candidum* for eleven of forty-eight patients with bronchopulmonary complications (25). These data would corroborate an endogenous etiology for *Geotrichum* infections. The report of an endemic geotrichosis involving five of eight members in a family (50) suggested a possible contagious mechanism. Usually, coexisting diseases such as tuberculosis, emphysema, bacterial and viral pneumonia and numerous other complications are predisposing to bronchopulmonary geotrichosis (53). Reports of disseminated or septisemic geotrichosis (11, 21, 24) invariably indicated predisposing or coexisting disease. *G. candidum* has been reported as causing tumefaction in the hand (22). The microorganism frequently is found in association with paronychial lesions, probably in a saprophytic rather than parasitic role.

Pityrosporum Folliculitis

Pityrosporum folliculitis exhibits itself as pilosebaceous follicular inflammatious vesiculopustular lesions usually on the upper back, shoulders and anterior chest. The frequent occurrence of *Pityrosporum ovale* blastospores in areas of inflammation strongly suggests a casual relationship between the microorganism and the disease process (23). Definitive data implicating *P. ovale* as the etiologic agent has not been presented. Possibly enhanced lipogenesis resulting from the pilosebaceous inflammation may simply attract the lipophilic yeast.

There appears to be no race or sex predilection or seasonal occurrence for the disease. Age preference is from twelve to sixty years. Clinically the disease can mimic acne, drug eruption, papular urticaria and less frequently herpes lesions, cutaneous candidiasis or cutaneous cryptococcosis (23).

Piedra

Piedra is characterized by the formation of concretions or nodules on the distal third of hair shafts caused by either *Trichosporon cutaneum* (white piedra) or the Ascomycete, *Piedraia hortai* (black piedra). The nodule, a tightly woven meshwork of hyphae, fragments into numerous ovoid arthrospores in the case of the former, and forms ascostroma in the latter. The disease causes little or no physiologic damage to the host and is generally eradicated by cropping the infected hair.

There is no age, sex or race predilection for either disease. The less frequent form, white piedra, generally is limited to temperate areas of the world, but is observed in tropical regions (39). Black piedra, on the other hand, is confined in its occurrence and limited almost entirely to tropical regions.

The exact source of either microorganism is unknown. It has been suggested that stagnant water in certain geographic areas may be the source of *P. hortai* (23). Kaplan (26) reported the disease occurred in lower primates but inferred no specific zoonotic implications. White piedra has been observed in lower primates and is not an uncommon infection of the equine, suggesting a zoonotic ramification. *T. cutaneum* also has been isolated from soil and plant residues. These may be the natural habitats for the microorganisms and provide the source for infection of human hair.

Tinea Versicolor

Tinea versicolor is a relatively common chronic, superficial infection of the skin. Involved epidermis usually appears normal, although slightly thickened. Characteristic lesions are usually apparent as hypochromic, furfuraceous, desquamating macules principally on the trunk.

The disease was first observed in 1846 and the microorganism was studied in histopathologic sections where similarity of the chains of yeast cells to the mosaic small spored ectothrix invasion at the base of the hair shaft by *Microsporuin audouinii* was observed. The microorganism was named *Microsporum furfur* (42). Baillon (4) examined similar tissue sections and recognized the blastogenic nature of the microorganism. He placed it in a new genus *Malassezia*, retaining the original species designation *furfur*. Further, convincing evidence was presented that *M. furfur* and *Pityrosporum orbiculare*, are one and the same (28).

The fungus appears to have its habitat in human skin, probably living in a quiescent state for a significant portion of the population. Burke (7) suggested that individuals exhibiting clinically apparent lesions probably possess a genetic predisposition for the disease. However, clinical disease occurs more frequently in the young and darker-pigmented individuals, consequently the disease is more common in tropical areas.

Tinea Nigra Palmaris

Tinea nigra palmaris is a chronic, asymptomatic disease usually occurring on the palms or palmar surfaces of the finger, and less frequently on the limbs, thorax, neck and soles. The disease is characterized by single or multiple dark-pigmented serpiginous macular lesions.

It was suggested that the dematiacous yeast-like fungus *Cladosporium werneckii* is the usual cause of tinea nigra palmaris in the Western Hemisphere while *C. mansoni* is responsible for the disease in the Orient (31). Less than four dozen cases have been reported in the Continental United States (48, 52). Those cases generally were limited to the Southeastern Seaboard states and Texas coastal areas. Cases also have been reported from Panama (46), Brazil (34), Puerto Rico (8), Cuba (38) and Great Britain (10). Castellani and Chalmers (9) indicated the disease is common in the Orient.

In the majority of cases in the Orient, lesions occurred on the neck and upper chest, while the palm was most often involved in patients from the Western Hemisphere (31).

The fungi presumably occur in soil and plant debris and are introduced into the epidermis via traumatization (38). Other reports of disease with familial associations would suggest a possible communicable mechanism (52). The disease has been reported in patients five to fifty-five years of age. However, the vast majority of patients observed in the United States are less than eighteen years old. The disease occurs predominantly in the lightly pigmented races, is about three times more common in the female than male and generally is limited to the less pigmented areas of the body.

Penicillosis

Penicillosis usually exhibits itself as a bronchopulmonary syndrome. Less frequently other complications, such as ear, eye, or urinary tract infections occur. At least eleven cases of bronchopulmonary disease have been substantiated by culture procedures (32). Eight of these cases were documented before the generalized use of antibiotics and five had no history of previous or concomitant disease. Clinical findings generally are compatible with pulmonary tuberculosis with occasional progression to cavitation. Implication of *Penicillium* species in ear infections also has been reported (41). Saprophytic fungi from 26 percent of patients with chronically infected, postoperative mastoid cavities were isolated (47). However, *Penicillium* species were implicated in only a small percentage of these infections. A fatal penicillosis with involvement of the ethmoid sinuses, orbit and cerebral arteries was recently reported (33). It is generally accepted that secondary penicillosis has increased considerably with widespread use of antibiotics, immunosuppressive drugs, antimetabolities and steroids. It is impossible to determine the importance of various *Penicillium* species in immediate hypersensitivity. Their significance in atopic dermatitis and respiratory allergy, however, has received considerable attention in recent years (20, 51).

Rhinosporidiosis

Rhinosporidiosis is a chronic granulomatous disease characterized by the formation of polypoid lesions on the nasal mucosa. Other sites, such as the eyes, ears, larynx, genitalia and skin may be involved secondarily (2). There also have been reports of disseminated viscereal involvement (1). Comprehensive review by Karunaratne (27) indicated the disease occurred predominantly in India and Ceylon. However, the first case was reported from Argentina in 1892 (54). The etiologic agent *Rhinosporidium seeberi* was described in 1896 but has never been cultured *in vitro*. Karunaratne (27) indicated the disease is most common in individuals who work or swim in stagnant sand or water from Indian streams. The male is infected at a much higher rate than the female, suggesting an occupational predisposition. All ages and races appear equally susceptible.

Adiaspiromycosis

The disease is described as a unique pulmonary disease common to rodents in the Southwestern United States (17). The etiologic agents generally were presented as *Emmonsia crescens* and *E. parva*. More recent reports (15, 19) indicate the disease is world wide in occurrence. Sparce reports of the disease in humans would indicate most cases present similar clinical pictures. However, Kodousek (29) reported observing *E. crescens* spherules in an infected appendix from a seven-year-old boy.

Mycotic Keratitis and Otitis

Mycotic infection of the eye is in reference to invasion of the corneal surface by a variety of usually innocuous fungal saprophytes. Invasion, if unchecked, can develop into an indolent corneal ulcer with extension into the anterior chamber and less frequently the posterior chamber with retinitis. Various species in the genera *Aspergillus, Penicillium, Fusarium, Geotrichum, Cladosporium, Rhodotorula,* routinely occur in the conjunctival sac (13). Newmark and Poack (35) indicated that *Fusarium, Aspergillus* and *Cephalosporium* species are most often incriminated in the disease process. Invasion apparently is predisposed to trauma, usually abrasion to the corneal surface and introduction of the fungal spores.

Prior to the advent and widespread use of antibiotics and steroids, most eye infections were caused by *Aspergillus fumigatus* (12). However, the antibiotic-steroid era has resulted in a wide variety of etiologies. Recent reports of infections by species of *Rhodotorula, Candida, Fusarium, Curvularia, Allescheria,* would confirm this conclusion (5, 36, 43, 56).

Review of the limited recent literature on mycotic infections of the ear reaffirm that, too often undefined pathology in otologic diagnosis is called *otomycosis* (54). Those rare instances of bona fide otomycosis invariably are associated with predisposing conditions such as trauma, surgery or prolonged use of immunosuppressives, steroids or antibiotics.

REFERENCES

1. Agrawal, S., Sharma, K. D., Shrivastava, J. B.: Generalized rhinosporidiosis with visceral involvement. *Arch Dermatol, 80*:22, 1959.
2. Allen, F. R. W. K., Dave, A. M.: The treatment of Rhinosporidiosis in man: Based on a study of sixty cases. *Ind Med Gaz, 71*:376, 1936.
3. Anderson, H. W.: Yeast-like fungi of the human intestinal tract. *J Infect Dis, 21*:341, 1917.

4. Baillon, E. H., Traite de botanique medicale cryptogamique. Paris, 1889.
5. Bakerspigel, A.: Fungi isolated from keratomycosis in Ontario, Canada. I. *Monosporium apiospermum (Allescheria boydii). Sabouraudia,* 9:109, 1971.
6. Belsan, I., Fragner, P.: Onychomycosen, hervorgerufen durch *Scopulariopsis brevicoulis. Hautarzt, 16*:258, 1965.
7. Burke, R. C.: Tinea Versicolor: Susceptibility factor and experimental infection in human beings. *J Invest Dermatol, 36*:389, 1961.
8. Carrion, A. L.: Yeast-like dematiaceous fungi infecting the human skin: Special reference to so-called hormiscium dermatitidis. *Arch Dermatol Syph (Chicago), 61*:996, 1950.
9. Castellani, A., Chalmers, A. S.: *Manual of Tropical Medicine.* London, Batlliere, Tindall and Cox, 1919.
10. Chadfield, H. W., Campbell, K.: A case of Tinea nigra in Britain. *Br J Dermatol, 87*:305, 1972.
11. Chang, W. W. L., Burger, W.: Disseminated geotrichosis; a case report. *Arch Int Med, 113*:365, 1964.
12. Chick, E. W., Conant, N. F.: Mycotic ulcerative keratitis: A review of 148 cases from the literature. *Invest Ophthal, 1*:419, 1962.
13. Cordero Moreno, R.: Etiologic factor in tropical eye disease. *Am J Ophthal, 75*:349.
14. Crissey, J. T., Rebell, G. C., Laskin, J. J.: Studies on the causative organism of Trichomycosis Axillaris. *J Invest Dermatol, 19*:187, 1952.
15. Doby, J. M., Boisseau Lebreuil, M. T., Rault, B.: L'Adiospiromycose par Emmonsia crescens chez les petits mammiferes sauvages in France. *Mycopath Mycol Appl, 44*:107, 1971.
16. Edebo, L., Jansson, L. E., Hallin, A.: A fatal case of Torulopsis fungaemia. *Acta Chir Scand, 131*:473, 1966.
17. Emmons, C. W., Ashburn, C. C.: The isolation of *Haplosporangum parvum* sp. n. and *Coccidioides immitis* from wild rodents. Their relationship to Coccidioidomycosis. *Pub Hlth Rep U S, 57*:1715, 1942.
18. Emmons, C. W., Joe, L. K., Eng, N. I. T., Pohaw, A., Kertopati, S., Van Der Meulen, A.: Basidiobolus and Cercospora from human infections. *Mycologia, 49*:1, 1957.
19. Emmons, C. W., Jellison, W. L.: *Emmonsia crescens* sp. n. and Adiaspiromycosis (Haplomycosis) in mammals. *N Y Acad Sci, 89*:91, 1960.
20. Fujisawa, S. Y., Ofuju, S.: Eczematous dermatitis produced by airebourne molds. *Arch Dermatol, 94*:413, 1968.
21. Ghamande, A. R., Landes, F. B., Snider, G. L.: Bronchial geotrichosis with fungemia complications bronchogenic carcinoma. *Chest, 59*: 98, 1971.

22. Goldman, S., Lipscome, P. R., Ulrich, J. A.: Geotrichum Tunefaction of the hand: Report of a case. *J Bone Joint Surg (A) Am, 51*:587, 1969.
23. Graham, J. H., Johnson, W. C., Helwig, E. B.: *Dermatology Pathology.* Hagerstown, Harper and Row, 1972.
24. Kaliski, S. R., Beene, M. L., Mattman, L.: Geotrichosis in the blood stream of an infant. *JAMA, 148*:1207, 1959.
25. Kanelskaya, V. Y.: Klinika, diagnostika i lechenie gribkoykh grainoritov (Clinical picture, diagnosis and treatment of fungal highmorites). *Vestn Otorinolaringol, 32*:49, 1970.
26. Kaplan, W. J.: Piedra in lower animals. *Am Vet Med Assoc, 134*:113, 1959.
27. Karunaratne, W. A. E.: *Rhinosporidiosis in Man.* London Athlone Press, 1964.
28. Keddie, F. M., Shadomy, S.: Etiological significance of *Pityrosporum orbiculare* in Tinea Versicolor. *Sabouraudia, 3*:21, 1963.
29. Kodousek, R.: Nalez izolovanych sferul houby ze skuping *Emmonsia crescens* v aperacin vzorku appendixu u 7 leteho. *Path Anatusb Lek Fak P U Olomouc, 8*:160, 1972.
30. Lodder, J., De Vries, N. F.· Some notes on *Torulopsis glabrata* (Anderson). *Mycopath Mycol Appl, 1*:98, 1938, 1939.
31. Lurie, H. I., Borok, R.: Tinea Nigra: A review of the literature and report of the first case in South Africa. *S Afr J Med Sci, 23*:201, 1958.
32. Maddaux, G. L., Mohr, J. A., Muchmore, H. J.: Pulmonary Penicilliosis. A case report and review of the literature. *J Okla State Med Assoc, 65*:418, 1972.
33. Morriss, F. H., Jr., Spock, A.: Intracranial aneurysm secondary to mycotic orbital and sinus infection. Report of a case implicating penicillium as an opportunistic fungus. *Am J Dis Child, 119*:357, 1970.
34. Neves, J. A., Costa, O. G.: Tinea Nigra. *Arch Dermatol, 55*:67, 1947.
35. Newmark, E., Polack, F. M.: Tetroploa keratomycosis. *Ophthalmology, 70*:1013, 1971.
36. Nityanada, K.: Sirasubramaniam, P., Ajello, L.: Mycotic keratitis caused by *Curvularia lunata*: A case report. *Sabouraudia, 2*:35, 1962.
37. Papadatos, C., Pavlalow, M., Alexion, D.: Cephalosporium Meningitis. *Pediatr, 44*:749, 1969.
38. Pardo Castello, V.: Keratomycosis Nigricans Palmaris. *Rev Argent Dermatosifo, 22*:255, 1938.
39. Patterson, J. C., Laine, S. L., Taylor, W. B.: White Piedra. *Arch Dermatol, 85*:534, 1962.

40. Pilheu, J. A., Negromi, R., Toppi, B.: Flora mecotica en eh aparato respiratorio. *Thorax, 17*:159-163, 1968.
41. Polyanskiy, L. N.: A case of otogenic abscess of the temporal lobe of the brain produced by penicillium. *Zhleshn nos Garl Bolezn, 15*: 138, 1938.
42. Robin, C.: *Histoiri Naturella des Vegetaux Parasites Qui Croessent sur L'homme et sur Animaux Vivants.* Paris, J. B. Billiere, 1853.
43. Romano, A., Segal, E., Ben Tovim: Epithelial keratities due to *Rhodotorula. Ophthal, 166*:353, 1973.
44. Sarkany, I., Taplin, D., Blank, H.: Incidence and bacteriology of Erythrasma. *Arch Dermatol, 85*:578, 1962.
45. Schnoor, T. G.: The occurrence of Monilia in normal stools. *Am J Trop Med, 19*:163, 1939.
46. Slepyan, A. J., Geuting, B. G.: Tinea Nigra Palmaris in Chicago area. *Arch Dermatol, 76*:570, 1957.
47. Smyth. G. D. L.: Fungal infection Otology. *Br J Dermatol, 76*:425, 1964.
48. Spiller, W. F., Mullins, F., Knox, J. S.: Tinea Nigra. *J Invest Dermatol, 27*:187, 1956.
49. Symmers, W. St. C.: Opportunistic infection. *Proc R C Med, 58*:341, 1965.
50. Thjotta, I., Urdal, K.: A family endemic of Geotrichosis Pulmonium. *Acta Pathol Microbiol Scand, 26*:673, 1949.
51. Tuft, L., Tuft, H. S., Heck, V. M.: Atopic dermatitis: 1 An experimental clinical study of the role of inhalant allergens. *J Allergy, 21*:181, 1950.
52. Van Velsor, H., Singletary, H.: Tinea Nigra Palmaris: A report of fifteen cases from Coastal North Carolina. *Arch Dermatol, 90*:59, 1964.
53. Webster, R. H.: Bronchopulmonary Geotrichosis. A review with report of four cases. *Dis Chest, 35*:273, 1959.
54. Wilson, T. W., Plunkett, O. A.: *The Fungus Disease of Man.* Berkeley, Univ. Calif., 1967.
55. Wurzel, B., Goldburg, P., Caroline, W., Bozza, A. T., Kozinn, P. J.: *Torulopsis glabrata* meningoencephalites treated with 5-fluorocytosine. *Ann Intern Med, 77*:814, 1972.
56. Zapater, R. C., De Arrechia, A., Guevara, V. H.: Kertomycosis due to *Fusarium dimerum. Sabouraudia, 10*:274, 1972.

Chapter 19

THE MEDICAL MYCOLOGICAL ICEBERG

LIBERO AJELLO

ANY ATTEMPT TO QUANTITATE the socioeconomic impact of the mycoses on the public is virtually doomed to failure. Since they are not classified among the notifiable diseases, hard data on their incidence and prevalence, as well as information on the morbidity and mortality they cause, are either fragmentary or simply not available.

The situation that confronts us can well be likened to an iceberg. The only visible portions of the vast bulk of the mycoses problem are a few peaks and crags. Even these are only dimly revealed at best by the scattered reports that are available on the incidence and prevalence of fungus infections.

Data on the number of persons affected by mycoses are not compiled regularly by any nation or organization. Information on the occurrence of mycoses is further obscured by commercial secrecy, which makes it difficult to obtain or to publish figures on the dollar and cents value of the antifungal pharmaceutical preparations marketed. Consequently, the public is apathetic, and public health organizations have not given any truly significant or sustained support to programs to control these diseases.

This report of the incidence and prevalence of mycoses was compiled from numerous case reports, reviews, and surveys published by investigators throughout the world.

Revised version of 1971 publication in HSMHA Health Reports, 86:437-448, 1971.

Cutaneous Mycoses

It should be obvious to all that the cutaneous mycoses do, indeed, constitute a serious public health problem. Their toll in terms of suffering, disability, man-hour losses, psychological trauma, and monetary expenditure is much greater than is generally realized. Among this group of diseases are some that approach dental caries and the common cold in both incidence and prevalence. Untold numbers of people throughout the world are afflicted by the specialized fungi that invade and destroy skin, hair, and nails.

Tinea versicolor

In tropical regions of the world, tinea versicolor is widespread. Millions of persons are infected in Africa, Asia, and Latin America. For example, in the Democratic Republic of the Congo, Vanbreuseghem (63) noted that this disease was the most prevalent of all the mycoses. The disease is rife among the inhabitants of the coastal areas of Mexico, the so-called tierras calientes, and Gonzalez-Ochoa (20) has observed a 50 percent rate of infection in the general population.

An equally high prevalence of this disease was encountered by Marples (42) in Western Samoa. A similar situation must exist throughout Melanesia and Polynesia. Indifference to tinea versicolor is universal; many victims are either unaware of their infection or are resigned to live with it because of limited financial resources and lack of medical facilities.

Although tinea versicolor is especially prevalent in the tropics, it occurs elsewhere as well. Stein's data (59) show that it is responsible for approximately 5 percent of the fungus infections in temperate regions. Certainly this disease is not uncommon in the United States.

Tinea pedis

Tinea pedis is another cosmopolitan disease; myriads of cases occur in all countries of the world. In contrast to tinea versicolor, this disease is more widespread in temperate than in tropical areas. As it happens, athlete's foot is virtually unknown in those regions where large numbers of inhabitants go without shoes because of the combined factors of warm climate and low income. In other areas, however, it may affect from 50 to 90 percent of the people in the course of their lives (36). English (15) estimated that up to 70 percent of the general population may have clinical signs of tinea pedis, however, a mycotic infection can be proven in only a small percentage of these people.

In certain population groups, however, the rate of confirmed cases may be high. Hulsey and Jordan (29) observed fungus infections in 63 percent of the university students they examined. During World War II, Hopkins and co-workers (28) found lesions in the feet of more than 80 percent of the men on an infantry post. Microscopic studies of the skin revealed fungus elements in 70 percent of those who had intertrigo of the toes and in more than 90 percent of those with dysidrotic lesions on the soles.

Blank and co-workers (7) reported that skin diseases among the American troops in Vietnam are the commonest cause of disability. In the Mekong Delta, for example, 77 percent of 209 men required hospitalization for foot infections. The most frequent etiologic agent of the dermatophyhosts was *Trichophyton mentagrophytes*.

Tinea capitis

Despite such optimistic statements as, "Ringworm of the scalp, a scourge of childhood for more than 2,000 years, has finally yielded to treatment with griseofulvin" (27), this disease still flourishes in many parts of the world (35, 47, 58). It is especially prevalent in the underdeveloped areas of Africa, Asia, and Latin America, where funds for specific medication with griseofulvin are not readily available. The prevalence of tinea capitis is directly related to the economic status of the families and of the country in which they live. For example, a survey by Vanbreuseghem (64) in Somalia showed a 36 percent prevalence among boys five to ten years of age. In the Sudan, Mahgoub (40) noted that 17 percent of the students in a boys' boarding school were infected.

The incidence of scalp infections is also high in the Middle East and parts of Asia. Rates reached 23 percent in a home for boys in Poona, India (46), and 10 percent in a school in Kashmir (32).

In general, scalp infections in Europe and the United States are relatively infrequent. As in other parts of the world, however, their prevalence is greatest among the socially deprived groups. Beginning in 1960, one of the most extensive surveys of tinea capitis in history was conducted in Yugoslavia (24). A total of 1,782,000 people were screened. Among them, 94,296 cases of tinea capitis were diagnosed, corresponding to an infection rate of 5.3 percent. In some villages, morbidity was as high as 8.6 percent. In Greece a survey (60) revealed a 1.4 percent level of infection among 4,701 children examined. However, in one village the incidence was 17 percent. A Washington, D. C. survey in 1959 (31) showed that 0.8 percent of the elementary school children were infected, and in an Atlanta, Georgia, study, 2.6 percent of 1,753 school children had tinea capitis (5).

Although the tineas are not usually disabling, they do constitute an important public health problem. In many countries, children with ringworm of the scalp are barred from school until they are cured. Thus, at a critical age in their lives, they are deprived of their educational rights. In addition, they may be subjected to psychological traumas by being forced to wear distinctive headwear and by being shunned by their peers and by neighborhood families.

Tinea imbricata

The social consequences of *Trichophyton concentricum* infections in Melanesia and Polynesia merit special attention. Tinea imbricata is well established in many islands in the southern part of the Pacific Ocean. Infection rates of 18 percent have been observed in some villages of Papua and New Guinea (37).

In a carefully conducted epidemiologic study in New Guinea (55), the social consequences stemming from tinea imbricata were discovered to be profound. The shunning of infected men as prospective husbands contributes to bachelorhood. Infected women are married at a later age than uninfected ones, and then most often they become the second wife of a polygamous husband. In addition, infected children and adults are discriminated against educationally and in employment. Lack of funds for mass treatment and control programs prevents reduction or elimination of the disease and its attendant social problems.

Tinea corporis

Tinea corporis and nail infections are quite prevalent throughout the world. Data on their frequency are not available, but the general opinion is that these conditions are not uncommon and some, such as nail infections, are increasing in prevalence (27).

An indirect estimate of the size of the cutaneous mycoses infections can be obtained through data on expenditures for antifungal preparations. Information obtained in 1960 (3), revealed that 25 million dollars had been spent for ringworm medications during the previous year. More recently, the Wall Street Journal of March 6, 1968, quoted the 1966 sales of griseofulvin at 6,700,000 dollars. If we assume, conservatively that 25 million dollars has been spent in the United States for ringworm medications every year since 1959, their dollar value to date in this country alone comes to 375 million dollars for the past fifteen years.

SUBCUTANEOUS MYCOSES

Under the heading of subcutaneous mycoses the following three diseases are discussed: chromomycosis, mycetomas, and sporotrichosis. The data on prevalence and incidence of these mycoses are even more fragmentary and incomplete than those on the cutaneous mycoses. Nevertheless, occasional surveys give fleeting glimpses of the dimly sensed bulk of their numbers.

Chromomycosis

Cases of chromomycosis are especially prevalent in Africa and Latin America. The disease also occurs with less frequency in Asia, Australia, Europe, United States, and Canada.

Every public health worker in Latin America and anyone who has visited hospitals there cannot fail to be impressed by the number of patients with chromomycosis in the wards and outpatient clinics. Data compiled by Romero and Trejos (51) reveal how common this crippling and disfiguring disease may be. In

Costa Rica they estimated that the case rate was approximately one per 24,000 inhabitants. The prevalence rate in the Republic of Malagasy is also high. During the four-year period, 1955 through 1959, Brygoo and Segretain (8) recorded 129 cases, signifying a case rate of one per 32,500 persons. In one district, the incidence reached an astounding rate of one per 7,000 inhabitants.

Such estimates, few and crude as they may be, provide an insight into the size of the problem that must exist in these and many other countries. Due to the therapeutic intractability of this infection and its high incidence, chromomycosis looms as a disease of considerable public health importance.

Mycetomas

Mycetomas occur with striking frequency and have a devastating effect on the health of their victims in the tropical regions of the world. A survey by Abbott (1) in the Sudan revealed that for a thirty-month period, 1,231 persons had been admitted to hospitals and "a great many more were seen in outpatient dements."

Studies carried out in other parts of Africa reveal that mycetomas are prevalent in Algeria, Cameroun, Chad, Malagasy, Niger, Somalia, Tanzania, and Uganda (41). Data by Rey (50) support the thesis that mycetoma prevalence rates comparable to those of the Sudan exist across Africa in a belt characterized by an annual rainfall of 250 to 500 mm.

In Latin America a survey by Mariat (41) documented a large number of cases in Argentina, Mexico, and Venezuela (41). By far the greatest number was registered in Mexico. Latapi, during a twenty-year period, compiled a list of 206 cases (41). Venezuela with sixty-eight cases, and Argentina with twenty-three, were the other countries with a relatively high frequency of mycetomas.

Mycetomas are less common in temperate regions. Green and Adams (23) supported the validity of reports of only sixty-three cases for the United States for the years 1896 to 1964 and less than one hundred cases had been reported in Europe up to 1960 (45).

Only a vague idea of the prevalence of mycetomas in Asia can be comprehended since actual reports are few in number. A spot survey of material filed in the pathology departments of five medical colleges in southern India brought to light 187 cases (33). This report gives an inkling of the true size of the problem as it must exist not only in this area of India but also throughout Asia as well.

Mycetomas are not as uncommon as currently available data indicate. They occur frequently in a broad zone around the world. The numerous victims lead lives of resigned desperation, because in the absence of medical services and effective chemotherapy, they face the inevitable and irreparable loss of limbs and a desolate future. These infections challenge public health workers everywhere to develop preventive programs and to establish centers for early diagnosis and prompt surgical intervention.

Sporotrichosis

In recent years, sporotrichosis has cropped up with surprising frequency in both temperate and tropical regions throughout the world. The greatest recorded outbreak of this or any other subcutaneous mycosis occurred in the deep subterranean gold mines of South Africa. During a period of twenty-eight months, 2,825 miners became infected after contact with timber overgrown with *Sporothrix schenckii* (25).

Sporotrichosis is well known as an occupational hazard for florists, pottery packers, and others who come in contact with sphagnum moss (13, 17), straw (19), and wood products (6). But the majority of infections occur sporadically, usually following some traumatic incident in which soil-engendered spores of *S. schenckii* enter a wound. In parts of Brazil, sporotrichosis is estimated to account for 0.5 percent of all the dermatoses (53). The disease is especially common in Mexico (34); in the city of Guadalajara, it is considered to be the most prevalent of the noncutaneous mycoses (2). So many cases go unreported, however, that its true incidence remains unknown.

The development and use of antigens for a skin test of sporotrichosis have begun to reveal the occurrence of widespread subclinical infections by *S. schenckii* in the general population. Small scale surveys made in Louisiana showed a sensitivity level of 11 percent among prison and hospital inmates. In contrast, high-risk workers in plant nurseries had a 33 percent sensitivity rate, and the levels rose to 58 percent among those who had been employed ten years or longer (54). In Arizona the same antigen elicited positive reactions in 10 percent of a group of 203 hospital patients (30). Sporothrixin prepared in Brazil elicited a 24 percent level of reactions in a small group of Brazilians and no reactions among fifty-five persons in Germany (66).

SYSTEMIC MYCOSES

Blastomycosis

At present, blastomycosis is known with certainty to be endemic only in the United States, Canada, and fourteen African countries: Algeria, Egypt, Libya, Malawi, Morocco, Mozambique, Nigeria, Republic of South Africa, Rhodesia, Tanzania, Tunisia, Uganda, Zaire, and Zambia (4, 38, 39, 52, 57, 65).

By far the greatest occurrence has been recorded in the United States. A total of 1,470 cases, dating from 1894 to 1968, were tabulated. A survey of the records of 170 Veterans Administration hospitals for the twelve-year period 1946 to 1957 disclosed reports on 198 proved cases or an average of close to seventeen a year (9).

Another survey (56) revealed that ninety-nine patients were hospitalized in the United States during the first six months of 1953. A study of mortality from selected nonnotifiable diseases showed 157 deaths attributed to blastomycosis, an average of fifteen a year for the ten-year period, 1960 to 1969 (11). Thus, the disease is a matter of considerable public health importance within the United States.

The prevalence of blastomycosis in Canada is relatively low compared with that in the United States. In the latest available compilation, 114 cases had been registered from 1906 to 1962, for a yearly average of 1.8 (22).

More time is needed before the nature and extent of blastomycosis in Africa can be assessed. So far, information on only twenty-nine diagnosed cases from Africa has been cited (65).

Coccidioidomycosis

Coccidioidomycosis is a disease of limited distribution. It is only known with certainty to occur in North, Central, and South America. In the endemic areas of the United States, coccidioidomycosis is a major disease. Some 35,000 new infections are said to occur yearly in California alone (16). For the entire endemic area in Arizona, California, New Mexico, Nevada, Texas, and Utah, the annual total is believed to be about 100,000 cases. An estimated one-third of these persons have overt signs of infection. The latest compilation of deaths attributed to coccidioidomycosis in the United States reveals a yearly average of 55.3 for a total of 553 cases during 1960 to 1969 (11). As Fiese (16) has pointed out, however, it is morbidity rather than mortality that makes coccidioidomycosis a serious disease. "In the most highly endemic areas—Bakersfield, California; Phoenix, Arizona, and El Paso, Texas—nearly 100 percent of the population will have been infected in a few years, and about a fifth of them will have had an illness severe enough to cause temporary incapacity and to warrant medical care."

Unfortunately, data on coccidioidomycosis in Latin America are much less complete than those from the United States. In Mexico, for example, results of a survey of reactions to skin tests have hinted at prevalence rates ranging from 5 to more than 50 percent in many states (21).

Endemic areas are small in Central America, appearing only in Guatemala and Honduras. Coccidioidin sensitivity levels of 26 percent were observed in the population of two villages in the Motagua Valley of Guatemala and 16 percent among the inhabitants of the Comayagua Valley in Honduras (43).

In South America, Venezuela and Argentina have the most extensive endemic areas. Coccidioidin sensitivity levels of 46 and 24 percent have been noted in Lara and Falcon (Venezuela) respectively (10).

In Santiago del Estero, Argentina, a sensitivity level of 19 percent was recorded among 2,213 children between the ages of six to sixteen (44). Only two surveys of coccidiodin have been carried out in Paraguay, and none have been made in Bolivia. The Paraguayan studies revealed reactivity among eighty-two

Indians (44%) (4) and less than 3 percent reactivity in the residents of the city of Asuncion (18).

Much remains to be done before the full extent of the coccidioidomycosis problem in Latin America becomes known.

Cryptococcosis

Cryptococcosis is one of the most serious and dreaded of the systemic mycoses. Cases of this disease have been recorded in virtually all parts of the world. They present a diagnostic challenge because the symptoms inducc clinical and pathological changes that resemble tuberculosis, neoplasms, brain tumors, and insanity. Failure to recognize this mimicry leads to delays in accurate diagnosis and prompt administration of specific therapy and has even resulted in commitment to mental institutions.

An accurate estimate of the prevalence of cryptococcosis and the morbidity that it causes is impossible to make at this time. Although cases are not required to be registered, other types of data indicate that this disease causes great suffering and that mortality is high. In the United States, 824 deaths have been attributed to cryptococcosis for the ten-year span 1960 to 1969, for a yearly average of eighty-two (11). No statistics of this kind are available for other countries.

A few years ago, Utz (62) estimated that 200 to 300 cases of cryptococcal meningitis occurred annually in the United States. This figure, although based on an educated guess, may not be too far from reality. If the annual average of deaths attributed to *C. neoformans* is eighty-two, and if we assume in this era of amphotericin B therapy that fewer than one-fourth of the cryptococcosis patients die, then about 330 clinical cases of this disease probably occur annually.

Last year the Fungus Immunology Branch of the Center for Disease Control's Mycology Division received 666 sera and spinal fluids from 478 patients with suspected cryptococcosis, and eighty-five of these specimens gave positive reactions to tests. If other diagnostic centers released or recorded similar information, the prevalence of cryptococcosis could be determined, not only in the United States, but also in the rest of the world.

It is the author's belief that cryptococcosis is the sleeping giant among the deep mycoses. When reporting and surveillance programs are established, the number of cases of cryptococcosis will prove to be astonishingly high.

Histoplasmosis

Information on the prevalence and incidence of histoplasmosis is extensive when compared with that available for the other mycoses. Much remains to be learned, however, before its impact on the welfare of human beings can be determined. Histoplasmosis cases have been diagnosed in virtually all parts of the world, but the frequency of infection varies considerably from region to region. Skin-tests surveys with histoplasmin have revealed many areas with high levels of infection among certain groups of persons. Reaction levels of at least 10 percent were discovered in one or more regions of twenty-five countries: Algeria, Argentina, Brazil, Burma, Canada, Colombia, Cuba, Democratic Republic of the Congo, Ecuador, French Guiana, Honduras, Italy, Liberia, Malaya, Mexico, New Guinea, Nicaragua, Pakistan, Panama, Paraguay, Puerto Rico, Ruanda-Urundi, Surinam, United States, and Venezuela (26).

Absence of reporting makes it impossible to cite morbidity and mortality data for histoplasmosis. In the United States estimated infections number in the millions. On the basis of one of the best planned and most extensive histoplasmin surveys ever carried out, it was determined that the sensitivity level of the populations in the forty-eight contiguous States averaged 20 percent (14). Using the latest U. S. Census Bureau estimate of 200,485,000 people for these States, and assuming that the yearly sensitization rate is constant and the histoplasmin reaction is specific, it can be calculated that approximately 40 million persons are infected. On the basis of earlier data, Furcolow estimated that approximately 200,000 cases of acute pulmonary histoplasmosis occur yearly in the United States (61). From 1960 to 1969, 719 deaths were attributed to this disease, for an annual average of seventy-two (11).

Information of this kind suggests the magnitude of the histoplasmosis problem. Additional attention is needed to insure that facilities are made generally available for the prompt and accurate diagnosis of the infection so that specific therapy can be initiated in the early and more responsive stages of the disease.

Paracoccidioidomycosis

Of all the systemic mycoses, paracoccidioidomycosis has the most restricted geographic distribution. As far as is currently known, this disease occurs only in Latin America. Its domain extends from Mexico to Argentina. Only Chile, Guyana, and Surinam in South America; British Honduras and Panama in Central America; and all the islands of the West Indies have no reported cases.

In the endemic areas, the incidence and prevalence vary greatly from country to country and from region to region within the countries. The greatest number of cases have been encountered in Brazil, Colombia, and Venezuela. In Brazil, 1,724 cases had been recorded (12), for a morbidity rate of 2.5 per 100,000 inhabitants. Venezuelan cases totaled 300, giving a rate of five per 100,000. From Colombia, 373 cases were cited (48). For all Latin America, 3,037 cases have been recorded. Such figures should be regarded as only an approximation of the true prevalence of paracoccidioidomycosis. The actual number of clinically manifest cases is probably much higher.

Until recently, lack of potent and specific antigens for skin tests prevented epidemiologic surveys from being used in determining the prevalence of infections and in locating endemic areas. Restrepo Morena, however, has now developed such an antigen. With it she and her collaborators (49) have begun population surveys. Among 3,938 persons tested, 10 percent were positive to a mycelial antigen and 6 percent to a yeast-form reagent. Variation among the counties in Colombia ranged from 6 to 13 percent.

The paracoccidioidin survey indicated that an asymptomatic benign form of paracoccidioidomycosis may occur in the endemic areas. There is an obvious need for more extensive field studies using standardized antigens. When these studies and surveillance programs are underway, a more objective picture of the extent of paracoccidioidomycosis can then be obtained.

Discussion

An attempt has been made to reveal the dimensions of the medical mycological iceberg. The information gathered, based on the meager data available and on educated guesses, incomplete as it may be, indirectly allows us to visualize and quantitate the dimensions of the infections. The author is convinced that the mycoses represent a greater health burden and challenge than is realized by the public or by its health officials. Morbidity and mortality associated with the pathogenic fungi have been continuously underreported.

It is well known that whenever properly trained and motivated persons begin to study mycological problems, many cases are discovered where none had been thought previously to occur. As a result of this phenomenon, geographic distribution maps and prevalence and incidence data are misleading. The records generally reflect the location and activities of an investigator rather than true distribution patterns of the disease. Many regions considered to be relatively free of mycotic infections can properly be said to lack medical mycologists rather than mycoses.

The medical mycological picture is not all bleak, however. In the United States the recent second National Conference on Histoplasmosis (Atlanta, Ga., Oct. 6 through 8, 1969) passed a resolution recommending that steps be taken by the Center for Disease Control to have the mycoses classified as notifiable diseases. The lengthy process for implementing this resolution has already been initiated.

At Buenos Aires in 1966 the fifteenth Pan American Congress on Tuberculosis and Pulmonary Diseases passed a resolution sponsored by the Union of Latin American Tuberculosis Societies, under the guidance of Dr. Jose I. Baldo, recommending that all member countries establish coordinating commissions for the study of mycoses at the national level. Several countries have already done this. All others should be urged to follow their example. Once the commissions start to function, reporting mechanisms will be developed and implemented. Conceivably, the work of these groups could be coordinated under the auspices of the World Health Organization and the Pan American Health

Organization. Global morbidity and mortality data would then be systematically collected, evaluated, and distributed to all persons interested in public health.

Until it can be shown that the apparent number of mycoses cases is deceptively small, that in reality the mycoses are common diseases and that the toll they take in misery and mortality is high, support cannot be expected in the development and implementation of control programs, research projects, and training courses.

REFERENCES

1. Abbott, P.: Mycetoma in the Sudan. Trans. *Roy Soc Trop Med Hyg, 50*:11, 1956.
2. Aceves Ortega, R., Aguirre Castillo, R., Sosto Peralta, F.: Esporotricosis. Analisis de 70 casos estudiados en la ciudad de Guadalajara. *Bol. Dermatol* (Mex.), *1*:15, 1961.
3. Ajello, L.: Geographic distribution and prevalence of the dermatophytes. *Ann N Y Acad Sci, 89*:30, 1960.
4. Ajello, L.: Comparative ecology of respiratory mycotic disease agents. *Bact Rev, 31*:6, 1967.
5. Ajello, L., Brumfield, G., Palmer, J.: Nonfluorescent Microsporum audouinii scalp infections. *Arch Dermatol (Chicago), 87*:605, 1963.
6. Balabanoff, V. A., Koevu, A., Stoynooski, V.: Sporotrichose bei arbeitern in einer papierfabrik. *Berufsdermatosen, 16*:261, 1968.
7. Blank, H., Taplin, D., Zaias, N.: Cutaneous Trichophyton mentagrophytes infections in Vietnam. *Arch Dermatol (Chicago)* 99:135, 1969.
8. Brygoo, E. R., Segretain, G.: Etude clinique, epidemiologique et mycologique de la chromoblastomycose a Madagascar. *Bull Soc Pathol Exot, 53*:443, 1960.
9. Busey, J. F.: Blastomycosis. I. A review of 198 collected cases in Veterans Administration hospitals. *Am Rev Respir Dis, 89*:659, 1964.
10. Campins, H.: Coccidioidomycosis in Venezuela. In Coccidioidomycosis, Ajello, Ed., Tucson, Univ. Arizona Press, 1967.
11. Center for Disease Control Annual Supplement, Summary, 1972. *Morbidity and Mortality Weekly Report, 21*:1, 1973.
12. Chirife, A. V., Del Rio, C. A.: Geopatologia de la blastomicosis sudamericana. *Presna Med Argent, 52*:54, 1965.
13. D'Alessio, D. J., Leavens, L. J., Strumpf, G. B., Smith, C. D.: An outbreak of sporotrichosis in Vermont associated with sphagnum moss as the source of infection. *N Engl J Med, 272*:1054, 1965.

14. Edwards, L. B., et al.: An atlas of sensitivity to tuberculin, PPD-B, and histoplasmin in the United States. *Am Rev Respir Dis, 99*:1, 1969
15. English, M. P.: Tinea pedis as a public health problem. *Br J Dermatol, 81*:705, 1969.
16. Fiese, M. J.: *Coccidioidomycosis*. Springfield, Thomas, 1958.
17. Gastineau, F. M., Spolyar, L. W., Haynes, E.: Sporotrichosis; report of six cases among florists. *JAMA, 117*:1047, 1941.
18. Gines, A. R., Gould, E., Melgarejo De Talavera, S.: Intradermorreaccion con coccidioidina. *Hoja Tisiol, 9*:255, 1949.
19. Gonzalez Benavides, J.: La esporotrichosis; enfermedad ocupacional de los alfareros. *Rev Hosp Univ (Monterrey, Mex.), 2*:215, 1952.
20. Gonzalez-Ochoa, A.: Pitiriasis versicolor. *Rev Med* (Mex.), *2*:81, 1956.
21. Gonzalez-Ochoa, A.: Coccidioidomycosis in Mexico. In *Coccidioidomycosis*, edited by L. Ajello, Ed., Tucson, Univ. Arizona Press, 1967.
22. Grandbois, J.: La blastomycose nord-americaine au Canada. *Laval Med, 34*:714, 1963.
23. Green, W. O., Adams, T. E.: Mycetoma in the United States; a review and report of seven additional cases. *Am J Clin Pathol, 42*: 75, 1964.
24. Grin, E. I.: Epidemiology and control of tinea capitis in Yugoslavia. Trans. *St. John Hosp Dermatol Soc, 47*:109, 1961.
25. Helm, M. A. F., Berman, C.: The clinical, therapeutic and epidemiological features of the sporotrichosis infections on the mines. In Sporotrichosis infection in mines of the Witwatersrand. Transvaal Chamber of Mines, Johannesburg, 1947.
26. Hickey, M. A., Todosijczuk, D.: Sensitivity and incidence of histoplasmosis reported in the literature up to and including 1965. Published by authors. Copyright 1968.
27. Hildick-Smith, G., Blank, H., Sarkany, I.: *Fungus Diseases and Their Treatment*. Boston, Little, Brown, 1964.
28. Hopkins, J. G., et al.: Treatment and prevention of dermatophytosis and related conditions. *Bull U S Army Med Dept, 77*:42, 1944.
29. Hulsey, S. H., Jordon, F. M.: Ringworm of toes as found in university students. *Am J Med Sci, 169*:267, 1925.
30. Ingrish, F. M., Schneidau, J. D.: Cutaneous hypersensitivity to sporotrichin in Maricopa County, Arizona. *J Invest Dermatol, 49*:146, 1967.
31. Kirk, J., Ajello, L.: Use of griseofulvin in the therapy of tinea capitis in children. *Arch Dermatol (Chicago), 80*:259, 1959.
32. Klokke, A. H.: Tinea capitis in Kashmir. *Arch Dermatol (Chicago), 90*:205, 1964.
33. Klokke, A. H., Swamidasan, G., Anguli, R., Verghese, A.: The causal agents of mycetoma in South India. Trans. *Roy Soc Trop Med Hyg, 62*:509, 1968.

34. Lavalle, P.: Aspectos clinicos immunologicos y epidemiologicos de la esporotricosis. Mem. 4 Cong. Mex. Dermatol., Mexico, 1968.

35. Le Franc, M.: La teigne en milieu scolaire urbain. *Alger Med, 54*: 446, 1950.

36. Lewis, G. M., Hopper, M. E., Wilson, J. W., Plunkett, O. A.: *An Introduction to Medical Mycology*. Chicago, Year Book Medical Publishers, Inc., 1958.

37. MacLennan, R., O'Keeffe, M. F.: Superficial fungal infections in an area of lowland New Guinea; clinical and mycological observations. *Aust J Dermatol, 8*:157, 1966.

38. Magalhaes, M. J. C.: Lepra associada ao primeiro caso de blastomicose norte-americana evidenciado em Mocambique. *Rev Port Doenca Hansen, 6*:1, 1967.

39. Magalhaes, M. C., Drouhet, E., Destombes, P.: Premier cas de blastomycose a Blastomyces dermatitidis observe au Mozambique; guerison per l'amphoterecine B. *Bull Soc Pathol Exot, 61*:210, 1968.

40. Mahgoub, S.: Ringworm infection among Sudanese schoolchildren. Trans. *Roy Soc Trop Med Hyg, 62*:263, 1968.

41. Mariat, F.: Sur la distribution geographique et al rapartition des agents de mycetomes. *Bull Soc Pathol Exot, 56*:35, 1963.

42. Marples, M. J.: The incidence of certain skin diseases in Western Samoa; a preliminary survey. Trans. *Roy Soc Trop Med Hyg, 44*: 319, 1950.

43. Mayorga, R.: Coccidioidomycosis in Central America. In *Coccidioidomycosis,* edited by L. Ajello, Ed., Tucson, Univ. Arizona Press.

44. Negroni, P., et al.: Estudio sobre el Coccidioides immitis Rixford et Gilchrist. XII Cuarta contribucion al estudio de la endemia Argentina. *Rev Argent Dermatol, 36*:269, 1952.

45. Nicolau, S. G., Avram, A.: *Micetomul Cutanat.* Acad Rep Pop Romine, Bucharest, Rumania, 1960.

46. Padhye, A. A., Sukapure, R. S., Thirumalachar, M. J.: A local outbreak of tinea capitis in Remand Home for Boys. *Poona Ind J Med Sci, 20*:786, 1966.

47. Rahim, G. F.: A survey of fungi causing tinea capitis in Iraz. *Br J Dermatol, 78*:213, 1966.

48. Restrepo Morena, A., Sigifredo Espinol, T. L.: Algunas consideraciones ecologicas sobre la paracoccidioidomicosis en Colombia. *Antioquia Med, 18*:433, 1968.

49. Restrepo Morena, A., et al.: Distribution of paracoccidioidin sensitivity in Colombia. *Am J Trop Med, 17*:25, 1968.

50. Rey, M.: *Les Mycetomes dans l'Ouest Africain.* Paris, R. Foulon & Cie, 1961.

51. Romero, A., Trejos, A.: La cromoblastomicosis en Costa Rica. *Rev Biol Trop, 1*:95, 1953.

52. Ross, M. D., Goldring, F.: North American blastomycosis in Rhodesia. *Cent Afr J Med, 12*:207, 1966.
53. Sampaio, S. A. P., Lacaz, C. S., Almeida, F.: Aspectos clinicos da esporotrichose em Sao Paulo. *Rev Hosp Clin Fac Med S Paulo, 9*:391, 1954.
54. Schneidau, J. D., Lamar, L. M., Hairston, M. A.: Cutaneous hypersensitivity to sporotrichin in Louisiana. *JAMA, 188*:371, 1964.
55. Schofield, F. D., Parkinson, A. D., Jeffrey, D.: Observations on the epidemiology, effects and treatment of tinea imbricata. *Trans Roy Soc Trop Med Hyg, 57*:214, 1963.
56. Schwarz, J., Goldman, L.: Epidemiologic study of North American blastomycosis. *Arch Dermatol (Chicago), 71*:84, 1955.
57. Segretain, G.: La blastomycose a Blastomyces dermatitidis; son existence en Afrique. *Maroc Med, 48*:25, 1968.
58. Sicault, G., Gaud, J., Salm, G., Faure, J.: Les teignes au Maroc. *Bull Inst Hyg Maroc, 11*:165, 1951.
59. Stein, C. A.: Beitrag uber die Mykosehaufigkeit im Oldenburger Raum und deren Behandlung an der Oldenburger Klinik. *Z Haut Geschlechtskr, 10*:51, 1951.
60. Trichopoulos, D., Marselou-Kinti, U.: L'epidemiologie des teignes du cuir chevelu chez les enfants en Grece. *Ann Soc Belg Med Trop, 46*:691, 1966
61. U. S. National Communicable Disease Center: Mycoses Surveillance, No. 1, April 1969.
62. Utz, J. P.: Deadly fungus found in several D. C. areas. Quoted by W. Grigg in The Evening Star, Washington, D. C., Nov. 16, 1964.
63. Vanbreuseghem, R.: Un probleme de mycologie medicale; le pityriasis versicolor. *Ann Inst Pasteur (Paris), 79*:798, 1950.
64. Vanbreuseghem, R.: Les teignes en Republique de Somalie. *Bull Acad Roy Med Belg, 6*:247, 1966.
65. Vandepitte, J., Gatti, F.: La blastomycose Nord-Americaine en Afrique son existence en Republique du Zaire. *Ann Soc Belge Med Trop, 52*:467, 1972.
66. Wernsdorfer, R., et al.: Imunologia da esporotricose. IV. A prova da esporotriquina na Alemanha e no Brasil, em pessoas sem esporotricose. *Rev Inst Med Trop S Paulo, 5*:217, 1963.

AUTHOR INDEX

SUBJECT INDEX

B

C

H

I

R